Practical Management of Cardiac Arrhythmias

Edited by

Nabil El-Sherif, MD

Professor of Medicine and Physiology
Director of Electrophysiology
Department of Medicine, State University of New York
Health Science Center at Brooklyn
and
Chief, Cardiology Division
The Veterans Administration Medical Center
Brooklyn, New York

and

Jean Lekieffre, MD

Professor of Cardiology
Chief, Cardiology A
Cardiology Hospital
Lille University Medical Center
Lille, France

Futura Publishing
Company, Inc.
Armonk, NY

Library of Congress Cataloging-in-Publication Data

Practical management of cardiac arrhythmias / edited by Nabil El
-Sherif, Jean Lekieffre.
     p.   cm.
    Includes bibliographical references and index.
    ISBN 0-87993-652-5 (alk. paper)
    1. Arrhythmia—Treatment. I. El-Sherif, Nabil, 1938–
II. Lekieffre, Jean.
    [DNLM: 1. Arrhythmia—therapy.   WG 330 P896 1997]
RC685.A65P696 1997
616.1′28—dc21
DNLM/DLC
for Library of Congress   96-36935
                                                 CIP

Copyright 1997
Futura Publishing Company, Inc.

Published by
Futura Publishing Company, Inc.
135 Bedford Road
Armonk, NY 10504-0418

LC#: 96-36935
ISBN#: 0-87993-652-5

Every effort has been made to ensure that the information in this book is
as up to date and as accurate as possible at the time of publication.
However, due to the constant developments in medicine, neither the
author, nor the editor, nor the publisher can accept any legal or any
other responsibility for any errors or omissions that may occur.

Printed in the United States of America.

This book is printed on acid-free paper.

Contributors

Etienne Aliot, MD
Professor of Cardiology
Service de Cardiologie
Hôpital Central
Nancy, France

F. Rosas Andrade, MD
Department of Cardiac Pacing and
 Electrophysiology
Hôpital Jean Rostand
Ivry sur Seine, France

P. Aouate, MD
Department of Cardiac Pacing and
 Electrophysiology
Hôpital Jean Rostand
Ivry sur Seine, France

Ahmed Abdel-Azziz, MD
VACOMED Research Group
Service de Cardiologie
Hôpital Charles Nicolle
Université de Rouen
Rouen, France

Michael Block, MD
Hospital of the Westfälische
 Wilhelms-University of Münster
Department of Cardiology/
 Angiology
Münster, Germany

Dirk Böcker, MD
Hospital of the Westfälische
 Wilhelms-University of Münster
Department of Cardiology/
 Angiology
Münster, Germany

Martin Borggrefe, MD
Hospital of the Westfälische
 Wilhelms-University of Münster
Department of Cardiology/
 Angiology
Münster, Germany

Günter Breithardt, MD
Hospital of the Westfälische
 Wilhelms-University of Münster
Department of Cardiology/
 Angiology
Münster, Germany

A. John Camm, MD, FRCP
Professor of Cardiology
Chairman of Cardiological Sciences
The Medical School
St. George's Hospital
London, United Kingdom

Ronald W.F. Campbell, MD
British Heart Foundation Professor
 of Cardiology
University of Newcastle upon Tyne
Department of Academic
 Cardiology,
Freeman Hospital
Newcastle upon Tyne, United
 Kingdom

Edward B. Caref, PhD
Cardiology Division
Department of Medicine
State University of New York
 Health Science Center and
 Veteran Affairs Medical Center
Brooklyn, New York
USA

Jacques Clémenty, MD
Professor, Chef de Service
Département d'Electrophysiologie
 et Stimulation
Hôpital Cardiologique de
 l'universite de Bordeaux
Bordeaux, France

Christian de Chillou, MD
Department of Cardiology
Hôpital Central
Nancy, France

Xavier Copie, MD
Department of Cardiologie
Hôpital Broussais
Paris, France

Philippe Delfaut, MD
Cardiology Department
Hôpital Cardiologique
CHU de Lille
University of Lille
Lille, France

Nabil El-Sherif, MD
Professor of Medicine and
 Physiology
Director of Electrophysiology
Department of Medicine,
State University of New York

Health Science Center at Brooklyn
 and Chief, Cardiology Division
The Veterans Administration
 Medical Center
Brooklyn, New York
USA

Kevin Ferrick, MD
Department of Medicine
Division of Cardiology
Arrhythmia Service
Albert Einstein College of Medicine
 and Montefiore Medical Center
Bronx, New York
USA

John D. Fisher, MD
Professor of Medicine and Chief
 Cardiovascular Montefiore
 Medical Center
Department of Medicine
Division of Cardiology
Arrhythmia Service
Albert Einstein College of Medicine
 and Montefiore Medical Center
Bronx, New York
USA

Bruno Fischer, MD
Département d'Electrophysiologie
 et Stimulation
Hôpital Cardiologique de
 l'université Bordeaux
Bordeaux, France

Guy Fontaine, MD, PhD
Director of Department of Cardiac
Pacing and Electrophysiology,
Hôpital Jean Rostand
Ivry sur Seine, France

Robert Frank, MD
Department of Cardiac Pacing and
  Electrophysiology
Hôpital Jean Rostand
Ivry sur Seine, France

Yves Gallais, MD
Hôpital Jean Rostand
Ivry sur Seine, France

Laurent Gencel, MD
Chef de Clinique
Centre Hospitalier Regional de
  Bordeaux
Hôpital Cardiologique de Haut-
  Leveque
Bordeaux, France

Irakli Giorgberidze, MD
Research Electrophysiologist
Eastern Heart Institute
Passaic, New Jersey
USA

Philippe Gosse, MD
Hôpital Cardiologique
Université de Bordeaux II
Bordeaux, France

Daniel Grandmougin, MD
Cardiovascular Surgery Department
Hôpital Cardiologique
CHU de Lille
University of Lille
Lille, France

Colette M-J. Guiraudon, MD
Professor of Surgery
University of Western Ontario
London, Ontario
Canada

Gerard M. Guiraudon, MD
Professor of Surgery
University of Western Ontario
London, Ontario
Canada

Louis Guize, MD
Department of Cardiology
Hôpital Broussais
Paris, France

Michel Haïssaguerre, MD
Professor, Département
  d'Electrophysiologie et
  Stimulation
Hôpital Cardiologique de
  l'universite Bordeaux
Bordeaux, France

Dieter Hammel, MD
Hospital of the Westfälische
  Wilhelms-University of Münster
Department of Cardiovascular
  Surgery and Institute of
  Arteriosclerosis
  Research
Münster, Germany

Jean-Luc Hennequin, MD
Cardiovascular Surgery Department
Hôpital Cardiologique
CHU de Lille
University of Lille
Lille, France

Mélèze Hocini, MD
Département d'Electrophysiologie
  et Stimulation
Hôpital Cardiologique de
  l'université Bordeaux
Bordeaux, France

Pierre Jaïs, MD
Chef de Clinique
Centre Hospitalier Regional de
  Bordeaux
Hôpital Cardiologique de Haut-
  Leveque
Bordeaux, France

Debra Johnston, RN
Department of Medicine
Division of Cardiology
Arrhythmia Service
Albert Einstein College of Medicine
  and Montefiore Medical Center
Bronx, New York
USA

Salem Kacet, MD
Cardiology Department
Hopital Cardiologique
CHU de Lille
University of Lille
Lille, France

Soo G. Kim, MD
Department of Medicine
Division of Cardiology
Arrhythmia Service
Albert Einstein College of Medicine
  and Montefiore Medical Center
Bronx, New York
USA

George Klein, MD
Professor of Medicine
Universiy of Western Ontario
Director of Arrhythmia Service
Division of Cardiology
University Hospital, London,
  Ontario
Canada

Didier Klug, MD
Cardiology Department
Hopital Cardiologique
CHU de Lille
University of Lille
Lille, France

Ryszard B. Krol, MD
Clinical Assistant Professor of
  Medicine
UMD-NJ Medical School
Newark, New Jersey
USA

Dominique Lacroix, MD
Cardiology Department
Hôpital Cardiologique de Lille
CHU de Lille
Lille, France

Gilles Lascault, MD
Department of Cardiac Pacing and
  Electrophysiology
Hôpital Jean Rostand
Ivry sur Seine, France

Thomas Lavergne, MD
Cardiologie A
Hôpital Broussais
Paris, France

Ralph Lazzara, MD
Professor of Medicine
Chief, Cardiovascular Section
The University of Oklahoma
  Health Science Center
Department of Medicine
Cardiovascular Diseases Section
Oklahoma City, Oklahoma

Jean Yves Le Heuzey, MD
Department of Cardiology
Hôpital Broussais
Paris, France

Jean Lekieffre, MD, FACC
Professor of Cardiology
Chief, Cardiology A
Cardiology Hospital
Lille University Medical Center
Lille, France

Philippe Le Métayer, MD
Hôpital Cardiologique
Université de Bordeaux II
Bordeaux, France

Brice Letac, MD
Professor of Cardiology
Chief, Department of Cardiology
University of Rouen
Hôpital Charles Nicolle
Rouen, France

Samuel Lévy, MD
Professor of Medicine
University of Marseille
Chief of the School of Medicine
Cardiology Division
Hôpital Nord
Marseille, France

Régis Logier, PhD
Biomedical Research Department
Hôpital Cardiologique
CHU de Lille
University of Lille, France

Richard M. Luceri, MD
Director, Florida Arrhythmia
    Consultants
Fort Lauderdale, Florida
Assistant Professor of Clinical
    Medicine
University of Miami
Miami Florida

Nandini Madan, MBBS, MD
Arrhythmia and Pacemaker Service
Eastern Heart Institute
Passaic, New Jersey
USA

Philip Mathew, MS
Engineering Associate
Arrhythmia and Pacemaker Service
Eastern Heart Institute
Passaic, New Jersey
USA

Anand Munsif, MD
Attending Electrophysiologist
Arrhythmia and Pacemaker Service
Eastern Heart Institute
Passaic, New Jersey

Mohan Nair, MD
VACOMED Research Group
Service de Cardiologie
Hôpital Charles Nicolle
Université de Rouen
Rouen, France

Jacky Ollitrault, MD
St. Joseph Hospital
Paris, France

Pierre L. Pagé
Associate Professor of Surgery
Department of Surgery
Université de Montréal and Staff
  Surgeon
Division of Cardiovascular and
  Thoracic Surgery
Hôpital du Sacré-Coeur de
  Montréal
Montréal, Canada

F. Poulain, MD
Department of Cardiac Pacing and
  Electrophysiology
Hôpital Jean Rostand
Ivry Sur Seine, France

Atul Prakash, MD
Research Electrophysiologist
The Arrhythmia and Pacemaker
  Service
Eastern Heart Institute
Passaic, New Jersey

Hervé Poty, MD
VACOMED Research Group
Service de Cardiologie
Hôpital Charles Nicolle
Université de Rouen
Rouen, France

Frank Robert, MD
Hôpital Cardiologique
Université de Bordeaux II
Bordeaux, France

Dan M. Roden, MD
Professor of Medicine and
  Pharmacology

Director, Division of Clinical
  Pharmacology
Vanderbilt University School of
  Medicine
Nashville, Tennessee
USA

James Roth, MD
Department of Medicine
Division of Cardiology
Arrhythmia Service
Albert Einstein College of Medicine
  and Montefiore Medical Center
Bronx, New York
USA

Nicolas Sadoul, MD
Service de Cardiologie
Hôpital Central
Nancy, France

Nadir Saoudi, MD
Professor of Cardiology
Service de Cardiologie
Hôpital Charles Nicolle
Université de Rouen
Rouen, France

Sanjeev Saksena, MD
Director, Arrhythmia and
  Pacemaker Service
Eastern Heart Institute, Passaic
Clinical Associate Professor of
  Medicine and Pediatrics
UMDNJ-NJ Medical School,
  Newark and Director, Pediatric
  Electrophysiology
Children's Hospital of New Jersey
Newark, New Jersey

Claude Sebag, MD
Service de Cardiologie du
  Professeur Motté
Hôpital Antoine Béclére
Clamart, France

Alistair K.B. Slade, MA, MRCP
Department of Cardiological
  Sciences
St. George's Hospital Medical
  School
London, United Kingdom

Richard Sutton, DSc Med
Consultant Cardiologist and
  Director of Pacing and
  Electrophysiology
Royal Brompton Hospital
London, England

Dipen Shah, MD, DNB
Hôpital Cardiologique de
  l'universite de Bordeaux
Bordeaux, France

Joelci Tonet, MD
Department of Cardiac Pacing and
  Electrophysiology
Hôpital Jean Rostand
Ivry Sur Seine, France

Gioia Turitto, MD
Assistant Professor of Medicine
Director, Coronary Care Unit and
  Electrophysiology Laboratory
Cardiology Division
Department of Medicine
State University of New York

Health Science Center and the
  Veterans Affairs Medical Center
Brooklyn, New York
USA

Henri Warembourg, MD
Cardiovascular Surgery Department
Hôpital Cardiologique
CHU de Lille
University of Lille
Lille, France

Daniel Weiss, MD
Attending Electrophysiologist
Florida Arrhythmia Consultants
Fort Lauderdale, Florida
USA

Raymond Yee, MD
Associate Professor
Department of Medicine
University of Western Ontario
London, Ontario
Canada

Zhi Zhang, MD
Department of Medicine
Division of Cardiology
Arrhythmia Service
Albert Einstein College of Medicine
  and Montefiore Medical Center
Bronx, New York
USA

Philip Zilo, MD
Attending Electrophysiologist
Florida Arrhythmia Consultants
Fort Lauderdale, Florida
USA

Introduction

Therapeutic strategies for cardiac arrhythmias are both simple and complex. Simple, because in addition to the large arsenal of pharmacological agents which have long been the basis of the therapeutic approach to these disorders, we now have a wide range of nonpharmacological options. Among these techniques are radiofrequency catheter ablation, antiarrhythmic surgical treatment, and electrical devices, including the implantable cardioverter defibrillator (ICD). Complex, because this wider range of therapeutic options implies careful case-by-case consideration of all the advantages and relative risks of each therapeutic decision and application.

The first part of this book deals with pharmacological treatment of ventricular and supraventricular arrhythmias, with particular emphasis on controversial topics. One fundamental question concerns the proper place of antiarrhythmic drugs in respect to other types of treatment. The efficacy of antiarrhythmic drugs is well established, but their side effects remain a major problem, as has been pointed out in many reports, including the CAST Study. When considering this mass of evidence, the legitimacy of further development of antiarrhythmic drugs might seem questionable, and the debate is taken up in this section of the book. This is accompanied by a review of the place of antiarrhythmic drugs in current practice, and of their uses in ventricular tachycardia (VT) in ischemic and nonischemic cardiopathy, and in both congenital and acquired long QT syndrome.

The second part of this book looks at some of the remarkable progress which has been made in the field of radiofrequency catheter ablation. The basic principles of this technique are reviewed in detail. Recently developed techniques which modulate atrioventricular conduction are particularly interesting, because they overcome the early difficulties of ablation which often required permanent electrosystolic pacing. Unexpected positive results were obtained with radiofrequency catheter ablation in patients suffering from either paroxysmal supraventricular tachycardias with accessory pathways or AV nodal reentrant tachycardia, with success in over 90 percent of cases. The use of these techniques in patients with atrial flutter has produced surprisingly positive results in the common type of flutter. Among the supraventricular arrhythmias, idiopathic atrial fibrillation remains one of our major concerns. The use of radiofrequency ablation techniques to convert atrial fibrillation to sinus rhythm is currently being actively investigated. Finally, current techniques for treatment of VTs with radiofrequency gives less favorable results, with certain exceptions such as fascicular VT. It seems unlikely in the near future that radiofrequency catheter ablation of reentrant tachycardia will be able to replace pharmacological treatment or even more radical treatments such as antiarrhythmic surgery or the ICD.

It is appropriate that the last section of this book deals with antiarrhythmic surgery and the ICD. Antiarrhythmic surgery has proven to be useful in treating recurrent VT of certain types. With sophisticated mapping and surgical techniques, antiarrhythmic surgery can offer a high success rate and low morbidity. On the other hand, the ICD has undergone many technical improvements, especially in regard to the size of the generator and the use of nonthorocotomy leads. This has allowed the expansion of the indications for ICD far beyond that of patients resuscitated from cardiac arrest. It is obvious, however, that the ICD does not totally resolve the problems of the quality of life of the patient, and it remains a purely palliative, although very successful, solution to arrhythmic death. This section closes with the discussion of the future role of the atrial defibrillator.

In summary, this book offers a concise, yet all-inclusive, review of the up-to-date strategies in the management of cardiac arrhythmias and does so in a practical and less didactic manner. It should prove to be a valuable reading for all those involved in this field of medical practice.

Nabil El-Sherif, M.D.
Jean Lekieffre, M.D.

Contents

PART I

Pharmacological Treatment of Supraventricular and Ventricular Tachycardias

Chapter 1

New Antiarrhythmic Drug Development:
Rationale and Approach

Dan M. Roden, MD

Current Status of Antiarrhythmic Therapy

The last 20 years has seen dramatic advances in the understanding of mechanisms underlying cardiac arrhythmias and their rational treatment. Thus, for example, the routine use of ablative techniques in atrioventricular (AV) nodal reentry has emerged, because, first, the arrhythmia was recognized to be macroreentrant in nature and, second, portions of the circuit at which radiofrequency lesions could be placed without perturbing normal AV nodal function were identified. Similarly, technological advances in circuit and lead design, and in the basic understanding of the determinants of ventricular defibrillation, have led to the increasing acceptance of the use of implanted cardioverter defibrillators (ICDs) in the treatment of patients with ventricular fibrillation or sustained ventricular tachycardia. Nonpharmacological approaches for other arrhythmias, including especially atrial fibrillation, remain under intensive development, but are not yet available.

Against this background has emerged the increasing recognition that currently available antiarrhythmic drugs are flawed by the lack of consistent efficacy and a high incidence of adverse effects. These adverse effects can generally be grouped into two broad categories: noncardiac effects; and cardiac effects. Most available drugs are quite nonspecific in their pharmacological effects; that is, they exert a wide range of effects which become manifest in many organs (the heart and others), thereby accounting for a high incidence

[1] Supported in part by a grant from the United States Public Health Service (HL46681). Dr. Roden is the holder of the William Stokes Chair in Experimental Therapeutics, a gift from the Daiichi Corporation.

of noncardiac side effects. Drugs whose pharmacological actions are confined to a single specific target (e.g., an adrenergic receptor or an ion channel) are much less likely to produce these nonspecific side effects.

The single greatest perceived liability of currently available antiarrhythmic drug therapy, is the potential for arrhythmia aggravation ("proarrhythmia"), and the last two decades have also seen great advances in our understanding of the mechanisms underlying this phenomenon. These advances include: recognition that proarrhythmia consists of a number of distinct clinical syndromes; delineation of their clinical features; and identification of the underlying mechanisms. This new knowledge has developed along with an increasing appreciation of the complex nature of the cardiac action potential. Specifically, information is now becoming available on the characteristics of individual ion currents which underlie the action potential, as well as how these currents result from the expression of individual genes whose identity and regulation is under intensive study.

Currently available antiarrhythmic therapy, thus, consists of a series of drugs developed in the 1970s or before, and newer mechanism-based therapies which are often "nonpharmacological." However, the last decade has seen tremendous increases in our understanding of the molecular and cellular basis for cardiac excitability. With this new knowledge could come the development of new drug entities targeting specific molecules, producing acceptable efficacy, and lacking proarrhythmic or other toxicity.

Empiricism in Antiarrhythmic Drug Development

The bark of the cinchona plant has been used to treat arrhythmias since at least the mid-18th century, and one important component of the cinchona, quinidine, was introduced into systematic antiarrhythmic therapy in the early 20th century. However, it was only in the 1950s that quinidine's important fundamental mechanisms of action, sodium channel block, and action potential prolongation, were identified.[1-3] Most currently available antiarrhythmics were designed with the idea of mimicking one or more of the important properties of quinidine and quinidine-like drugs. This mimicry has fallen into two broad categories: (1) drugs which refine the sodium channel blocking actions of quinidine, procainamide, and lidocaine. These include agents such as encainide and flecainide which were synthesized in programs designed to discover more potent procainamide analogs; and (2) drugs such as dofetilide, E4031, and ibutilide which were the products of synthetic programs designed to uncover more potent action potential, prolonging analogs of N-acetyl-procainamide and sotalol, to which they bear some structural similarities. These medicinal chemistry efforts were undertaken virtually in the absence of any detailed knowledge of the specific ion channels that these drugs might block, of the important time and voltage dependence of that block, and, most importantly, in the face of only rudimentary understanding of the mechanisms underlying the arrhythmias these drugs are supposed to treat. Thus, in contrast to many other areas in contemporary therapeutics, the drug treatment of cardiac arrhythmias and indeed, the development of new antiarrhythmic drugs has been largely empiric.

A number of preclinical and clinical investigations have raised questions about the safety of sodium channel block as an antiarrhythmic mode of action, especially in patients with ischemic heart disease. Primary among these investigations was the Cardiac Arrhythmia Suppression Trial (CAST), in which the potent sodium channel blocking drugs encainide and flecainide increased mortality two to threefold in patients convalescing from myocardial infarction.[4] While the mechanisms underlying this effect are unknown, an interaction between conduction slowing by sodium channel block and recurrent ischemia is one leading possibility. Indeed, patients in CAST with non-Q wave myocardial infarction, a subset thought to be at an especially high risk of recurrent ischemia, had a very strikingly increased risk of dying during flecainide or encainide therapy, 8.7-fold compared to placebo-treated patients, as opposed to those with Q wave myocardial infarctions where the relative risk was 1.7-fold.[5] Moreover, preclinical studies support the idea that acute ischemia during treatment with sodium channel blocking drugs, results in an increased incidence of ventricular fibrillation and a decreased ability to defibrillate the heart.[6]

Singh and Vaughan Williams proposed that, beyond sodium channel block and antiadrenergic effects, a useful "third mode" of antiarrhythmic action might be action potential prolongation.[7,8] Since refractoriness in many tissues is determined largely by the voltage-dependent recovery of sodium channels from inactivation during phase 3 of the action potential, prolongation of the action potential, by whatever mechanism, prolongs refractoriness. It is prolongation of refractoriness, particularly prolongation that results in decreased heterogeneity of refractoriness, that is the likely antiarrhythmic effect of action potential prolonging drugs. This effect was initially identified in studies with amiodarone and with sotalol, both of which possess prominent antiadrenergic effects. More recently, drugs which "purely" prolong cardiac action potentials, usually by inhibiting one or more repolarizing potassium currents, have been shown to produce a range of desirable actions: they are effective in some animal models of ischemic ventricular fibrillation; they render the heart more difficult to fibrillate; they decrease defibrillation energy requirement; and they increase contractility.[9] A common liability of many action potential prolonging drugs (amiodarone appears to be an exception[10,11]) is the occasional, and often unpredictable, development of exaggerated QT prolongation and torsades de pointes. Thus, the development of an action potential-prolonging compound that does not produce torsades de pointes might represent an important advance in antiarrhythmic therapy. The remainder of this chapter is devoted to a description of available knowledge that might impact on such a drug development strategy.

The Physiology of Cardiac Repolarization

Substantial advances have been made recently in the cellular electrophysiology of cardiac repolarization, as well as the molecular biology of ion channels which support it. These may be important both in refining our understanding of repolarization and its variability, as well as in understanding how best to accomplish action potential prolongation as an antiarrhythmic mode of action, while minimizing any risks associated with this approach. The maintenance of a relatively stable voltage during the plateau of the cardiac action potential is attributable to what has been referred to as the "delicate balance" between inward and outward currents. Even small changes in this balance can result in substantial alterations in action potential duration. Recent molecular genetic studies[12,13] in the congenital long QT syndrome have elegantly confirmed that action potential prolongation can result from either increased inward, or decreased outward current. In some families, the disease is caused by a failure of sodium channel inactivation (with augmented inward current[14]) whereas in others, the cause is an abnormal potassium channel, and decreased outward current.[15]

The major inward current during the plateau phase of most cardiac cells is carried through L-type calcium channels. Under some conditions, inward currents may also be carried through sodium channels, T-type calcium channels, or the electrogenic sodium-calcium exchange mechanism. Enhancement of any of these inward currents would prolong the duration of the cardiac action potential. The magnitude of these currents in an individual cell is determined by how many channel molecules are present in the cell, how large a current flows through each channel when it is open, and the likelihood that the channel is open at any instant in time. The latter, in turn, is reflected by rates at which the channel opens and at which it inactivates (inactivation being the process whereby a current, once activated, spontaneously decreases despite a constant membrane potential). Thus, a drug could increase an inward current by increasing the probability that a single channel would open, by decreasing the rate of inactivation, or by increasing the number of functional channels. Multiple outward currents controlled by similar mechanisms are described below.

Ion Channel Molecular Biology

The first ion channel gene to be cloned, was the ion channel gene encoding the sodium channel of the electric organ of the electric eel.[16] Sodium and calcium channels in other tissues, including human heart, all share structural similarities to this original clone: they are large proteins (molecular weight 200–250,000) with four roughly homologous domains, each consisting of six membrane-spanning segments.[17] The first potassium channel cDNA was isolated in 1987 from a mutant of the fruit fly *Drosophila melanogaster* which, when exposed to ether, developed abnormal shaking behavior in its flight muscles.[18] The encoded proteins resemble a single domain of a sodium or calcium channel, with six membrane-spanning segments. Thus, these proteins are thought to assemble in groups of four (tetramers) to form functional ion channels.[19] *Shaker*-like cDNAs have also been isolated from rat heart and human heart, as well as from mammalian brain and pancreas. A common nomenclature has been adopted, Kv1.4 and Kv1.5 appear to be the major *Shaker*-like channels found in the human heart,[20] although it is not clear, their expression is myocyte specific.[21] Other members of an extended *Shaker* super family that may play a role in cardiac repolarization include Kv2.1 and Kv4.2. In addition, other potassium channel cDNAs have been isolated which have no structural similarity to those of the *Shaker* super family. These include a small cDNA, minK, that may encode the slowly activating, delayed rectifier I_{Ks},[22,23] described further below, as well as members of an inward rectifier family which conceivably represent truncated versions of a *Shaker* channel.[24] In early 1995, molecular genetic studies in the long QT syndrome identified mutations in *HERG*,[25] a gene that is now recognized to encode the rapidly activating cardiac delayed rectifier I_{Kr}.[13,26]

The identification of multiple ion currents which control cardiac repolarization has led to refinements in understanding mechanisms of drug action which might cause increased action potential duration. A difficulty in studying drug action in cardiac myocytes is that multiple overlapping currents are frequently present. Thus, systems in which a single current can be studied in isolation from others, are required for studies of the mechanisms of drug-channel interactions. These systems may include native myocytes, cultured cells, and ordinarily nonexcitable cells which have been transected with ion channel RNA or cDNA. It is, however, critical to recognize that the cardiac action potential is the highly integrated product of the voltage- and time-dependent activities of multiple ion channels. Thus, even drugs which specifically target only a single ion channel, may nevertheless, cause sufficient changes in the trajectory of the cardiac action potential to alter the time- and voltage-dependent function of other repolarizing currents. Indeed, as described below, this appears to be a common underlying mechanism for the genesis of torsades de pointes.

An important problem in contemporary ion channel biology, is the correspondence between individual ion channel genes and individual ion currents. This is all the more complicated by the recognition that the faithful replication of an individual ion current in a heterologous expression system, often requires expression of two or more different genes (i.e., ion channels may be multiprotein structures). The most extensive studies with cloned channels have been conducted with the human Kv1.5 (hKv1.5) expressed in mouse fibroblasts (L-cells). In this system, quinidine, quinine, imipramine, clofilium, perhexilene, verapamil, and terfenadine all appear to be open-state blockers.[27-32] Expression of a single ion current in isolation from others in experimental models such as this, also allows some inferences as to mechanisms of block. A common mechanism of a block of hKv1.5, is a block of open channels by a charged form of a drug acting from the inside of the membrane, at a site that is approximately 20% within the electric field of the membrane. It is thought that this site may reside in the permeation pore and that the presence of a drug in this site of action, may be stabilized by long hydrophobic side chains, which interact with adjacent portions of the ion channel protein molecule.[32]

Variability in Cardiac Action Potentials

It is increasingly recognized that ion currents recorded in the heart may vary as a function of region, autonomic tone, development, or disease. The cloning of cDNAs encoding ion channel proteins provides an important new tool in studies of the mechanisms underlying these differences in repolarization among cardiac cells. For example, it is well-recognized that action potentials recorded from atrial tissue are much shorter than those in the ventricle tissue, that endocardial cells lack a distinct phase 1 "notch," whereas, a prominent notch is seen in epicardial cells, and that action potentials in the Purkinje network (and in M-cells, isolated from the mid-myocardium of a number of species) are much longer than those in the ventricle.[33] Presumably, such differences reflect differences in the number or function of ion channels in a given cell. As well, it is now increasingly recognized that, in disease, the number or function of ion channels contributing to cardiac repolarization may be altered. For example, transient outward current is markedly decreased in cells from the border zone of recent myocardial infarction in dogs.[34] In hypertensive cats, T-type calcium current appear to be increased.[35] In ventricular cells isolated from humans with heart failure, I_{TO} appears to be reduced.[36] The molecular mechanisms underlying these changes are only now beginning to be addressed. These changes are important not only to understand the long-term arrhythmogenic consequences of diseases such as ischemia or hypertension, but also point out that responses to antiarrhythmic drug therapy might be quite different in patients with and without these diseases.

Drugs that Prolong Cardiac Action Potentials

Among antiarrhythmic drugs available or under investigation, only ibutilide acts by increasing inward current.[37] Ibutilide shares some structural similarity with I_{Kr} blockers such as E4031 and dofetilide, and recent studies indicate that it too is a potent I_{Kr} blocker.[38] Action potential prolongation may also augment contractility and a number of positive inotropic drugs do produce such an effect, which may contribute to their clinical actions in heart failure. Examples include OPC-18790 (which blocks I_{Kr}[39]) and BDF-9148 (which activates I_{Na}[40,41]).

It appears that most currently available drugs which prolong cardiac action potentials do so by blocking multiple potassium currents. Sotalol blocks I_{Kr},[42] and may block I_{TO} in some tissues.[43] Amiodarone blocks I_{Ks}, I_{Kr}, and I_{K1}.[24,44,45] Similarly, quinidine blocks I_{TO}, I_{Ks}, and I_{K1}.[45–47] Interestingly, these effects are most apparent at quinidine concentrations > 5–10 μM; at lower concentrations, quinidine is a blocker of I_{Kr},[48–50] as well as sodium current.[51] The specific potassium currents blocked by procainamide or disopyramide have not been identified. Flecainide is clearly a blocker of I_{Kr}[52] as well as of I_{TO},[53] and propafenone similarly appears to block I_{TO}.[54]

A number of drugs which specifically target the delayed rectifier have been tested in clinical trials.[9] These include E4031, dofetilide, and almokalant. These specific I_{Kr} blockers are highly effective in preventing ischemic ventricular fibrillation in some animal models, and appear to suppress some atrial and ventricular arrhythmias. However, they can cause early afterdepolarizations (EADs) and triggered activity *in vitro*, and torsades de pointes in some patients. In general, these drugs appear to be open channel blockers (i.e., block increases as a function of time at plateau potentials[38,48]). Thus, these agents should block I_{Kr} to a greater extent in rapidly driven tissues than in slowly driven tissues. Nevertheless, specific I_{Kr} blockers generally prolong action potentials to a greater extent at *slow* rates rather than *fast* rates, a phenomenon that has been termed "reverse use-dependence" and that may contribute to torsades de pointes.[55] The explanation for this paradox likely lies in the multifactorial nature of action potential control.[56] In rapidly driven tissues, I_{Kr} is but one of many repolarizing currents (including I_{Ks} as well as a current due to electrogenic sodium-potassium pumping), so its block is unlikely to have major effects on action potential duration. On the other hand, in slowly driven tissues, I_{Ks} may be completely deactivated, and pump current while absent;

under these conditions, I_{Kr} block may produce marked action potential prolongation. Recent reports also indicate that elevated extracellular potassium developing during tachycardia may reverse drug block of I_{Cr}, thereby providing a second mechanism for "reverse use-dependence."[50] Although some differences in the kinetics of onset of and recovery from block have been described for I_{Kr} blockers, it is not known whether these subtle differences are important in determining differences in efficacy, or in torsades de pointes toxicity.

Given the primacy of I_{Ks} deactivation at rapid rates, an I_{Ks} blocker might be expected to prolong action potentials to a greater extent at rapid rates than at slow rates, a desirable effect. Azimilide (NE-10064), an agent now in clinical trials, was originally thought to be a relatively specific I_{Ks} blocker, but more recent investigations have indicated that it also blocks other currents, including I_{TO} and I_{Kr}.[57] Modulation of I_{Ks} by β-adrenergic stimulation represents a potential liability of I_{Ks} block: the extent of residual I_{Ks} might be highly dependent on the extent of adrenergic activation, at any point in time. On the other hand, the coadministration of an I_{Ks} blocker and a β-adrenergic receptor blocker might circumvent this difficulty. In atrial tissue, flecainide produces the interesting effect of prolonging action potentials to a greater extent at rapid rates than at slow rates.[58] While the exact mechanism is unknown, block of outward current has not been implicated; rather, sodium channel block resulting in decreased intracellular sodium loading at rapid rates, with resultant inhibition of the electrogenic sodium-potassium pump, has been suggested.[59]

Torsades de Pointes

Given the complexities of action potential control, it is not surprising that the prediction of the effects of blocking a specific current are difficult. This is rendered all the more difficult by the time-dependency of many of the currents such as I_{TO}, $_{ICR}$, and I_{Ks} that underlie the action potential; the time- and voltage-dependent block of those currents by drugs; autonomic modulation of ion currents and modulation of autonomic effects by drugs. Preclinical and clinical data described above strongly supports the idea that action potential prolongation may be a valuable approach to antiarrhythmic therapy, particularly if combined with antiadrenergic interventions. The "class" toxicity which appears to be the greatest obstacle to the widespread use of action potential prolonging drugs is torsades de pointes. When action potentials are recorded from canine cardiac Purkinje fibers studied under conditions mimicking those seen in torsades de pointes (low potassium, slow drive rates, action potential-prolonging drug), EADs, and triggered activity are frequently observed.[51,60-62] Similar triggered activity has also been reported in M-cells.[33] These and other findings support the idea that EAD-mediated triggering provides at least the initiating mechanism for torsades de pointes. The mechanisms underlying the maintenance of torsades de pointes, its polymorphic nature, and its frequent termination remain speculative. Although many animal models for this arrhythmia have been proposed, very few actually reproduce the marked QTU lability, and prolongation and the "short-long-short" series of cycle length, changes prior to initiation of typical drug-induced torsades de pointes. Interestingly, electrocardiographically typical torsades de pointes does occur in rabbits treated with the α-agonist methoxamine plus an I_{Kr} blocker[63] ; additive suppression of I_{TO} (by methoxamine) and I_{Kr} seems likely. Theories which have been advanced to explain the maintenance of the arrhythmia include: based on heterogenous repolarization times; drifting scroll or spiral wave reentry within the myocardium; or nonreentrant activity, driven by repetitive-triggered beats either from a single focus or from multiple foci within the conducting system and/or M-cells.

Understanding the mechanisms underlying EADs and resultant-triggered activity would be useful in minimizing the incidence of torsades de pointes, or in developing drugs lacking this toxicity. By definition, an EAD represents a transient increase in net inward current during the repolarization phase of an action potential. Such a net increase could result from either an exaggerated decrease in net outward current (perhaps I_{K1} block) or an actual increase in an inward current during terminal repolarization. Both experimental and computer modeling studies suggest the latter mechanism.[64] If the trajectory of repolarization is sufficiently slow, the action potential may enter a voltage range in which inward current may flow through reactivated L-type or T-type calcium channels. Such calcium channel "windows" would certainly account for EADs and, in fact, could also account for the triggered upstroke arising from EADs.[65] Alternatively, it has been suggested that action potential prolongation might result in a prolonged intracellular calcium transient, which in turn would increase sodium-calcium exchange.[66] Since this exchange is electrogenic (3 Na^+ in exchange for 1 Ca^{2+}), a net inward current would result. These potential mechanisms point out the highly interdependent nature of the time- and voltage-dependent behavior of individual ion currents during the action potential. Thus, even drugs which "specifically" block a single potassium current such as I_{Kr}, may well result in these secondary changes in inward currents which form the basis of their major toxicity. The question of why amiodarone only rarely produces torsades de pointes is unanswered; inhibition of calcium-recurrent reactivation or greater action potential-prolonging effects on ventricular cells than on Purkinje or M-cells, or an antireentry effect are all possibilities.

Summary and Future Directions

The major attraction of action potential-prolonging agents as antiarrhythmics is their potential antifibrillatory activity. An effect against ventricular fibrillation may only be detected in studies using large populations at risk for spontaneous ventricular fibrillation. Two agents, dofetilide and d-sotalol, have been evaluated in large clinical trials, in patients with coronary artery disease deemed to be at a high risk for sudden death. The d-sotalol trial (SWORD) was stopped because of excess mortality in drug-treated patients, while the dofetilide trial (DIAMOND) is continuing as of January 1996. The outcome of these trials, presumably depends on the drugs' antifibrillatory actions in the populations chosen for study and the risk that, at the doses chosen for study, they produce torsades de pointes or other arrhythmic toxicity. Further investigation of the molecular and cellular physiology and pharmacology of cardiac repolarization will not only increase our understanding of the sources of variability in repolarization and its response to drugs, but also will allow the rational identification of molecular targets for pharmacological intervention. These could include not only ion channels themselves, but also the mechanisms that regulate their expression in health and disease. Action potential prolongation without torsades de pointes seems a possible goal.

References

1. Hoffman BF. The action of quinidine and procaineamide on single fibers of dog ventricle and specialized conducting system. *An da Acad Brasileira de Ciencias* 1957; 29:365–368.
2. Johnson EA, McKinnon MG. The differential effect of quinidine and pyrilamine on the myocardial action potential at various rates of stimulation. *J Pharmacol Exp Ther* 1957;120:460–468.
3. Vaughan Williams EM. The mode of action of quinidine on isolated rabbit atria interpreted from intracellular potential records. *Br J Pharmacol* 1958;13:276–287.
4. Echt DS, Liebson PR, Mitchell LB. Mortality and morbidity in patients receiving encainide, flecainide, or placebo. *N Engl J Med* 1991;324:781–788.
5. Akiyama T, Pawitan Y, Greenberg H, Kuo CS, Reynolds-Haertle RA, The CAST Investigators. Increased risk of death and cardiac arrest from encainide and flecainide in patients after non-Q-wave acute myocardial infarction in the Cardiac Arrhythmia Suppression Trial. *Am J Cardiol* 1991;68:1551–1555.
6. Nattel S, Pedersen DH, Zipes DP. Alterations in regional myocardial distribution and arrhythmogenic effects of aprindine produced by coronary artery occlusion in the dog. *Cardiovasc Res* 1981;15:80–85.
7. Singh BN, Vaughan Williams EM. A third class of anti-arrhythmic action: effects on atrial and ventricular intracellular potentials and other pharmacologic actions of MJ1999. *Br J Pharmacol* 1970;39:675–689.
8. Singh BN, Vaughan Williams EM. The effect of amiodarone, a new anti-anginal drug, on cardiac muscle. *Br J Pharmacol* 1970;39:657–667.

9. Roden DM. Current status of class III antiarrhythmic therapy. *Am J Cardiol* 1993; 72:44B-49B.

10. Mattioni TA, Zheutlin TA, Sarmiento JJ, Parker M, Lesch M, Kehoe RF. Amiodarone in patients with previous drug-mediated Torsade de Pointes. *Ann Intern Med* 1989;111:574–580.

11. Lazzara R. Amiodarone and torsades de pointes. *Ann Intern Med* 1989;111: 549–551.

12. Wang Q, Shen J, Splawski I, et al. *SCN5A* mutations associated with an inherited cardiac arrhythmia, long QT syndrome. *Cell* 1995;80:805–811.

13. Curran ME, Spiawski I, Timothy KW, Vincent GM, Green ED, Keating MT. A molecular basis for cardiac arrhythmia: *HERG* mutations cause long QT syndrome. *Cell* 1995;80:795–803.

14. Bennett PB, Yazawa K, Makita N, George AL Jr. Molecular mechanism for an inherited cardiac arrhythmia. *Nature* 1995;376:683–685.

15. Sanguinetti MC, Curran ME, Spector PS, Keating MT. Spectrum of HERG K^+ channel dysfunction in an inherited cardiac arrhythmia. *Proc Natl Acad Sci USA* 1996 (In Press).

16. Noda M, Shimizu S, Tanabe K, et al. Primary structure of *Electrophorus electricus* sodium channel deduced from cDNA sequence. *Nature* 1984;312:121–127.

17. Catterall WA. Structure and function of voltage-sensitive ion channels. *Science* 1988;242:50–61.

18. Papazian DM, Schwarz TL, Tempel BL, Jan YN, Jan LY. Cloning of genomic and complementary DNA from Shaker, a putative potassium channel gene from Drosophila. *Science* 1987;237:749–753.

19. Roberts SL, Knoth KM, Po S, et al. Molecular biology of the voltage-gated potassium channels of the cardiovascular system. *J Cardiovasc Electrophysiol* 1993; 4:68–80.

20. Tamkun MM, Knoth KM, Walbridge JA, Kroemer H, Roden DM, Glover DM. Molecular cloning and characterization of two voltage-gated K^+ channel cDNAs from human ventricle. *FASEB J* 1991;5:331–337.

21. Barry DM, Trimmer JS, Merlie JP, Nerbonne JM. Differential expression of voltage-gated K^+ channel subunits in adult rat heart. Relation to functional K^+ channels? *Circ Res* 1995;77:361–369.

22. Takumi T, Ohkubo H, Nakanishi S. Cloning of a membrane protein that induces a slow voltage-gated potassium current. *Science* 1988;242:1042–1045.

23. Folander K, Smith JS, Antanavage J, Bennett C, Stein RB, Swanson R. Cloning and expression of the delayed rectifier IsK channel from neonatal rat heart and diethylstilbestrol-primed rat uterus. *Proc Natl Acad Sci USA* 1990;87:2975–2979.

24. Wible BA, De Biasi M, Majumder K, Taglialatela M, Brown AM. Cloning and functional expression of an inwardly rectifying K^+ channel from human atrium. *Circ Res* 1995;76:343–350.

25. Warmke J, Drysdale R, Ganetzky B. A distinct potassium channel polypeptide encoded by the *Drosophila eag* locus. *Science* 1991;252:1560–1562.

26. Sanguinetti MC, Jiang C, Curran ME, Keating MT. A mechanistic link between an inherited and an acquired cardiac arrhythmia: *HERG* encodes the I_{Kr} potassium channel. *Cell* 1995;81:299–307.

27. Snyders DJ, Knoth KM, Roberds SL, Tamkun MM. Time-, voltage-, and state-dependent block by quinidine of a cloned human cardiac potassium channel. *Mol Pharmacol* 1992;41:322–330.

28. Yang T, Prakash C, Roden DM, Snyders DJ. Mechanism of block of a human cardiac potassium channel by terfenadine racemate and enantiomers. *Br J Pharmacol* 1995;115:267–274.
29. Rampe D, Wible B, Fedida D, Dage RC, Brown AM. Verapamil blocks a rapidly activating delayed rectifier K^+ channel cloned from human heart. *Mol Pharmacol* 1993;44:642–648.
30. Rampe D, Wang Z, Fermini B, Wible B, Dage RC, Nattel S. Voltage- and time-dependent block by perhexiline of K^+ currents in human atrium and in cells expressing a Kv1.5-type cloned channel. *J Pharmacol Exp Ther* 1995;274:444–449.
31. Rampe D, Wible B, Brown AM, Dage RC. Effects of terfenadine and its metabolites on a delayed rectifier K^+ channel cloned from human heart. *Mol Pharm* 1993;44:1240–1245.
32. Snyders DJ, Yeola SW. Determinants of antiarrhythmic drug action electrostatic and hydrophobic components of block of the human cardiac hKv1.5 channel. *Circ Res* 1995;77:575–583.
33. Antzelevitch C, Sicouri S, Lukas A, et al. Clinical implications of electrical heterogeneity in the heart: the electrophysiology and pharmacology of epicardial, M, and endocardial cells. In: Podrid PJ, Kowey PR (eds): *Cardiac Arrhythmia: Mechanisms, Diagnosis, and Management.* Baltimore, MD: William & Wilkins, 1995, pp 88–107.
34. Lue W, Boyden P. Abnormal electrical properties of myocytes from chronically infarcted canine heart. *Circulation* 1992;85:1175–1188.
35. Nuss HB, Houser SR. T-type Ca^{2+} current is expressed in hypertrophied adult feline left ventricular myocytes. *Circ Res* 1993;73:777–782.
36. Beuckelmann D, Näbauer M, Erdmann E. Alterations of K^+ currents in isolated human ventricular myocytes from patients with terminal heart failure. *Circ Res* 1993;73:379–385.
37. Lee KS. Ibutilide, a new compound with potent class III antiarrhythmic activity, activates a slow inward Na^+ current in guinea pig ventricular cells. *J Pharmacol Exp Ther* 1992;262:99–108.
38. Yang T, Snyders DJ, Roden DM. Ibutilide, a methanesulfonanilide antiarrhythmic, is a potent blocker of the rapidly-activating delayed rectifier K^+ current (I_{Kr}) in AT-1 cells: concentration-, time-, voltage-, and use-dependent effects. *Circulation* 1995;91:1799–1806.
39. Yang T, Snyders DJ, Roden DM. Cardiac K^+ channel blocking activity of the versnarinone analog OPC-18790. *Circulation* 1994;90:I-146 (Abstract).
40. Doggrell S, Hoey A, Brown L. Ion channel modulators as potential positive inotropic compound for treatment of heart failure. *Clin & Exp Pharmacol & Physiol* 1994;21:833–843.
41. Amos GJ, Ravens U. The inotropic agents DPI 201–106 and BDF 9148 differentially affect potassium currents of guinea-pig ventricular myocytes. *Naunyn-Schmiedebergs Arch Pharmacol* 1994;350:426–433.
42. Sanguinetti MC, Jurkiewicz NK. Two components of cardiac delayed rectifier K^+ current: differential sensitivity to block by class III antiarrhythmic agents. *J Gen Physiol* 1990;96:195–215.
43. Carmeliet E. Electrophysiologic and voltage clamp analysis of the effects of sotalol on isolated cardiac muscle and Purkinje fibers. *J Pharmacol Exp Ther* 1985;232:817–825.
44. Colatsky TJ, Follmer CH, Starmer CF. Channel specificity in antiarrhythmic drug action. Mechanism of potassium channel block and its role in suppressing and aggravating cardiac arrhythmias. *Circulation* 1990;82:2235–2242.

45. Balser JR, Bennett PB, Hondeghem LM, Roden DM. Suppression of time-dependent outward current in guinea pig ventricular myocytes. Actions of quinidine and amiodarone. *Circ Res* 1991;69:519–529.
46. Balser JR, Roden DM, Bennett PB. Single inward rectifier potassium channels in guinea pig ventricular myocytes. Effects of quinidine. *Biophys J* 1991;59:150–161.
47. Imaizumi Y, Giles WR. Quinidine-induced inhibition of transient outward current in cardiac muscle. *Am J Physiol* 1987;253:H704-H708.
48. Carmeliet E. Use-dependent block of the delayed K^+ current in rabbit ventricular myocytes. *Cardiovasc Drugs Ther* 1993;7(Suppl 3):599–604.
49. Woosley RL, Chen Y, Freiman JP, Gillis RA. Mechanism of the cardiotoxic actions of terfenadine. *JAMA* 1993;269:1532–1536.
50. Yang T, Roden DM. Extracellular potassium modulation of drug block of I_{kr}: implications for Torsades de Pointes and reverse use-dependence. *Circulation* 1996(In Press).
51. Roden DM, Hoffman BF. Action potential prolongation and induction of abnormal automaticity by low quinidine concentrations in canine Purkinje fibers. Relationship to potassium and cycle length. *Circ Res* 1985;56:857–867.
52. Follmer CH, Cullinan CA, Colatsky TJ. Differential block of cardiac delayed rectifier current by class Ic antiarrhythmic drugs: evidence for open channel block and unblock. *Cardiovasc Res* 1992;26:1121–1130.
53. Wang Z, Fermini B, Nattel S. Effects of flecainide, quinidine, and 4-aminopyridine on transient outward and ultrarapid delayed rectifier currents in human atrial myocytes. *J Pharmacol Exp Ther* 1995;272:184–196.
54. Duan D, Fermini B, Nattel S. Potassium channel blocking properties of propafenone in rabbit atrial myocytes. *J of Pharmacol Exp Ther* 1993;264:1113–1123.
55. Hondeghem LM, Snyders DJ. Class III antiarrhythmic agents have a lot of potential, but a long way to go: reduced effectiveness and dangers of reverse use-dependence. *Circulation* 1990;81:686–690.
56. Jurkiewicz NK, Sanguinetti MC. Rate-dependent prolongation of cardiac action potentials by a methanesulfonanilide class III antiarrhythmic agent: specific block of rapidly activating delayed rectifier K^+ current by dofetilide. *Circ Res* 1993;72: 75–83.
57. Fermini B, Jurkiewicz NK, Jow B; et al. Use-dependent effects of the class III antiarrhythmic agent NE-10064 (azimilide) on cardiac repolarization: block of delayed rectifier potassium and L-type calcium currents. *J Cardiovasc Pharmacol* 1995;26:259–271.
58. Wang ZG, Pelletier LC, Talajic M, Nattel S. Effects of flecainide and quinidine on human atrial action potentials. Role of rate-dependence and comparison with guinea pig, rabbit, and dog tissues. *Circulation* 1990;82:274–283.
59. Wang Z, Fermini B, Nattel S. Mechanism of flecainide's rate-dependent actions on action potential duration in canine atrial tissue. *J Pharmacol Exp Ther* 1993; 267:575–581.
60. Strauss HC, Bigger JT, Hoffman BF. Electrophysiological and beta-receptor blocking effects of MJ 1999 on dog and rabbit cardiac tissue. *Circ Res* 1970;26: 661–678.
61. Dangman KH, Hoffman BF. In vivo and in vitro antiarrhythmic and arrhythmogenic effects of N-acetyl procainamide. *J Pharmacol Exp Ther* 1981;217:851–862.
62. Brachmann J, Scherlag BJ, Rosenshtraukh LV, Lazzara R. Bradycardia-dependent triggered activity: relevance to drug-induced multiform ventricular tachycardia. *Circulation* 1983;68:846–856.

63. Carlsson L, Almgren O, Duker G. QTU-prolongation and Torsades de Pointes induced by putative class III antiarrhythmic agents in the rabbit: etiology and interventions. *J Cardiovasc Pharmacol* 1990;16:276–285.
64. Zeng J, Rudy Y. Early afterdepolarizations in cardiac myocytes: mechanism and rate dependence. *Biophysical Journal* 1995;68:949–964.
65. January CT, Riddle JM. Early afterdepolarizations: mechanism of induction and block: a role for L-type Ca^{2+} current. *Circ Res* 1989;64:977–990.
66. Szabo B, Sweidan R, Rajagopalan CB, Lazzara R. Role of $Na^{+}:Ca^{2+}$ exchange current in Cs^{+}-induced early afterdepolarizations in Purkinje fibers. *J Cardiovasc Electrophysiol* 1994;5:933–944.

Chapter 2

Antiarrhythmic Agents in Paroxysmal Atrial Fibrillation:
When and How?

Samuel Lévy, MD

Introduction

Atrial fibrillation is the most commonly sustained arrhythmia seen in clinical practice. In the Framingham study, the incidence is estimated to be 2% to 4% of the general population above 65 years of age.[1] The incidence is even higher in patients with underlying heart disease.[2] Atrial fibrillation may be associated with hemodynamic impairment, occasionally disabling symptoms, and a decrease in life expectancy. In advanced heart failure, atrial fibrillation is common and was found to be a marker for increased risk of death.[3] The most important concern with atrial fibrillation relates to its embolic manifestations that, in 75% of instances, are complicated by cerebrovascular accidents.[4,5]

Atrial fibrillation is generally subdivided into two forms: paroxysmal atrial fibrillation; and established or chronic atrial fibrillation. Chronic atrial fibrillation may be the end result of paroxysmal fibrillation in about 30% of the latter. However, in most patients, the arrhythmia presents as chronic fibrillation.

Pharmacological therapy remains by far, the most common treatment for restoring or maintaining sinus rhythm, for prevention of recurrences or for control of heart rate. Therapeutic strategy in paroxysmal atrial fibrillation is not uniform, as it should take into account patient symptoms, duration, and frequency of attacks. The therapeutic end-point is twofold: suppression of symptoms; and reduction of embolic risk. Selection of antiarrhythmic agents should take into account the end-point to be achieved, the underlying heart disease, and the status of myocardial function.

From *Practical Management of Cardiac Arrhythmias* edited by Nabil El-Sherif, and Jean Lekieffre. Futura Publishing Co., Armonk, NY, © 1997.

Antiarrhythmic Agents in Atrial Fibrillation: How?

The definitions used were those proposed by Lévy et al[6] and the French Society of Cardiology.[7] Pharmacological therapy may be indicated to restore sinus rhythm if the attack of atrial fibrillation is persistent and, to prevent recurrences or to slow heart rate in order to suppress patient symptoms.

Restoring Sinus Rhythm

Pharmacological treatment dates back over 200 years, although the modern era commenced in 1918 when Frey used quinidine to terminate atrial fibrillation of recent onset. Today, quinidine is less used for this indication, as its safety has been questioned based on reported cases of sudden death.[8,9] A number of other antiarrhythmic agents have been given orally for this indication, including procainamide, disopyramide, and oral amiodarone. However, there is no control trial demonstrating the safety and efficacy of such use, and amiodarone is not approved for this indication. More recently, oral flecainide or propafenone has been used in atrial fibrillation of recent onset in order to restore sinus rhythm.[10,11] Success rates as high as 91% were recently reported[10] with a single oral dose of 300 mg of flecainide. This was significantly higher than the success rates with placebo (48%) during an observation period of 8 hours. In other reports,[12,13] the success rates with flecainide ranged between 67% and 95%. Studies with oral propafenone (600 mg as a single dose) showed success rates as high as 81% at 12 hours, which was significantly better than placebo (33%) or the combination of oral quinidine and intravenous digoxin (50%).[11]

Pharmacological conversion of atrial fibrillation of recent onset or prolonged episodes of paroxysmal atrial fibrillation, is routinely attempted in hospital practice using intravenous injection of an antiarrhythmic agent. Intravenous digoxin (0.5–1 mg in the absence of ongoing digitalis therapy) is commonly used, although the efficacy of the drug and the mechanism of action are still uncertain. Furthermore, controlled studies have suggested that the conversion rate to sinus rhythm is no better than with placebo,[14,15] although the effect of digoxin to slow the ventricular response during atrial fibrillation is unquestioned. Intravenous amiodarone 5 mg/kg over 10 to 30 minutes followed by an infusion of 500 mg over 24 hours has been reported to be associated with a high success rate,[16,17] although there is no controlled study.

Newer antiarrhythmic agents have been used for this indication. Intravenous flecainide (1.5 mg/kg), intravenous propafenone (2 mg/kg), and intravenous cibenzoline (1.5 mg/kg) have been reported to be successful in recent onset of atrial fibrillation, with a wide range of good results related at least in part, to differences in the patient population.[18,19] In established atrial fibrillation, the results are less impressive than in paroxysmal or recent onset atrial fibrillation. Comparing intravenous propafenone (2 mg/kg) and intravenous flecainide over 10 minutes in atrial fibrillation of less than 6 months duration, Suttorp et al[20] reported a better result (18 of 20 patients or 90%) with flecainide than with propafenone (11 of 20 patients or 55%). Pharmacological conversion with Na-channel blockers carries the risk of converting atrial fibrillation to atrial flutter and ventricular proarrhythmia, as the slowing of atrial rate may allow 1:1 propagation through the atrioventricular node. This phenomenon may be facilitated by the anticholinergic action of certain Na-channel blockers like quinidine and disopyramide.

Prevention of Recurrences of Atrial Fibrillation

Following pharmacological or electrical cardioversion, recurrences of atrial fibrillation are common, and only 25% of patients taking placebo are in sinus rhythm at 1 year versus 50% of patients when quinidine is administered.[8] Therefore, pharmacological therapy is needed to prevent recurrences of atrial fibrillation.

Induction of atrial fibrillation may be precipitated by premature atrial depolarizations or, less commonly, by premature ventricular depolarizations through appropriately-timed retrograde conduction to the atria, or by changes in heart rate related to increases in sympathetic or parasympathetic tone. To date, only a limited number of cases of vagally induced fibrillation have been reported.[21]

The concepts recently developed by the Sicilian Gambit Group[22,23] have been helpful for selecting the appropriate antiarrhythmic agent adapted to the therapeutic end-point (Tables 1 and 2). To prevent recurrences of atrial

Table 1

Mechanism of Arrhythmia	Reentry
Vulnerable Parameters	Atrial refractoriness
Therapeutic Choice	Increase atrial refractoriness
	Increase wavelength
Cibles	Na- and K-channel blockers
Antiarrhythmic Agent	

—Na channel blockers: quinidine, disopyramide, propafenone, flecainide, cibenzoline.
—K-channel blockers: amiodarone, sotalol.

Table 2

Mechanism of Arrhythmia	Random reentry
Vulnerable Parameters	Atrial refractoriness; sympathetic tone
Therapeutic Choice	1. increase atrial refractoriness
	2. decrease sympathetic tone
	3. decrease vagal tone
Targets	1. Na channel and/or K channels
	2. β-adrenergic receptors
	3. muscarinic receptors
Drugs	1. Na- and K-channel blockers
	2. β-antagonist
	3. vagolytic agents

fibrillation, one may choose to suppress the trigger mechanism of premature atrial depolarizations and premature ventricular depolarizations, or to modify the atrial substrate by modifying atrial refractoriness, which may be another vulnerable parameter. An increase in atrial refractoriness may be achieved by Na-channel blockers, such as quinidine, procainamide, disopyramide, propafenone, or flecainide, which prolong inactivation of Na channels, or by antiarrhythmic agents whose major electrophysiological effect is to prolong action potential duration and refractoriness, such as amiodarone or sotalol. In selected cases of catecholamine-induced atrial fibrillation, the therapeutic option may be to decrease the sympathetic tone. The target in this particular situation is constituted by β-adrenergic receptors and the logical antiarrhythmic agent is a β-blocking agent.

The antiarrhythmic agents used in the prevention of recurrences following cardioversion of persistent or chronic atrial fibrillation are the same than those used to prevent recurrences of paroxysmal atrial fibrillation. In most studies paroxysmal and chronic atrial fibrillation are lumped together. Only few studies have dealt specifically with paroxysmal atrial fibrillation. Most studies have used as a model prevention of recurrences of atrial fibrillation following cardioversion. We have selected few studies which we feel are important and have shaped our thinking about the strategy of atrial fibrillation. Quinidine has been and probably is in some countries, the most used agent in the prevention of recurrences of atrial fibrillation. Jüul-Moller et al[24] compared the efficacy of quinidine (600-mg bid) and sotalol (80-mg or 160-mg bid) following cardioversion of atrial fibrillation. The study included 174 patients, 95 on sotalol and 79 on quinidine. At 6 months, sinus rhythm was present in 49 patients (52%) on sotalol and in 38 patients (48%) on quinidine. Side effects were observed in 28% of patients on sotalol and 50% of patients on quinidine. Proarrhythmic ventricular event was observed in one patient on sotalol (torsades de pointes), and one patient on quinidine (ventricular fibrillation cardioverted) and was associated with no death. The conclusion was that sotalol was as efficient as quinidine in maintaining sinus rhythm and was better tolerated than quinidine.

Another important study was reported by Crijns[25] and included 127 patients who underwent successful cardioversion of atrial fibrillation. They used a stage-care approach including flecainide (stage 1), sotalol or quinidine (stage 2), and amiodarone (stage 3). Stages 2 and 3 were only used in case of recurrence. This approach resulted at 2 years with an increase in the percentage of patients; they were free from arrhythmia from 31% to 63%. The number of patients requiring stage 2 and stage 3 was 53 and 34, respectively. Among the factors predictive of refractoriness to therapy were: age; number of previous recurrences; duration of arrhythmia and mitral valve disease.

Reimold et al[26] compared propafenone with sotalol following cardioversion of atrial fibrillation. Their study included 100 patients with paroxysmal or chronic atrial fibrillation. At 12 months, 30% of patients were on sinus rhythm on propafenone (775 mg); and 37% on sotalol (320 mg); and the difference was not statistically significant. Two patients died during the study on sotalol and nine on propafenone. Ventricular proarrhythmia occurred in two patients on propafenone and three on sotalol. Gastrointestinal side effects were observed in eight patients on propafenone and nine on sotalol.

Pharmacological Therapy of Paroxysmal Atrial Fibrillation: When?

Following the Sicilian Gambit approach, the vulnerable parameter is atrial refractoriness. The increase in atrial refractoriness may be achieved by the above-mentioned Na- and K-channel blockers. However, the problem remains in which patient, and when to use an antiarrhythmic agent. Atrial fibrillation is quite heterogeneous in its clinical presentation. In paroxysmal atrial fibrillation, the attacks may differ in their duration, frequency, and functional tolerance. The wide spectrum of clinical aspects associated with atrial fibrillation may account for the difficulty in evaluating the effects of antiarrhythmic agents given to prevent recurrences.

Paroxysmal atrial fibrillation was subdivided into three classes.[6] Class I included a first attack of paroxysmal atrial fibrillation, either with spontaneous termination (Ia) or requiring pharmacological or electrical cardioversion (Ib). Class II referred to recurrent attacks of atrial fibrillation with three subgroups: IIa—no symptoms during the attack; IIb— an average of < 1 symptomatic attack every 3 months ; IIc— > 1 symptomatic attack every 3 months. Class III included symptomatic attacks of recurrent atrial fibrillation in patients treated with antiarrhythmic agents for the prevention of recurrences (sodium or potassium channel blockers) including amiodarone. Class III consisted also of three subgroups: IIIa—no symptoms ; IIIb—< 1 symptomatic attack per 3-month period ; and IIIc— > 1 symptomatic attack per 3-month period.

In the new classification system described in this study, three clinical aspects of paroxysmal atrial fibrillation were isolated in such a way as to have implications for therapy. In the first attack of atrial fibrillation (class I), the frequency of recurrences cannot be determined and therefore, pharmacological treatment for the prevention of recurrences may not be justified. Recurrent atrial fibrillation (class II) may be asymptomatic, and recorded by Holter monitoring (IIa), or symptomatic and categorized in the subgroups IIb or IIc according to the frequency of attacks. In class IIa, the role of pharmacological treatment to prevent asymptomatic recurrences and stroke is not established. In class IIb, episodic treatment to terminate or slow the rate of the attack may be an option as opposed to long-term treatment for the prevention of recurrences. In class IIc, prevention of recurrences with sodium-channel blockers or potassium-channel blockers may be warranted.

Atrial fibrillation resistant to antiarrhythmic drug therapy (class III) may lead to further investigations to uncover a possible mechanism on the atrio-ventricular node (e.g., calcium-blockers, beta-blockers, digitalis) in order to slow the ventricular rate or consideration of atrioventricular node modification or ablation.

The evaluation of antiarrhythmic agents in patients with paroxysmal atrial fibrillation is difficult. The approach used by Anderson et al[27] is particularly interesting. These authors used transtelephonic monitoring to evaluate the effect of the largest tolerated dose of flecainide on prevention of recurrences. The patients were randomized to flecainide or to placebo with a crossover. Two parameters were assessed: the time to first recurrence; and the interval between attacks. Flecainide (300 mg daily) increased significantly ($p < 0.001$), the time to first recurrence (14.5 days), compared to placebo (3 days), as well as the time between attacks (from 6.2 days for placebo and 27 days for flecainide). In the 55 patients included, the drug was discontinued for side effects in seven. Cardiac arrest occurred in one patient on flecainide.

A stage-care approach was used by Antman et al,[28] in 109 patients with chronic (53 patients) or paroxysmal (56 patients) atrial fibrillation who failed a median of 2 (range 1–5) type IA drugs. Propafenone (791 ± 176 mg) was used as stage 1 and sotalol (537 ± 242 mg) as stage 2. Propafenone resulted in a successful prevention at 5.6 months in 34 patients. Of the 75 failures, 48 patients completed stage 2 (sotalol) and resulted in 26 successful results (at 3.9-month mean follow-up) and 22 failures. At 6 months, 39% of patients were free of recurrence on propafenone and 50% on sotalol. Intolerable side effects requiring discontinuation of therapy ranged from 7% to 8%.

Safety of Antiarrhythmic Agents

Quinidine is the antiarrhythmic agent with the most wide-spread application in prevention of atrial fibrillation recurrences. A recent meta-analysis[8] has shown that 50% of patients taking quinidine were in sinus rhythm at 1 year versus 25% of controls. However, the mortality in the quinidine group was 2.9% versus 0.8% in the placebo group, suggesting that proarrhythmia may be responsible for the excess mortality. This was echoed by a report derived from the Stroke Prevention in Atrial Fibrillation study[29] showing that the mortality in patients with atrial fibrillation and having a history of congestive heart failure, was 4.7 times higher during antiarrhythmic therapy than in patients not taking antiarrhythmic agents. However, there was a better outcome during antiarrhythmic therapy in those patients without heart failure. These studies highlight the importance of the patient's overall cardiovascular status in determining the outcome of drug therapy.

Whether K-channel blockers are safer than Na-channel blockers in the prevention of recurrences of atrial fibrillation is not established. A recent study has shown that sotalol is as effective as quinidine, and better tolerated.[24] At 1 year, 52% of patients were in sinus rhythm in the sotalol group versus 48% in the quinidine group. Recent reports[30] have shown that low-dose amiodarone treatment is effective (38% to 65% in sinus rhythm) and associated with very few side effects at 1 year. However, there have been no controlled or comparative studies, particularly, regarding the long-term mortality with amiodarone or its long-term safety in atrial fibrillation. Therefore, except for selected indications, amiodarone is not recommended as a first-line drug for preventing recurrences of atrial fibrillation. As suggested by Feld,[31] knowledge about the prevention of arrhythmia recurrences with antiarrhythmic agents needs to be reevaluated in light of long-term safety.

Control of Heart Rate

In case of paroxysmal symptomatic atrial fibrillation refractory to sodium-channel blockers, or potassium-channel blockers, or in whom their use is associated with intolerable side effects, control of patient symptoms may be obtained by slowing heart rate.

Selecting the Antiarrhythmic Agent

A convenient and vulnerable parameter for achieving control of ventricular rate is the atrioventricular nodal action potential. To facilitate block of atrioventricular nodal conduction, the target is the L-type calcium channel

Table 3

Vulnerable Parameter	Atrioventricular nodal (Ca-dependent) refractoriness and propagation
Target	I_{ca-L}
Drugs	Calcium-channel blockers (e.g., verapamil, diltiazem)
Alternatives	β-adrenergic blockers; digitalis

(Table 3). Calcium-channel blockers such as verapamil and diltiazem are appropriate drugs. These agents both slow atrioventricular nodal conduction and prolong the nodal-effective refractory period.

Conduction through the atrioventricular node may also be slowed and refractoriness prolonged through another target, (i.e., β-adrenergic receptors.) The appropriate drugs are β-adrenergic blockers that control ventricular rate both at rest and during exercise. The prototype, propranolol, has been extensively studied for this indication. The drawbacks of β-adrenergic blockers are their negative inotropic effects, and their contraindications in conditions such as bronchial asthma or peptic ulcer.

Digoxin is still, in most centers, the first-line drug in patients having atrial fibrillation with a rapid ventricular response and/or congestive heart failure. Digoxin has a direct effect, as well as an indirect effect mediated by the vagus. Digoxin exerts its direct effects on the atria and the atrioventricular node, and in the atria, tends to increase the refractory period. However, the vagotonic actions of digitalis appear to be of far greater importance than its direct actions in the setting of atrial fibrillation. The vagotonic action results in apparent sensitization to the effects of acetylcholine. This, in turn, induces the slowing of atrioventricular nodal conduction, and the prolongation of the atrioventricular nodal refractory period. The effect on the atrioventricular node represents the major action of digoxin relied on by the clinician to slow the ventricular rate in atrial fibrillation. Finally, digoxin-positive inotropic effect makes it the drug of choice in patients with atrial fibrillation associated with heart failure.

Clinical Use of Antiarrhythmic Agents

The prototype calcium channel blocker used is verapamil, which has been administered for more than two decades to slow the ventricular rate in chronic atrial fibrillation.[32] However, verapamil is not effective in restoring sinus rhythm. Control of the ventricular response in atrial fibrillation is observed both at rest and during exercise. Diltiazem has also been shown to be effective in controlling ventricular rate in chronic atrial fibrillation.

β-adrenergic receptor blockers are also useful in controlling heart rate both at rest and during exercise. The β-blocking agents associated with bradycardia such as propranolol and nadolol seem to be more effective than β-blocking agents with intrinsic sympathetic activity such as acebutolol or pindolol.

Digoxin was the first agent to be used for slowing the ventricular response in patients with atrial fibrillation. However, there have been a few studies showing that ventricular rate is consistently reduced during exercise. Digoxin is of particular value in patients with atrial fibrillation associated with heart failure or in patients with depressed left ventricular function.

In patients in whom the ventricular response may not be controlled by pharmacological agents, alone or in combination, radiofrequency modification or ablation of the His bundle may be recommended. Finally, oral anticoagulant therapy is indicated in patients at risk of embolic complications.

Conclusion

Atrial fibrillation is a common arrhythmia which presents the frightening risk of embolic complications which in more than two-thirds of cases result in cerebrovascular accidents. Pharmacological therapy is the most commonly used to restore sinus rhythm, to maintain sinus rhythm by preventing recurrences, or to control heart rate. Paroxysmal atrial fibrillation is quite heterogenous in its clinical presentation. Attacks of paroxysmal atrial fibrillation may differ in their duration, frequency, and functional tolerance.

In the new classification system described, three clinical aspects of paroxysmal atrial fibrillation were isolated in such a way as to have implications for therapy. In the first attack of atrial fibrillation (class I), the frequency of recurrences cannot be determined and therefore pharmacological treatment for prevention of recurrences may not be justified. Recurrent atrial fibrillation (class II) may be asymptomatic, and recorded by Holter monitoring (IIa), or symptomatic and categorized in the subgroups IIb or IIc according to the frequency of attacks. In class IIa, the role of pharmacological treatment to prevent asymptomatic recurrences and stroke is not established. In class IIb, episodic treatment to terminate or slow the rate of the attack may be an option as opposed to long-term treatment for prevention of recurrences. In class IIc, prevention of recurrences with sodium-channel blockers or potassium-channel blockers may be warranted.

It seemed appropriate to separate patients with recurrent paroxysmal atrial fibrillation into those who were untreated (class II), and those who failed one or more antiarrhythmic agents aimed at prevention of recurrences (class III). Selection of the appropriate agents may be based on the concepts recently developed by the Sicilian Gambit Group and on the clinical experience gained over the years with the use of antiarrhythmic agents.

References

1. Kannel WB, Abbott RD, Savage DD, MacNamara PM. Epidemiologic features of atrial fibrillation. The Framingham Study. *N Engl J Med* 1982;306:1018–1022.
2. Zipes D. Cardiac arrhythmias. In: Braunwald W (ed). *Heart Diseases*. Philadelphia, PA: W.B. Saunders, 1984, pp 669–670.
3. Kulbertus HE. Antiarrhythmic treatment of atrial arrhythmias. *J Cardiovasc Pharm* 1991;17 (Suppl 6):S32–S35.
4. Cabin HS, Clubb KS, Hall C, Perlmutter RA, Feinstein AR. Risk for systemic embolization of atrial fibrillation without mitral stenosis. *Am J Cardiol* 1990;61 : 714–717.
5. Rawles J. *Atrial Fibrillation*. London: Springer-Verlag, 1992, pp 181–197.
6. Lévy S, Novella P, Ricard Ph, Paganelli F. Paroxysmal atrial fibrillation: a need for classification. *J Cardiovasc Electrophysiol* 1995;6:69–74.
7. Lévy S, Attuel P, Fauchier JP, Medvedowsky JL. Nosologie de la fibrillation auriculaire. Essai de clarification. *Arch Mal Coeur* 1995;88:1035–1038.
8. Coplen SE, Antman EM, Berlin JA, Hewitt P, Chalmers TC. Efficacy and safety of quinidine therapy for maintenance of sinus rhythm after cardioversion. A meta-analysis of randomized control trials. *Circulation* 1990;82 :1106–1016.
9. Cramer G. Early and late results of conversion of atrial fibrillation with quinidine: a clinical and hemodynamic study. *Acta Med Scand* 1968; 490:5–102.
10. Capucci A, Tiziano L, Boriani G et al. Effectiveness of loading oral flecainide for converting recent-onset atrial fibrillation to sinus rhythm in patients without organic heart disease or with only systemic hypertension. *Am J Cardiol* 1992;70: 69–72.
11. Capucci A, Rubino I, Boriani G, Della Casa S, Sanguinetti M, Magnani B. A placebo controlled study comparing oral propafenone or quinidine plus digoxin in conversion of recent onset atrial fibrillation. *Eur Heart J* 1990;12:338.
12. Goy JJ, Kaufmann L, Kappenberger L, Sigwart U. Restoration of sinus rhythm with flecainide in patients with atrial fibrillation. *Am J Cardiol* 1988;62:38D-40D.
13. Suttorp MJ, Kingma HJ, Jessurun ER, Lie-A-Huen L, Van Hemel NM, Lie KI. The value of class 1C antiarrhythmic drugs for acute conversion of paroxysmal atrial fibrillation or flutter to sinus rhythm. *J Am Coll Cardiol* 1990;16:1722–1727.
14. Falk RH, Knowlton AA, Bernard SA, Gotlieb NE, Battinelli NJ. Digoxin for converting recent-onset atrial fibrillation to sinus rhythm. A randomized double-blinded trial. *Ann Intern Med* 1987;106:503–506.
15. Falk RH, Leavitt JL. Digoxin for atrial fibrillation: a drug whose time has gone ? *Ann Intern Med* 1991;14:573–575.
16. Faniel R, Schoenfeld PH. Efficacy of i. v. amiodarone in converting rapid atrial fibrillation and flutter to sinus rhythm in intensive care patients. *Eur Heart J* 1983;4:180–185.
17. Halpern SW, Ellrodt G, Singh BN, Mandel WJ. Efficacy of intravenous procainamide infusion in converting atrial fibrillation to sinus rhythm. Relation to left atrial size. *Br Heart J* 1980;44:589–595.
18. Suttorp MJ, Kingma HJ, Jessurun ER, Lie-A-Huen L, Van Hemel NM, Lie KI. The value of class1C antiarrhythmic drugs for acute conversion of paroxysmal atrial fibrillation or flutter to sinus rhythm. J Am Coll Cardiol 1990;16:1722–1727.

19. Lacombe P, Cointe R, Metge M, Bru P, Gérard R, Lévy S. Intravenous flecainide in the management of acute supraventricular tachyarrhythmias. *J Electrophysiol* 1988;2:19–22.
20. Suttorp MJ, Kingma HJ, Lie-A-Huen L, Mast EG. Intravenous flecainide versus verapamil for acute conversion of paroxysmal atrial fbirillation or flutter to sinus rhythm. *Am J Cardiol* 1989;63:693–696.
21. Coumel P, Attuel P, Lavallée JP, Flammang D, Leclercq JF, Slama R. Syndrome d'arythmie auriculaire d'origine vagale. *Arch Mal Coeur* 1978;71:645–656.
22. Schwartz PJ, Zaza A. The Sicilian Gambit revisited. Theory and practice. *Eur Heart J* 1992;13(Suppl F) : 23–29.
23. The Sicilian Gambit. A new approach to the classification of antiarrhythmic drugs based on their actions on arrhythmogenic mechanisms. Task force of the working group on arrhythmias of the European Society of Cardiology. *Circulation* 1991; 84:1831–1851. (Simultaneously published in *Eur Heart J* 1991;12:1112–1131.)
24. Jüul-Moller S, Edvardsson N, Rehnqvist-Ahlberg N : Sotalol versus quinidine for the maintenance of sinus rhythm after direct current conversion of atrial fibrillation. *Circulation* 1990;82:1932–1939.
25. Crijns HJGM. Drugs after cardioversion to prevent relapses of chronic atrial fibrillation or flutter. In: Kingman JH, et al (ed). Atrial fibrillation, a treatable disease? Netherlands: Kluwer Academic Publishers, 1992, pp 105–148.
26. Reimold SC, Cantillon CO, Friedman PL, et al. Propafenone versus sotalol for suppression of recurrent symptomatic atrial fibrillation. Am J Cardiol 1993;71: 558.
27. Anderson JL, Gilbert EM, Alpert BL, et al. Prevention of symptomatic recurrences of paroxysmal atrial fibrillation in patients initially tolerating antiarrhythmic therapy. *Circulation* 1989;80:1557–1570.
28. Antman EM, Beamer AD, Caytillon C, et al. Long term oral propafenone therapy for suppression of refractory symptomatic atrial fibrillation and atrial flutter. *J Am Coll Cardiol* 1988;12:1005–1011.
29. Flaker GC, Blackshear JL, McBride R, et al. Antiarrhythmic drug therapy and cardiac mortality in atrial fibrillation. *J Am Coll Cardiol* 1992;20:527–532.
30. Lévy S, Lauribe Ph, Dolla E, et al. A randomized comparison of external and internal cardioversion of chronic atrial fibrillation.*Circulation* 1992;86:1415–1420.
31. Feld GK. Atrial fibrillation: is there a safe and highly effective pharmacological treatment ? *Circulation* 1990;82:2248–2250.
32. Lundstrom T, Ryden L. Ventricular rate control and exercise performance in chronic atrial fibrillation: effects of diltiazem and verapamil. *J Am Coll Cardiol* 1990;16:89–90.

Chapter 3

Is There an Effective Pharmacological Treatment in the Prevention of Vasovagal Syncope?

Richard Sutton, DSc Med

Summary

This chapter has reviewed the published literature on the pharmacological prevention of vasovagal syncope. Many studies have claimed successful treatment in open formats with a wide variety of drugs. However, when pharmacological therapy has been subjected to rigorous clinical trial, to date, no drug has shown any real benefit. In order to qualify this negative statement, it is necessary to add that the means of gauging successful treatment leave much to be desired. These means are repeat tilt testing, reported symptoms, analysis of syncopal burden in a population, and the time to syncopal recurrence. The disadvantages of any assessment parameter derived from tilt testing, is that, the reproducibility of tilt positivity is open to question and other aspects such as tilt duration before syncope have not been adequately investigated. With respect to symptom recurrence, there are potential limitations, because of the well-known occurrence of vasovagal syncope in clusters and the long time-frame that it is necessary for the trial because of relatively infrequent attacks. Furthermore, there appears to be a placebo effect of the initial investigation of this type of syncope which tends to delay the first syncopal recurrence. The first large trials are now either under way or in the planning phase, and it is hoped that they may offer a pharmacological method of prevention of vasovagal syncope, which is both effective in significant numbers of patients and acceptable from the point of view of side effects.

From *Practical Management of Cardiac Arrhythmias* edited by Nabil El-Sherif, and Jean Lekieffre. Futura Publishing Co., Armonk, NY, © 1997.

Introduction

Pharmacological treatment for the prevention of vasovagal syncope has been undertaken for decades, but its administration was always empirical and not subjected to any kind of scientific appraisal. A drug such as etilefrine has been on the market for approximately 40 years and is sold over the counter in Germany. This weak alpha and beta agonist was found to offer amelioration of hypotensive syndromes by many German physicians and has, therefore, been widely used in that country. However, its introduction occurred before the need for elaborate trials of clinical efficacy that are the norm today. With the advent of tilt testing in the mid-1980s,[1] it became possible to diagnose vasovagal syncope in the clinical laboratory. Thus, a new insight into unexplained syncope was afforded and this diagnostic capability prompted therapeutic efforts. There followed a large variety of pharmacological strategies which can be grouped under the following headings:

1. Vagolytics
2. Beta blockers
3. Fluid retaining agents
4. Alpha agonists
5. Adenosine antagonists
6. Negative inotropic agents
7. Selective serotonin reuptake inhibitors.

All of these categories of drugs can be argued to have a role to play in the management of the complex phenomenon that is vasovagal syncope. However, it is only in the recent past that attempts have been made to apply scientific appraisal of their efficacy by the performance of randomized double-blind clinical trials.

Pharmacological Therapy— Uncontrolled Studies

Vagolytics

This group of drugs includes scopolamine, disopyramide, and atropine, which may be expected to act by antagonizing the vagal component of the vasovagal syncopal reaction. One study using atropine administered intravenously, demonstrated that this drug was not always effective in preventing vasovagal syncope.[2] Scopolamine administered transcutaneously received an enthusiastic report,[3] but this drug is no longer manufactured. Disopyramide also appeared to be promising, but its action is only weakly vagolytic and it was claimed to be acting more as a negative inotropic agent.[4]

Beta-Blockers

This group of drugs has been studied more than any other; the use of propranolol,[2,5] metoprolol,[6-12] atenolol[13,14] and esmolol[15] has been reported. The rationale behind their use is antagonism of the well-documented rise in plasma epinephrine that occurs prior to the development of the vasovagal reaction. Of these, the greatest experience has been with metoprolol with the longest follow-up. Achievement of a negative tilt test has ranged from 25%[2] to 100%,[6,8] and recurrence of syncope in follow-up has varied between 0% over 21 months in four patients[8] to 25% over 33 months in 138 patients.[12] These are sufficiently encouraging results to provide the possibility of valuable therapy and show an adequate performance in a controlled trial. The data also points toward a circulatory antagonism of epinephrine, rather than dependence on a cerebral action as the majority of the drugs used does not cross the blood-brain barrier.

Fluid Retaining Agents

The only drug used in this category is fludrocortisone,[3,6,10,13] but experience has been small, amounting to little more than 30 patients with a modest result in 21 patients; 48% tilt negativity and 10% recurrent syncope over 20 months.[10] Initially, advice was given to measure the blood volume to identify which patients to treat with this agent[2] although this is not widely praticed.

Fludrocortisone, by retaining fluid, should attenuate the effect of the loss of central blood volume that occurs in the adoption of the erect posture, and in so doing, has a similar effect to that of support stockings which are sometimes a beneficial physical maneuver. They may be best in combination, and this physicopharmacological strategy may need to be used in tandem with another treatment.

Alpha Agonists

These drugs might be expected to achieve their effect, by raising the blood pressure and maintaining it in the face of developing hypotension in vasovagal syncope. Etilefrine, phenylephrine, pseudoephedrine, and ephedrine, fall into this group of drugs and all have been subjected to uncontrolled trials.[2,12,15] Results have shown promise for etilefrine with 100% tilt negativity and no syncopal recurrence over 12 months in 7 patients. In the study of Strieper and Campbell,[15] phenylephrine was used intravenously to test the acute effect on the early repeat tilt test with a 94% rate of negative tilts and pseudoephedrine was used as the oral medication in follow-up; a 6% recurrence over 11 months. Natale et al's experience with ephedrine was not so encouraging with only 40% negative tilt tests.[12]

Adenosine Antagonists

The only adenosine antagonist for which there is any experience is theophylline[12,16] with modest results in terms of tilt conversion from negative 49% to 82% with minimal follow-up data.

Negative Inotropic Agents

Disopyramide should be considered in this category and, perhaps, betablockers. The theory of action in this case hinged upon the triggering of left ventricular baroreceptors in a paradoxical fashion, by the vigorously contracting myocardium, thus, bringing about the intense and inappropriate vagal outflow. [17] It was thought that by depressing left ventricular function, the paradoxical triggering could be avoided. However, the more recent documentation of positive tilt tests in patients who have received orthotopic heart transplants,[18] has cast much doubt on that theory.[19,20] The experience with disopyramide has been variable with the first report, showing very good results [4] with a 90% negative tilt rate and only a 10% recurrence rate over 20 months of follow-up. This was, however, in a group of only 10 patients. Further experience[6,8,12,21] has shown when any appreciable numbers have been included to vary from 57% to 94% tilt negativity with minimal follow-up data.

Selective Serotonin Reuptake Inhibitors

Two drugs of this type have been studied by one group of workers.[22,23] The role of serotonin, a neurotransmitter, in cardiac arrhythmias,[24] and in migraine,[25] has called into question,whether it may also facilitate vasovagal syncope. Serotonin reuptake inhibitors lead to the down regulation of serotonin receptors[26] and the efferent reflex arc involved in the vasovagal reaction may include a serotonergic component.[27] With this background, Grubb and colleagues[22,23] studied fluoxetine and sertraline in a total of 33 patients. Those who subsequently had negative tilt tests were only 53%, but syncopal recurrences were not recorded on either drug during 19 and 12 months, respectively, of follow-up.

Parameters for Assessment of Successful Therapy in Vasovagal Syncope

Given that tilt testing is the only means of laboratory diagnosis of vasovagal syncope at present, it is tempting to employ this as a tool to evaluate the possible beneficial effect of a pharmacological treatment and to add this to the benefit afforded by the drug in clinical terms.

However, this may not be a correct use of tilt testing. Reproducibility of tilt has come under considerable scrutiny with rates quoted in the range of 64% to 90% over periods, from 1 day to 4 years for initially positive tilts in a wide variety of patient ages[2,18,28-33] and with a wide variety of tilt protocols. It can be seen that the reproducibility leaves more than a little to be desired and that this must taint the value of tilt testing as an indicator of therapeutic success. The reasons for this are probably twofold. First, tilt testing is, when positive, very unpleasant for the patient and, being a test which is potentially open to supratentorial input, the patient may be able to influence its outcome. Second, study of the natural history of vasovagal syncope has revealed that attacks tend to occur in clusters.[20] These may or may not have an identifiable cause, but clearly, if the test is performed during a cluster, it is most likely to be positive, but at other times it may be negative. It appears that the reproducibility of tilt testing is most high in very symptomatic patients.[34] Therefore, some circumspection is required. Other possible parameters such as the duration of tilt prior to the onset of the vasovagal reaction, have not been prospectively evaluated for their meaning in terms of therapeutic efficacy, and cannot presently be used.

Occurrence of symptoms is the mainstay of the assessment of therapeutic benefit, but even this demands careful appraisal. Investigation of syncope has a definite placebo effect which has not been characterized for its intensity or duration. Moreover, the infrequent nature of symptoms in this apparently benign disease, determines long follow-up periods to provide sufficient time for them to have occurred in a 'natural' way, as well as allowing the evaporation of the placebo effect of the initial investigation.

The time until symptom recurrence may also be a valid approach to assess drug efficacy, but this has not received full attention yet in the literature. One study of the benefits of pacing therapy examined the total syncopal burden per prepacing year and compared it with that of per postpacing year,[35] which seems attractive, and the detailed assessment of incidence of postpacing symptoms provided by Sheldon and colleagues[36] require more widespread appraisal.

In summary, the assessment of drug efficacy in vasovagal syncope is fraught with pitfalls.

Pharmacological Therapy—Controlled Studies

Controlled studies are few in number, and have not all been well-designed and have, in some cases, depended largely on tilt testing to assess therapeutic efficacy. Of the seven categories of drugs discussed above in the context of uncontrolled studies, three have not been represented so far in controlled trials, fluid retaining agents, adenosine antagonists, and serotonin reuptake inhibitors. However, two new drugs have been included in trials that do not fall into any of the seven categories; these are dihydroergotamine and domperidone. Instead of considering the results of trials by drug category, in view of the small number of studies, each will be individually discussed.

The four studies that are available, show no significant therapeutic benefit for any of the drugs used. In that of Brignole et al,[37] 30 patients who demonstrated reproducible tilt positivity, had therapy selected by the results of these initial tilts. Because of the wide variety of drugs employed, including atenolol, dihydroergotamine, domperidone, and cafedrine, there were small numbers receiving each. The acute phase of the study evaluated response to therapy by tilt testing with no demonstrable differences between drugs and placebo. Therefore, the chronic phase, where atenolol and cafedrine were each compared with placebo, is of greatest interest. The observation period for the two drugs was 10.7 ± 7.3 months versus that for placebo of 9.3 ± 6.7 months. The end-point was syncopal recurrence and this occurred in 29% of the atenolol group (7 patients), 100% of the single cafedrine-treated patients and in 27% of the 15 placebo-treated patients. Clearly, there were no significant differences favoring either drug.

The study by Fitzpatrick and colleagues[38] also suffered from small numbers including 13 patients with vasodepressor syncope as many had received dual-chamber pacing systems to control the cardioinhibitory component. The study protocol was complex involving a triple blind multiple cross-over format. The drugs included were atenolol, clonidine, and scopolamine plus a placebo period: each treatment phase was 3 months with end-points being tilt positivity, time to tilt positivity, or recurrence of syncope. By this method, none of the drugs was significantly better than placebo. Not only can this study be criticized for its small numbers, but also for its short treatment phases.

Improved methods followed these early trials: that of Morillo et al,[39] investigated disopyramide both acutely, by tilt testing, and chronically, over more than 2 years by reports of syncopal recurrence. In the acute study, disopyramide and placebo were given intravenously, which involved a heavy multitilt protocol for which the reproducibility is not well-known. Twelve of 15 patients who received disopyramide were tilt positive after the drug, versus 13 of 15 placebo-treated patients and in the chronic phase 8 of the 11 at 1 week became tilt negative on disopyramide compared with 9 of the 11 on placebo. After more than 2 years (24.5 months disopyramide and 30.3 placebo), syncope had recurred in 27% of the actively treated patients and in 30% of the placebo group. None of these results acquired any statistical significance. Again, the numbers of patients were small, but the follow-up duration cannot be criticized. It is important to note that all these studies have shown a diminution of frequency of attacks during the observation period.

The fourth and most recent trial to become available is that of Moya and coworkers.[40] They compared etilefrine with placebo in a study using repeat tilt testing and recurrence of symptoms as end-points. They included 30 patients in each group with 1 year of follow-up and significant differences were revealed in either parameter. These workers may be criticized for choosing a rather low dose of etilefrine 10 mg, three times daily as higher doses are advised for the over-the-counter prescription in Germany and were also used by Raviele et al[2] in their early study.

Thus, all the published controlled trials leave something to be desired in terms of methodology and numbers of patients included. Despite these reservations, no pharmacological treatment has so far shown any benefit when subjected to close appraisal.

Pharmacological Treatment as a Cause of Vasovagal Syncope

Since vasovagal syncope is a physiological phenomenon that can probably occur in any person, given sufficiently adverse circumstances, it may be possible for a pharmacological treatment to render this tendency manifest in some patients. This is most likely to occur during vasodilator therapy and nitroglycerin syncope is well-known. Other vasodilators may behave in a similar fashion. Figure 1 shows a patient referred for investigation of severe and frequent vasovagal syncope. He was being treated with calcium antagonists for chest pain which had been considered to be of cardiac origin. The initial tilt test shown in the upper panel was positive. Thereafter, the calcium antagonists were discontinued and a subsequent exercise stress test was negative for myocardial ischemia. The follow-up tilt test was also negative (see lower panel of Figure 1) and the patient remains free of syncope over 6 months of observation. No formal studies in this field have yet to be reported. The possibility that the drugs chosen for treatment of vasovagal syncope may actually exacerbate the condition, and this should also be borne in mind. Thus, pharmacological treatment should not be considered a cause of vasovagal syncope, but as potentially exposing an innate tendency.

Future of Pharmacological Treatment of Vasovagal Syncope

The difficulties in assessing therapeutic benefit of any medication for vasovagal syncope determine that placebo-controlled randomized trials are

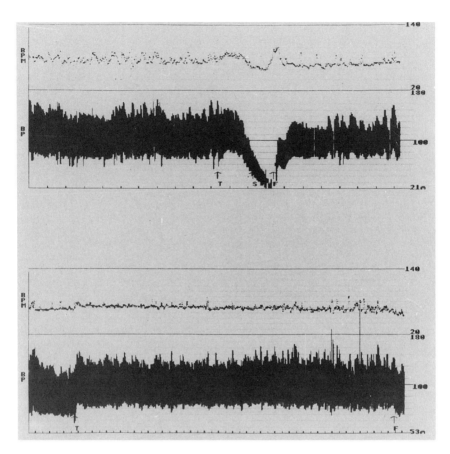

Figure 1. In the **upper panel** a tilt test is shown recorded at a very slow speed with each vertical bar denoting 1 minute. The heart rate obtained from the electrocardiogram is displayed above the arterial pressure which is derived from digital plethysmography. T indicates tilt upright. After a few minutes the heart rate and blood pressure fall in parallel and the patient becomes symptomatic [S]. F denotes tilt back to supine position. This was a positive tilt test of VASIS type 1.[41,42] The **lower panel** has a similar format and labeling, but the test shows no hypotension or bradycardia and is a negative tilt test. These two tilt tests were performed 1 week apart on the same patient: in the first tilt; a calcium antagonist was being prescribed; and in the second; there was no medication.

necessary. It is also clear that tilt testing may not be an adequate means of challenging the patients who participate in these trials. Since it is essential to rely heavily on the effect of the drug on symptom recurrence, long observation periods are required to take the patients beyond the placebo effect of the initial investigation.

There is one large trial in hand, the vasovagal syncope international study (VASIS) which has enrolled more than 80 patients and had a goal of 200 enrollments by mid-1996. The protocol has been published:[41] it has two arms with the drug study using etilefrine in a dose of 25 mg, three times daily versus placebo, and includes patients with mixed cardioinhibitory and vasodepressor, moderately severe cardioinhibitory, and pure vasodepressor categories.[42] The very severe cardioinhibitory patients are being included in the other arm of the study, where dual-chamber pacing with rate hysteresis is compared with no treatment. For each arm, the follow-up period is 1 year and includes symptoms, the time to symptom recurrence, and tilt testing results.

Conclusions

Pharmacological treatment for the complex pathophysiological problem that is vasovagal syncope has addressed many different aspects of the reflex arc, but hitherto, no medication has been shown to have any benefit over placebo. In the future, controlled trials are needed and possibly, should be based more precisely on the hemodynamic alterations which occur in different groups of patients.

References

1. Kenny RA, Bayliss J, Ingram A, Sutton R. Head-up tilt: a useful test for investigating unexplained syncope. *Lancet* 1986;1:1352–1354.
2. Raviele A, Gasparini G, DiPede F, Delise P, Bonso A, Piccolo E. Usefulness of head-up tilt test in evaluating patients with syncope of unknown origin and negative electrophysiologic study. *Am J Cardiol* 1990;65:1322–1327.
3. Abi-Samra F, Maloney JD, Fouad-Tarazi FM, Castle LW. The usefulness of head-up tilt testing and hemodynamic investigations in the workup of syncope of unknown origin. *PACE* 1988;11:1202–1214.
4. Milstein S, Buetikofer J, Dunnigan A, Benditt DG, Gornik C, Reyes WJ. Usefulness of disopyramide for prevention of upright tilt-induced hypotension-bradycardia. *Am J Cardiol* 1990;65:1330–1344.
5. Theodorakis GN, Kremastinos DT, Stefanakis GS, et al. The effectiveness of beta-blockade and its influence on heart rate variability in vasovagal patients. *Eur Heart J* 1993;14:1499–1507.
6. Grubb BP, Temesy-Armos P, Hahn H, Elliot L. Utility of upright tilt-table testing in the evaluation and management of syncope of unknown origin. *Am J Med* 1991;90:6–10.
7. Sra JS, Anderson AJ, Sheikh SH, et al. Unexplained syncope evaluated by electro-

physiological studies and head-up tilt testing. *Ann Intern Med* 1991;114: 1013–1019.

8. Grubb BP, Temesy-Armos P, Moore J, Wolfe D, Hahn H, Elliot L. Head-upright tilt-table testing in evaluation and management of the malignant vasovagal syndrome. *Am J Cardiol* 1992;69:904–908.

9. Muller G, Deal BD, Strasburger JF, Benson DW. Usefulness of metoprolol for unexplained syncope and positive responses to tilt testing in young persons. *Am J Cardiol* 1993;71:592–595.

10. Grubb BP, Temesy-Armos P, Moore J, Wolfe D, Hahn H, Elliot L. The use of head-upright tilt table testing in the evaluation and management of syncope in children and adolescents. *PACE* 1992;5:742–748.

11. Tonnessen GE, Haft JI, Fulton J, Rubinstein DG. The value of tilt table testing with isoproterenol in determining therapy in adults with syncope and presyncope of unknown origin. *Arch Intern Med* 1994;4:1613–1617.

12. Natale A, Sra J, Dhala A, et al. Efficacy of different treatment strategies for neurocardiogenic syncope. *PACE* 1995;8:655–662.

13. Perry JC, Garson A. Jr. The child with recurrent syncope: autonomic function testing and beta-adrenergic hypersensitivity. *J Am Coll Cardiol* 1991;17: 1168–1171.

14. Blanc JJ, Corbel C, Mansourati J, Genet L. Evaluation of beta-blocker therapy in vasovagal syncope reproduced by the head-up tilt test. *Arch Mal Coeur* 1991; 84:1453–1457.

15. Strieper MJ, Campbell RM. Efficacy of alpha-adrenergic agonist therapy for prevention of pediatric neurocardiogenic syncope. *J Am Coll Cardiol* 1993;22: 594–597.

16. Nelson SD, Stanley M, Love CJ, Coyne KS, Schaal SF. The autonomic and hemodynamic effects of oral theophylline in patients with vasodepressor syncope. *Arch Intern Med* 1991;151:2425–2429.

17. Thoren P. Role of cardiac vagal C-fibers in cardiovascular control. *Rev Physiol Biochem Pharmacol* 1979;86:1–94.

18. Fitzpatrick AP, Theodorakis G, Vardas P, Sutton R. Methodology of head-up tilt in patients with unexplained syncope. *J Am Coll Cardiol* 1991;17:125–130.

19. Dickinson CJ. Fainting precipitated by collapse firing of venous baroreceptors. *Lancet* 1993;342:970–972.

20. Sutton R, Petersen MEV. The clinical spectrum of neurocardiogenic syncope. *J Cardiovasc Electrophysiol* 1995;6:569–576.

21. Kelly PA, Mann DE, Adler SW, Fuenxalida CE, Reiter MJ. Low dose disopyramide often fails to prevent neurogenic syncope during head-up tilt testing. *PACE* 1994;17:573–576.

22. Grubb BP, Wolfe DA, Samoil D, Temesy-Armos P, Hahn H, Elliot L. Usefulness of fluoxetine hydrochloride for prevention of resistant upright tilt induced syncope. *PACE* 1993;16:458–464.

23. Grubb BP, Samoil D, Kosinski D, Kip K, Brewster P. Use of sertraline hydrochloride in the treatment of refractory neurocardiogenic syncope in children and adolescents. *J Am Coll Cardiol* 1994;24:490–494.

24. Verrier R. Neurochemical approaches to the prevention of ventricular fibrillation. *Federation Proc* 1986;45:2191–2196.

25. Silberstein SD. Serotonin [5HT] and migraine headache.Headache 1994;34: 408–417.

26. Rickels K, Schweitzer E. Clinical overview of serotonin reuptake inhibitors. *J Clin Psychiatry* 1990;51:9–12.
27. Abboud FM. Neurocardiogenic syncope. *N Engl J Med* 1993;328:1117–1119.
28. Chen XC, Chen MY, Remole S, et al. Reproducibility of head-up tilt table testing for eliciting susceptibility to neurally mediated syncope in patients without structural heart disease. *Am J Cardiol* 1992;69:755–760.
29. Fish FA, Strasburger JF, Benson DW. Reproducibility of a symptomatic response to upright tilt testing in young patients with unexplained syncope. *Am J Cardiol* 1992;70:605–609.
30. Blanc JJ, Mansourati J, Maheu B, Boughaleb D, Genet L. Reproducibility of a positive passive upright tilt test at a seven-day interval in patients with syncope. *Am J Cardiol* 1993;72:469–471.
31. Grubb BP, Wolfe D, Temesy-Armos P, Hahn H, Elliot L. Reproducibility of head upright tilt table test results in patients with syncope. *PACE* 1992;15:1477–1481.
32. Sheldon R, Splawinski J, Killam S. Reproducibility of upright tilt-table tests in patients with syncope. *Am J Cardiol* 1992;69:1300–1305.
33. Petersen MEV, Price D, Williams T, Jensen N, Riff K, Sutton R. Short AV interval VDD pacing does not prevent tilt induced vasovagal syncope in patients with cardioinhibitory vasovagal syndrome. *PACE* 1994;17:882–891.
34. Sutton R, Petersen MEV. Invasive tilt testing; the search for a new sensor to permit earlier pacing therapy in vasovagal syncope. In: Raviele A (ed): Cardiac Arrhythmias 1995. Milano, Italy: Springer-Verlag Italia, 1995, pp 132–133.
35. Petersen MEV, Chamberlain-Webber R, Fitzpatrick AP, Ingram A, Williams T, Sutton R. Permanent pacing for cardioinhibitory malignant vasovagal syndrome. *Br Heart J* 1994;71:274–281.
36. Sheldon RS, Rose S, Flanagan P, Koshman ML, Killam S. Multivariate predictors of syncope recurrence in drug-free patients following a positive tilt table test. *Circulation* 1994;90:I-54(Abstract).
37. Brignole M, Menozzi C, Gianfranchi L, Lolli G, Bottoni N, Oddone D. A controlled trial of acute and long-term medical therapy in tilt-induced neurally mediated syncope. *Am J Cardiol* 1992;70:339–342.
38. Fitzpatrick AP, Ahmed R, Williams S, Travill C, Sutton R. A randomised trial of medical therapy for vasodepressor vasovagal syncope. *Eur J Cardiac Pacing Electrophysiol* 1991;1:99–102.
39. Morillo CA, Leitch JW, Yee R, Klein GJ. A placebo controlled trial of intravenous and oral disopyramide for prevention of neurally mediated syncope. *J Am Coll Cardiol* 1993;22:1843–1848.
40. Moya A, Permanyer-Miralda G, Sagrista-Sauleda J, et al. Limitations of head up tilt test for evaluating the efficacy of therapeutic interventions in patients with vasovagal syncope: results of a controlled study of etilefrine versus placebo. *J Am Coll Cardiol* 1995;25:65–69.
41. VASIS. Vasovagal international study. *Eur J Cardiac Pacing Electrophysiol* 1993;3:164–172.
42. Sutton R, Petersen M, Brignole M, Raviele A, Menozzi C, Giani P. Proposed classification for tilt induced vasovagal syncope. *Eur J Cardiac Pacing Electrophysiol* 1992;2:180–183.

Chapter 4

Nonsustained Ventricular Tachycardia in Ischemic Heart Disease:
Risk Stratification and Management Strategies

Nabil El-Sherif, MD, Gioia Turitto, MD,
Edward B. Caref, PhD

Introduction

Nonsustained ventricular tachycardia (NSVT), defined as three or more consecutive ventricular premature beats (VPBs) at a rate of > 120 beats per minute, and lasting less than 30 seconds, continues to present a formidable challenge for risk stratification and management. Nonsustained ventricular tachycardia is not uncommon in the absence of organic heart disease, and it seems not to be associated with an increased risk.[1] However, in the presence of organic heart disease including ischemic heart disease (IHD), especially in the postinfarction period, NSVT is associated with an increased risk for sudden cardiac death (SCD)[2-4] and possibly for nonsudden cardiac death as well.[5-7] Although ventricular tachyarrhythmias are implicated in most cases of SCD, there has been no evidence to suggest a cause and effect relationship between NSVT and SCD. Following the results of the Cardiac Arrhythmia Suppression Trial (CAST),[8] the widespread empirical use of antiarrhythmic drugs to suppress VPBs and NSVT with the goal of reducing the incidence of SCD is no longer acceptable. Several noninvasive and invasive tests have been utilized, individually and in combination, to identify patients with IHD and NSVT at high risk for malignant tachyarrhythmias and to provide guidelines for effective management.[9,10] Although at present, there is no consensus as to the best strategy in this regard, ongoing multicenter clinical trials may

From *Practical Management of Cardiac Arrhythmias* edited by Nabil El-Sherif, and Jean Lekieffre. Futura Publishing Co., Armonk, NY, © 1997.

eventually provide such guidelines. A brief review of these issues will be presented.

Identification of High-Risk Patients

Many studies have shown that NSVT in patients with a recent myocardial infarction (MI)[2-7] or chronic heart failure and remote MI,[11,12] identifies a group at increased risk for SCD. In three major studies[5-7] NSVT was shown to significantly influence both sudden and nonsudden cardiac mortality. The treatment of such patients, however, remains a major challenge, in part because of the lack of an effective strategy for identifying high-risk patients who would benefit the most from treatment. Several noninvasive and invasive tests have been utilized for arrhythmia risk stratification in patients with IHD with or without NSVT. These include, the ambulatory long-term electrocardiogram (ECG) Holter recording, left ventricular ejection fraction (LVEF), the signal-averaged ECG (SAECG), heart rate variability (HRV), measurements of QT interval and QT dispersion, T wave alternans, and programmed ventricular stimulation (PVS).

Ambulatory Holter Recording

The finding of NSVT on a Holter recording is not specific enough to define individual patients who are likely to benefit from antiarrhythmic therapy.[13] In addition, most patients with NSVT after MI have infrequent episodes.[14] This is in addition to the fact that spontaneous variation from day to day in incidence of NSVT makes interpretation of the results of therapy guided by Holter recording subject to large errors. A more difficult question that remains unanswered at present is the relationship of asymptomatic ventricular ectopy to symptomatic ventricular tachyarrhythmia. It is not clear whether these two factors are related mechanically, and therefore whether alterations in spontaneous ectopy by antiarrhythmic therapy will impact on the prognosis.[13]

Left Ventricular Ejection Fraction (LVEF)

Left ventricular function is one of the best predictors of cardiac mortality in patients with IHD, particularly after an acute MI.[2,3,15,16] For example, in the Multicenter Postinfarction Research Group, patients with LVEF of < 20% had an approximately 45% 1-year mortality rate compared with a 4% rate in patients with a LVEF > 40%.[15] Similarly, in patients with IHD and NSVT, the degree of left ventricular dysfunction is among the most powerful predictors of outcome.[16] Therefore, left ventricular function should be assessed in all patients with NSVT. Results of other tests, such as the SAECG and PVS are influenced by the extent of left ventricular dysfunction.[9,17]

Signal-Averaged ECG

The SAECG appears to be useful in risk stratification of patients with IHD.[17-19] Late potentials have been shown to predict future arrhythmic events.[17-19] However, recent studies have shown that time-domain SAECG indices of late potentials do not provide the best prediction criteria for serious arrhythmic events in the first year post-MI.[20] The SAECG has some limitations: although it appears to have an excellent negative predictive value, both its sensitivity and positive predictive value are low.[20] In addition, it cannot be used to follow the course of treatment, since it is not consistently affected by antiarrhythmic drugs.

The Need for Different Criteria of Time-Domain SAECG

Time-domain SAECG criteria reflecting the presence of late potentials (i.e., RMS40 and/or LAS40) are usually most predictive for spontaneous and/or inducible sustained ventricular tachycardia (VT).[21] The electrophysiological rationale for the predictive value of these criteria is that late potentials represent slowed and disorganized conduction of localized myocardial zones that could provide the anatomic-electrophysiological substrate for reentrant VT. It does not necessarily follow that these criteria would also be predictive in the post-MI period, where the majority of serious arrhythmic events are fatal ventricular tachyarrhythmias rather than nonfatal sustained VT. The above concept is justified by the results of a recent multicenter NIH-sponsored study that was conducted to define the best predictive criteria of time domain SAECG in the post-MI period.[20] A large study group of 1160 patients were followed for an average of 10.3 ± 3.2 months. Forty-five patients (4.3%) suffered serious arrhythmic events (42 sudden cardiac deaths judged to be due to arrhythmias, and 3 nonfatal sustained VT). The SAECG parameters were found to be independently predictive of arrhythmic events and a filtered QRSD of ≤ 120 ms provided the best predictive criterion. The incidence of an abnormal SAECG in the study group was 12%. The positive, negative, and total predictive accuracy of a 40 Hz QRSD ≤ 120 ms was 17%, 98%, and 88%, respectively. The electrophysiological rationale as to why an abnormally long signal-averaged QRSD best predicts fatal arrhythmic events in the first year post-MI is not clear. However, it is possible that this may reflect slowed and nonhomogeneous conduction of a "larger mass" of ventricular myocardium. Such hearts may be more vulnerable to rapid ventricular tachyarrhythmias.

Frequency-Domain SAECG

Current techniques for TD late potential analysis have some limitations. There is a lack of standardization as to the optimal filter characteristics, as well as to the best numerical criteria of abnormality. The numerical measurements are sensitive to the specific algorithm used for determining QRS termination.[22] In the presence of intraventricular conduction defect and/or bundle branch block, which many patients at potential risk have, interpretation of late potentials may be difficult. Several authors have reported promising results employing frequency analysis techniques for VT risk assessment.[23] Because of the limitations of the traditional FFT technique, several investigators utilized a spectrotemporal technique.[24] The rationale for this technique is the observation that the QRS, late potentials, and ST segment waveforms in the SAECG have different spectral characteristics or, in other words, that the ECG signal has a time-varying spectrum. However, some techniques that utilize a "normality factor" analysis were shown to be nonreproducible primarily because of sensitivity of the measurement to QRS offset localization.[25]

Our group has described a frequency-domain analysis technique that overcomes some of the disadvantages of both TD late potential analysis and previously advocated methods of frequency analysis (Figure 1).[26] In the technique of spectral turbulence (ST) analysis, the hallmark of an arrhythmogenic abnormality is postulated to be frequent and abrupt changes in the frequency signature of QRS wavefront velocity as it propagates throughout the ventricle around and across areas of abnormal conduction, resulting in a high degree of ST. The technique was shown to provide a more accurate marker for the anatomical-electrophysiological substrate of reentrant tachyarrhythmias.[14] However, recent studies from this laboratory suggest that the ST criteria for the prediction of inducible sustained VT may not apply for risk stratification of post-MI patients, and that a different set of criteria in these patients is required.[27]

Combined Time and Frequency-Domain Analysis of SAECG

One of the limitations of TD late potentials analysis of the SAECG is that partial obscuring of late potentials may occur if the abnormal myocardial region is activated relatively early during the QRS complex. This occurs more often with anterior wall (AW) MI than inferior wall (IW) MI and may partially explain the higher incidence of false-positive abnormal recordings in patients with IWMI. On the other hand, there is a higher incidence of abnormal ST in AWMI compared with IWMI, leading to a high incidence of false-positive abnormal test results in patients with AWMI.[27] A recent study from this laboratory investigated the hypothesis that combined TD and ST analysis of

TIME DOMAIN LATE POTENTIAL ANALYSIS

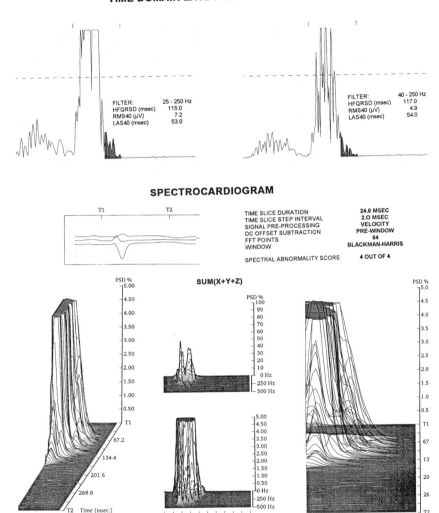

SPECTROCARDIOGRAM

Figure 1. Time-domain plots **(top)** and spectral plots **(bottom)** of the signal-averaged electrocardiogram of a patient with anterior wall myocardial infarction. The spectrocardiogram is displayed in different views: an oblique view **(left)**; a horizontal view at both low and high gains **(middle)**; and a transparent view **(right)**. Note the presence of late potentials in the time-domain plots and an abnormal spectral turbulence score of 4 in the spectral plots. The patient had sudden arrhythmic death 4 weeks following myocardial infarction.

the SAECG could improve its predictive accuracy in post-MI patients.[27] The total predictive accuracy of combined TD + ST (92%) was higher than TD (87%), while ST had the lowest total predictive accuracy of 78%. The negative predictive accuracy of all three analyses was high (96%–97%). On the other hand, the positive predictive accuracy of TD (28%) was higher than ST (14%). Combined TD + ST significantly improved the positive predictive accuracy of the test to 35% in the total group and to 40% in patients with first AWMI or IWMI. The best results were obtained in patients with first AWMI, where the positive predictive accuracy of combined analysis was 50%.

Heart Rate Variability

Heart rate variability (HRV) had been used to study sympathovagal balance.[28,29] Methods to analyze HRV employ both time and frequency domain measurements that quantify periodicities in the data. Prognostic information to risk-stratify patients for future ventricular arrhythmias or other cardiac events leading to premature death may be possible by quantifying HRV. Kleiger et al,[30] reported a weak correlation between time and frequency domain measures of HRV and more traditional risk predictors. Farrell et al,[31] analyzed risk stratification for arrhythmic events in post-MI patients utilizing HRV, ambulatory ECG variables, SAECG and left ventricular function, and found that impaired HRV was most predictive of future arrhythmic events. However, when impaired HRV was combined with the presence of late potentials on the SAECG, the sensitivity was only 58%. Baroreflex sensitivity assessed with phenylephrine injection weakly correlated with HRV.

Two major questions concerning HRV remain to be clarified. First, many methods to measure HRV have been reported, and it is very difficult to conclude which one is most appropriate for establishing normal values and for particular patient subgroups. There is a need to standardize the measurement of HRV and to quantify normal values under various circumstances, including patient age and gender. A recent effort in this regard, is the report of the task force of the European Society of Cardiology and the North American Society of Pacing and Electrophysiology.[32] Newer analytical techniques, (e.g., regression of log [power] on log [frequency] for R-R interval fluctuations), may prove to be excellent predictors of death of any cause and arrhythmic death after MI.[33] Second, the sensitivity, specificity, and predictive accuracy of various HRV parameters require much more prospective investigation. Prospective multicenter studies should be undertaken to determine the sensitivity, specificity, and predictive accuracy of HRV in various situations, particularly in patients with post-MI. Correlation of HRV with other risk stratification measurements will be necessary to evaluate its independent predictive value.

QT Interval and QT Dispersion

Previous studies have shown that prolongation of the QT interval is a risk factor for ventricular arrhythmias and sudden death in patients with a previous MI,[34,35] but there has been some controversy as to the predictive accuracy of the prolonged QT interval.[36] QT dispersion may be a more powerful predictor of susceptibility to ventricular tachyarrhythmias, suggesting that inhomogeneity of repolarization is more closely associated with arrhythmic risk than is prolongation of repolarization itself.[37] Spatial dispersion of recovery times may be a fundamental electrophysiological substrate for the genesis of reentrant arrhythmias. Previous studies on the relation between QT dispersion and arrhythmic susceptibility were performed in patients with the long QT syndrome,[38] hypertrophic cardiomyopathy,[39] congestive heart failure,[40] in mixed patient populations with IHD,[41] and in patients with torsades de pointes induced by antiarrhythmic drugs.[42]

Measurement of the variability in QT interval duration among the different leads of the standard 12-lead ECG (i.e., QT dispersion) has been proposed as a noninvasive method for detecting the inhomogeneity of ventricular recovery times.[37] Several recent studies suggest that increased QT dispersion is related to susceptibility to reentrant ventricular tachyarrhythmias, independent of the degree of left ventricular dysfunction or clinical characteristics of the patient.[43,44] Thus, a simple noninvasive measurement of this interval from a standard 12-lead ECG may contribute to identifying patients at risk for life-threatening arrhythmias after a previous MI.

T Wave Alternans

Alternation of the configuration and/or duration of the repolarization wave of the ECG, usually referred to as T wave alternans, is seen under diverse experimental and clinical conditions.[45] Interest in repolarization alternans is attributed to the hypothesis that it may reflect underlying dispersion of repolarization in the ventricle, a well-recognized electrophysiological substrate for reentrant ventricular tachyarrhythmias. Although overt T wave alternans in the ECG are not common, in recent years digital signal-processing techniques capable of detecting subtle degrees of T wave alternans have suggested that the phenomenon may be more prevalent than previously recognized, and could represent an important marker of vulnerability to ventricular tachyarrhythmias.

T wave alternans in vivo may be so subtle as to preclude visual detection, yet be statistically significant and easily measurable with digital signal processing techniques.[46] In a recent study, signal-processing techniques to measure electrical alternans at a microvolt level was utilized to establish the prognostic importance of electrical alternans in a group of 83 patients referred for diagnostic electrophysiological testing.[47] Irrespective of left ventricular mechanical function, subtle alternation of the ST segment of the T wave was an independent marker of vulnerability to inducible ventricular arrhythmias and clinical arrhythmic events. The maximum level of T wave alternans recorded in this study was only 116 μV, indicating the need for sensitive signal processing techniques and explaining why alternans is not commonly recognized on standard ECG tracings. In this study, alternans was measured during atrial pacing in order to eliminate any possible influence of heart rate or beat-to-beat variability in heart rate on measured T wave alternans.

To make the measurement of repolarization alternans a suitable test for ambulatory patients, improvements in the algorithm is required to compensate for the fluctuations in heart rate associated with sinus rhythm. Recent technical improvements allow the detection of microvolt T wave alternans during sinus rhythm with the heart rate moderately elevated using bicycle exercise (Figure 2). In a preliminary multicenter study,[48] alternans voltage > 1.0 μV at rest or > 1.9 μV during exercise, and alternans ratio > 3 were required for a positive alternans test. Arrhythmia vulnerability was defined by clinical or induced sustained VT or ventricular fibrillation (VF). The positive and negative predictive values of T wave alternans in this group of patients were 85% and 100%, respectively. Further studies will be required to evaluate the test as a noninvasive index of vulnerability to ventricular tachyarrhythmias and to compare its sensitivity and specificity to other indices of sudden cardiac electrical death.

Programmed Ventricular Stimulation

Several studies examined the results of PVS in patients with IHD and NSVT.[9,49–51] The rationale was that inducible sustained VT by PVS identifies patients at high risk for future arrhythmic events. In spite of several shortcomings, published studies seem to demonstrate that patients without inducible sustained VT have a very low rate of SCD and do not appear to require specific antiarrhythmic therapy. In addition, because SCD rates were low in patients with LVEF > 40%, regardless of induced arrhythmias, patients with NSVT with LVEF > 40%, would likely be a relatively "low yield" population to screen for risk of SCD.[13] PVS can identify those patients with low LVEF who are not likely to benefit from antiarrhythmic therapy (those without inducible sustained VT). However, the positive predictive value of inducible sustained VT in patients with LVEF ($\leq$ 40%) remains unknown. Moreover, the ability of antiarrhythmic therapy guided by electrophysiological testing to prevent SCD in this population has not been proven. Several studies that did not have a randomized control group suggest that antiarrhythmic therapy

Electrocardiogram

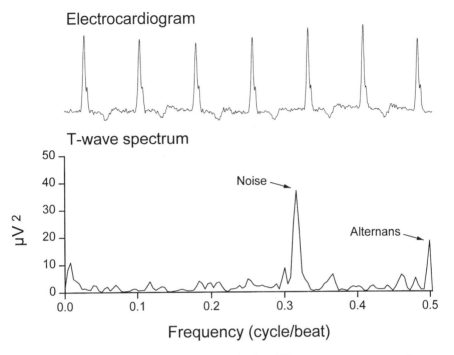

Figure 2. Surface Electrocardiogram (ECG) lead and T wave power spectrum from a patient with resuscitated cardiac arrest and inducible fast ventricular tachyarrhythmia who later received an implantable cardioverter defibrillator. The ECG and T wave spectrum were obtained during bicycle exercise that increased the heart rate to approximately 100 beats per minute. The spectrum shows a large noise peak at 0.33 cycles per beat reflecting the noise artifact associated with the bicycle pedaling rate. A second peak at 0.5 cycles per beat illustrates the presence of T wave alternans. Note the absence of any visible beat-to-beat alternation of T wave in the surface ECG lead.

guided by PVS in this group is associated with a lower rate of SCD compared to empirical therapy.[9,51]

Management Strategies

At present, it remains uncertain how to manage patients with IHD, reduced LVEF, and NSVT. Although a combination of algorithms that utilize several noninvasive and invasive tests may provide better risk stratification, there is still no consensus as to what is the best way to characterize a patients' arrhythmic risk and whether anti-ischemic measures, antiarrhythmic pharmacological therapy, an implantable cardioverter defibrillator (ICD), or a combi-

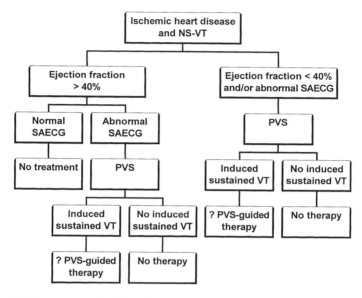

Figure 3. Management algorithm for patients with ischemic heart disease and spontaneous nonsustained ventricular tachycardia (NSVT). PVS: programmed ventricular stimulation; SAECG: signal-averaged electrocardiogram.

nation of measures, represent the best management strategy. Several randomized controlled studies are currently under way to answer these questions.

While waiting for the results of ongoing multicenter randomized controlled studies, our group has followed an algorithm based on the results of the SAECG, LVEF, and PVS as follows (Figure 3)[9]:

(1) Patients with normal SAECG and LVEF ≥ 40% do not require PVS or long-term antiarrhythmic therapy, since the incidence of induced sustained monomorphic VT and SCD are low in this subgroup.

(2) Patients with normal SAECG but with LVEF < 40% as well as patients with abnormal SAECG should be recommended for electrophysiological evaluation, since the incidence of induced sustained monomorphic VT is high in those subgroups. Based on the results of PVS, patients with no inducible sustained monomorphic VT may be followed off antiarrhythmic therapy. If VT is induced, however, those patients should be enrolled in one of the ongoing randomized studies to assess the value of antiarrhythmic therapy in preventing SCD. If this is not feasible, inducible patients should probably receive antiarrhythmic ther-

apy (possibly a type III drug), with the understanding that the value of antiarrhythmic therapy has yet to be definitely established. Although the empiric use of amiodarone has been shown in some trials to reduce cardiac mortality in post-MI patients with complex ventricular ectopy,[52,53] the results from large multicenter randomized trials seem to show no significant benefits.[54,55]

Two of the multicenter randomized trials for the management of NSVT in the post-MI patients deserve mentioning. These are the Multicenter Automatic Defibrillation Implantation Trial (MADIT)[56] and the Multicenter Unsustained Tachycardia Trial (MUSTT).[13] A preliminary report of the results of MADIT have recently been published.[56] MADIT was designed to determine if prophylactic implantation of an ICD in high-risk coronary patients with asymptomatic NSVT would improve survival when compared to conventional medical therapy. Over the course of 5 years, 196 patients with one or more prior MIs, ejection fraction (EF) $\leq$ 0.35, NYHA class I-III, a documented episode of NSVT, and inducible, nonsuppressible VT or VF were randomized to either ICD (n = 95) or conventional medical therapy (n = 101). MADIT was terminated early by the Safety Monitoring Committee because of significantly improved survival in patients randomized to the ICD arm. The baseline characteristics of the two groups were similar. At one month after randomization, amiodarone therapy was used in 80% of conventional therapy and 2% of ICD patients. There were 15 deaths in the ICD group and 39 deaths in the conventional group (hazard ratio = 0.46; 95% CI = 0.6 to 0.82; P = 0.009.) There was no evidence that amiodarone or any other antiarrhythmic therapy had significant influence on the hazard ratio. It was concluded that prophylactic implantation of an ICD in high-risk patients with asymptomatic NSVT saves lives.

At present, however, there is no available data on the best management strategy of patients with IHD, NSVT, low LVEF but noninducible sustained VT, nor on the outcome of those patients with inducible VT who are followed on drugs shown to suppress inducibility. Some of these data, however, may be provided by the other ongoing studies, especially MUSTT.[13] This study enrolls patients with IHD, NSVT, and LVEF < 40% to determine the role of PVS-guided therapy. Patients with inducible sustained monomorphic VT are randomly assigned to either PVS-guided antiarrhythmic therapy or no therapy. The role of the ICD is also being evaluated. Because half of the patients with inducible VT in MUSTT will be given no antiarrhythmic therapy, the study will be able to ascertain the true risk of sudden death in this patient population without the influence of these agents.

Summary

NSVT is not uncommon both in the presence and absence of organic heart disease and in the latter situation, is usually not associated with an increased risk. However, in patients with IHD, especially in the post-MI period, NSVT is associated with an increased risk of sudden, and possibly nonsudden, cardiac death. Several noninvasive and invasive tests have been utilized, individually or in combination, to risk stratify those patients. Noninvasive electrophysiological risk stratifiers such as the SAECG, QT dispersion, T wave alternans, as well as PVS and LVEF have been utilized singly and in combination to identify those patients at high risk for malignant tachyarrhythmias and to evaluate the potential benefit from antiarrhythmic management strategies. At present, however, there is no consensus as to the best strategy to identify and treat high-risk patients. Several ongoing multicenter clinical trials may eventually provide such guidelines.

References

1. Kennedy HL, Whitlock JA, Sprague MK, Kennedy LJ, Buckingham TA, Goldberg RJ. Long-term follow-up of asymptomatic healthy subjects with frequent and complex ventricular ectopy. N Engl J Med 1985;312:193–197.
2. Moss AJ, Davis HT, DeCamilla J, Bayer LW. Ventricular ectopic beats and their relation to sudden and nonsudden cardiac death after myocardial infarction. Circulation 1979;60:998–1003.
3. Bigger JT, Fleiss JL, Kleiger R, Miller JP, Rolnitzky LM, and the Multicenter Post-Infarction Research Group. The relationships among ventricular arrhythmias, left ventricular dysfunction and mortality in the 2 years after myocardial infarction. Circulation 1984;69:250–258.
4. Mukharji J, Rude FE, Poole K, and the Myocardial Infarction LIS Study Group. Risk factors for sudden death after acute myocardial infarction: two-year follow-up. Am J Cardiol 1984;54:31–36.
5. Anderson KP, DeCamilla J, Moss AJ. Clinical significance of ventricular tachycardia (3 beats or longer) detected during ambulatory monitoring after myocardial infarction. Circulation 1978;57:890–897.
6. Bigger JT, Weld FM, Rolnitzky LM. Prevalence, characteristics, and significance of ventricular tachycardia (3 or more complexes) detected with ambulatory electrocardiographic recording in the late hospital phase of acute myocardial infarction. Am J Cardiol 1981;48:815–823.
7. Kleiger HE, Miller JP, Thanavaro S, Province MA, Martin TF, Oliver GC. Relationship between clinical features of acute myocardial infarction and ventricular runs 2 weeks to 1 year after infarction. Circulation 1981;63:64–70.
8. The Cardiac Arrhythmia Suppression Trial (CAST) Investigators. Preliminary report: effect of encainide and flecainide on mortality in a randomized trial of arrhythmia suppression after myocardial infarction. N Engl J Med 1989;321: 406–412.
9. Turitto G, Fontaine JM, Ursell S, Caref EB, Bekheit S, El-Sherif N. Risk stratification and management of patients with organic heart disease and non-sustained

ventricular tachycardia: role of programmed stimulation, left ventricular ejection fraction, and the signal averaged electrocardiogram. *Am J Med* 1990;88:35N-41N.

10. Pires LA, Huang SKS. Nonsustained ventricular tachycardia: identification and management of high-risk patients. *Am Heart J* 1993;126:189–200.

11. Follansbee WP, Michelson EL, Morganroth J. Nonsustained ventricular tachycardia in ambulatory patients: characteristics and association with sudden cardiac death. *Ann Intern Med* 1980;92:741–747.

12. Holmes J, Kubo SH, Cody RJ, Kligfield P. Arrhythmias in ischemic and nonischemic dilated cardiomyopathy: prediction of mortality by ambulatory electrocardiography. *Am J Cardiol* 1985;55:146–151.

13. Buxton AE, Fisher JD, Josephson ME et al. Prevention of sudden death in patients with coronary artery disease: the multicenter unsustained tachycardia trial (MUSTT). *Prog Cardiovasc Dis* 1993;36:215–226.

14. Denes P, Gillis AM, Pawitan Y, et al. Prevalence, characteristics and significance of ventricular premature complexes and ventricular tachycardia detected by 24-hour continuous electrocardiographic recording in the Cardiac Arrhythmia Suppression Trial. *Am J Cardiol* 1991;68:887–896.

15. The Multicenter Post-Infarction Research Group. Risk stratification and survival after myocardial infarction. *N Engl J Med* 1983;309:331–336.

16. Hammill SC, Trusty JM, Wood DL, et al. Influence of ventricular function and presence or absence of coronary artery disease on results of electrophysiologic testing for asymptomatic nonsustained ventricular tachycardia. *Am J Cardiol* 1990; 65:722–728.

17. Gomes JA, Winters SL, Stewart D, Horowitz S, Milner M, Barreca P. A new noninvasive index to predict sustained ventricular tachycardia and sudden death in the first year after myocardial infarction: based on signal-averaged electrocardiogram, radionuclide ejection fraction and Holter monitoring. *J Am Coll Cardiol* 1987;10:349–357.

18. Kuchar DL, Thornburn CW, Sammel NL. Prediction of serious arrhythmic events after myocardial infarction: signal averaged electrocardiogram, Holter monitoring and radionuclide ventriculography. *J Am Coll Cardiol* 1987;9:531–538.

19. El-Sherif N, Ursell SN, Bekheit S, et al. Prognostic significance of the signal averaged ECG depends on the time of recording in the postinfarction period. *Am Heart J* 1989; 118:256–264.

20. El-Sherif N, Denes P, Katz R, et al. Definition of the best prediction criteria of the time-domain signal-averaged electrocardiogram for serious arrhythmic events in the postinfarction period. *J Am Coll Cardiol* 1995;25:908–914.

21. Turitto G, Fontaine JM, Ursell SN, Caref EB, Henkin R, El-Sherif N. Value of the signal-averaged electrocardiogram as a predictor of the results of programmed stimulation in non-sustained ventricular tachycardia. *Am J Cardiol* 1988;61: 1272–1279.

22. Turitto G, Mansoor S, Rao S, Caref EB, El-Sherif N. A comparative analysis of commercial software for signal averaged electrocardiography. *J Noninvas Electrocardiogr* 1996;1(2 Pt. 1):147–150.

23. Cain ME, Ambos HD, Witkowski FX, Sobel BE. Fast Fourier transform analysis of signal averaged ECGs for identification of patients prone to sustained ventricular tachycardia. *Circulation* 1984;69:711–720.

24. Haberl R, Jilge G, Putler R, Steinbeck G. Spectral mapping of the electrocardi-

ogram with Fourier transform for identification of patients with sustained ventricular tachycardia and coronary artery disease. *Eur Heart J* 1989;10:316–322.

25. Malik M, Kulakowski P, Poloniecki J, et al. Frequency versus time-domain analysis of signal-averaged electrocardiograms. I. Reproducibility of the results. *J Am Coll Cardiol* 1992; : 127–134.

26. Kelen GJ, Henkin R, Starr A-M, Caref EB, Bloomfield D, El-Sherif N. Spectral turbulence analysis of the signal-averaged electrocardiogram and its predictive accuracy for inducible sustained monomorphic ventricular tachycardia. *Am J Cardiol* 1991;67:965–975.

27. Ahuja RK, Turitto G, Ibrahim B, Caref EB, El-Sherif N. Combined time-domain and spectral turbulence analysis of the signal-averaged electrocardiogram improve its predictive accuracy in post-infarction patients. *J Electrocardiol* 1994;27(Suppl): 202–206.

28. Lombardi F, Sandrone G, Pernpruner S, et al. Heart rate variability as an index of sympathovagal interaction after acute myocardial infarction. *Am J Cardiol* 1987; 60:1239–1245.

29. Saul JP, Arai Y, Berger RD, Lilly LS, Colucci WS, Cohen RJ. Assessment of autonomic regulation in chronic congestive heart failure by heart rate spectral analysis. *Am J Cardiol* 1988;61:1292–1299.

30. Kleiger RE, Miller JP, Bigger JT Jr, Moss AJ, and the Multicenter Post-Infarction Research Group. Decreased heart rate variability and its association with increased mortality after acute myocardial infarction. *Am J Cardiol* 1987;59:256–262.

31. Farrell TG, Bashir Y, Cripps T, et al. Risk stratification for arrhythmic events in postinfarction patients based on heart rate variability, ambulatory electrocardiographic variables and the signal-averaged electrocardiogram. *J Am Coll Cardiol* 1991;18:687–697.

32. Task Force of the European Society of Cardiology and the North American Society of Pacing and Electrophysiology. Heart rate variability. Standards of measurement, physiological interpretation, and clinical use. *Circulation* 1996;93: 1143–1165.

33. Bigger JT, Steinman RC, Rolnitzky LM, Fleiss JL, Albrecht P, Cohen RJ. Power law behavior of RR-interval variability in healthy middle-aged persons, patients with recent acute myocardial infarction, and patients with heart transplants. *Circulation* 1996;93:2142–2151.

34. Ahnve S, Gilpin E, Madsen EB, Froelicher V, Henning H, Ross J. Prognostic importance of QT interval at discharge after acute myocardial infarction: a multicenter study of 865 patients. *Am Heart J* 1984;108:395–400.

35. Wheelan K, Mukharji J, Rude RE, et al. Sudden death and its relation to QT-interval prolongation after acute myocardial infarction: two-year follow-up. *Am J Cardiol* 1986;57:745–750.

36. Pohjola-Sintonen S, Siltanen P, Haapakoski J. Usefulness of QT-interval on the discharge electrocardiogram for predicting survival after acute myocardial infarction. *Am J Cardiol* 1986;57:1066–1068.

37. Higham PD, Campbell RWF. QT dispersion. *Brit Heart J* 1994;71:508–510.

38. Linker NJ, Colonna P, Kekwick CA, Till J, Camm AJ, Ward DE. Assessment of QT dispersion in symptomatic patients with congenital long QT syndromes. *Am J Cardiol* 1992;69:634–638.

39. Buja G, Miorelli M, Turrini P, Melacini P, Nava A. Comparison of QT dispersion in hypertrophic cardiomyopathy between patients with and without ventricular arrhythmias and sudden death. *Am J Cardiol* 1993;72:973–976.

40. Barr CS, Naas A, Freeman M, Lang CC, Struthers AD. QT dispersion and sudden unexpected death in chronic heart failure. *Lancet* 1994;343:327–329.
41. Zareba W, Moss AJ, le Cessie S. Dispersion of ventricular repolarization and arrhythmic cardiac death in coronary artery disease. *Am J Cardiol* 1994;74: 550–553.
42. Hii JTY, Wyse DG, Gillis AM, Duff HJ, Solylo MA, Mitchell LB. Precordial QT interval dispersion as a marker of torsades de pointes. Disparate effects of class la antiarrhythmic drugs and amiodarone. *Circulation* 1992;86:1376–1382.
43. Pye M, Quinn AC, Cabbe SM. QT interval, a noninvasive marker of susceptibility to arrhythmias in patients with sustained ventricular arrhythmias? *Br Heart J* 1994;71:511–514.
44. Perkiomaki HS, Koistinen MG, Yli-Mayry S, Huikuri HV. Dispersion of QT interval in patients with and without susceptibility to ventricular tachyarrhythmias after previous myocardial infarction. *J Am Coll Cardiol* 1995;26:174–179.
45. El-Sherif N. T wave alternans. A marker of vulnerabilty to ventricular tachyar-rhythmias. In: Raviele A (ed). *Cardiac Arrhythmias 1995*. Milano, Italy: Springer, 1996, pp 12–16.
46. Smith JM, Clancy EA, Valeri CR, et al. Electrical alternans and cardiac electrical instability. *Circulation* 1988;77:110–121.
47. Rosenbaum DS, Jackson LE, Smith JM, et al. Electrical alternans and vulnerability to ventricular arrhythmias. *N Engl J Med* 1994;330:235–241.
48. Estes MNA, Zipes DP, El-Sherif N, et al: The value of T-wave alternans and signal averaged electrocardiogram as predictors of arrhythmia vulnerability. *PACE* 1995;18:796 (Abstract).
49. Gomes JAC, Hariman HI, Kang PS, Chowdry I, Lyons J, El-Sherif N. Pro-grammed electrical stimulation in patients with high-grade ectopy: electrophysio-logic findings and prognosis for survival. *Circulation* 1984;70:43–51.
50. Buxton AE, Marchlinski FE, Flores BT, Miller JM, Doherty JV, Josephson ME. Nonsustained ventricular tachycardia in patients with coronary artery disease: role of electrophysiologic study. *Circulation* 1987;75:1178–1185.
51. Wilber DJ, Olshansky B, Moran JF, Scanlon PJ. Electrophysiological testing and nonsustained ventricular tachycardia: use and limitations in patients with coronary artery disease and impaired ventricular function. *Circulation* 1990;82:350–358.
52. Burkart F, Pfisterer M, Kiowski W, Follath F, Burckhard D. Effect of antiarrhyth-mic therapy on mortality in survivors of myocardial infarction with asymptomatic complex ventricular arrhythmias: Basel Antiarrhythmic Study of Infarct Survival (BASIS). *J Am Coll Cardiol* 1990;16:1711–1718.
53. Cairns JA, Connolly SJ, Gent M, Roberts R. Post-myocardial infarction mortality in patients with ventricular premature depolarization: Canadian amiodarone myo-cardial infarction arrhythmia trial pilot study. *Circulation* 1991;84:550–557.
54. Singh SN, Fletcher RD, Fisher SG, et al. Amiodarone in patients with congestive heart failure and asymptomatic ventricular arrhythmia. Survival Trial of Antiar-rhythmic Therapy in Congestive Heart Failure. *N Engl J Med* 1995;333(2): 121–122.
55. Camm AJ, Julian D, Janse G, et al: The European Myocardial Infarct Amiodarone Trial (EMIAT). Am J Cardiol 1993;72:95F–98F.
56. Moss AJ, Hall J, Cannon DS, et al: Multicenter Automatic Defibrillator Implanta-tion Trial. *Circulation* 1996;94:I-567 (Abstract).

Chapter 5

Postinfarction-Sustained Ventricular Tachycardias:
The Role of Drugs and Methods for Assessing Antiarrhythmic Efficacy

Ronald W.F. Campbell, MD

Introduction

The processes of damage and repair associated with myocardial infarction are very complex. In the late phase of postinfarction, cells will either have survived the event or will by that stage, be dead and replaced by fibrous tissue. It is the architecture of the damaged area which has implications for mechanical performance and for disturbances of electrical activity. The postinfarction situation is further complicated by the distinct possibility of further ischemic events and by what may be a precariously balanced hemodynamic state. For instance, a normal heart may tolerate a quite rapid ventricular tachyarrhythmia, with only a minimal risk of deterioration to ventricular fibrillation. In the diseased heart, however, a ventricular tachyarrhythmia may so reduce cardiac output as to create ischemia with rapid and profound consequences for electrical organization in the myocardium. These and a myriad of other factors create a complex scenario for postinfarction arrhythmogenesis, making it difficult to establish consensus guidelines for management.[1]

Sustained Ventricular Tachycardias Postinfarction

The classical ventricular tachyarrhythmic complication of late infarction is sustained monomorphic ventricular tachycardia (VT). This arrhythmia occurs in particular situations. Patients who have suffered extensive anterior

Academic Cardiology is supported by the British Heart Foundation.

From *Practical Management of Cardiac Arrhythmias* edited by Nabil El-Sherif, and Jean Lekieffre. Futura Publishing Co., Armonk, NY, © 1997.

myocardial infarction, often in the setting of single vessel coronary artery disease and who develop a ventricular aneurysm are those most likely to be affected. It may appear as early as 4 or 5 days after the acute infarct event, or years may elapse after the index infarction before its first occurrence. Recurrences are common, necessitating a long-term management strategy.

Postinfarction-sustained monomorphic VT was the first ventricular tachyarrhythmia to be examined by programmed stimulation. This showed an almost universal easy inducibility and termination by critically timed stimuli.[2] The inference was that this was a reentrant arrhythmia. Subsequent surgical strategies for dealing with the arrhythmia have revealed more information. When mapped peroperatively, postinfarction-sustained monomorphic VT often appears to arise from a point source as though microreentry is the basic mechanism. More sophisticated mapping studies are now revealing that it is probably a macroreentrant circuit involving slender fibers of surviving muscle cells embedded in fibrous sheets.[3] Surgical management has also revealed that the majority of these arrhythmias can be controlled by endocardial resection.[4] This raises the possibility that in some way the His-Purkinje system might be involved in the arrhythmia, but this has never been clearly established. The easy inducibility and termination of sustained monomorphic VT has been the basis for using electrophysiological testing to determine the utility of administered antiarrhythmic drug therapy.

Apart from ventricular fibrillation, no other postinfarction ventricular tachyarrhythmias are sustained. Polymorphic VT is seen principally in the early phase of infarction and is probably due to triggered activity. It is uncommon for this arrhythmia to persist into the late postinfarction phase and even if it does, it is rarely sustained.[5]

Electrophysiological Testing

The remarkable control offered by programmed stimulation for investigating postinfarction-sustained monomorphic VT has lead to its use for evaluating antiarrhythmic drug therapy. Natural history reports have clearly indicated that patients affected by such VTs have bad outcomes.[6] Even if life is not immediately threatened, each episode is distressing and it is almost universal that some form of prophylaxis or treatment is needed. When electrophysiological induction of a sustained monomorphic VT is no longer possible after antiarrhythmic drug administration, that drug is likely to provide benefits for the patient.[7] The benefits include reduced arrhythmia recurrences and improved prognosis. For over 15 years, there has been considerable enthusiasm for this strategy, but electrophysiological testing does not select drug therapy. It merely tests how administered drugs modify the inducibility of a ventricular tachyarrhythmia.

The selection of drugs to test remains a considerable problem. Do all drugs need to be tested in all patients? Are there short cuts? Can a representative drug be taken from each Vaughan Williams class and subclass? In the event of the failure of one drug, does that provide information about the next best drug? None of these questions is satisfactorily answered at the present time, resulting in many different protocols. Some explore antiarrhythmic drugs in detail, others offer early recourse to other strategies. Some patients are disadvantaged by multiple drug tests. This coupled with an antiarrhythmic drug efficacy of a little more than 40% has not encouraged enthusiasm for antiarrhythmic drugs.

The concept of electrophysiological testing of drugs for sustained monomorphic VT has significant weaknesses. While in the electrophysiological investigation of an accessory pathway, it would be near unthinkable not to have catheters close to that pathway, most ventricular stimulation for sustained monomorphic VT is performed in the right ventricle. It is possible that some administered drugs merely affect the conduction characteristics of myocardium between the catheter position and the reentrant circuit without necessarily affecting the reentrant circuit itself. The results would then erroneously suggest a useful effect of the agent. The level of aggression of the stimulation protocol is also hotly debated. Should a protocol be repeated merely to the point at which, previously, a ventricular tachyarrhythmia was provoked or should the protocol reach a predefined end-point (e.g., a specific cycle length and a specific number of extrastimuli?)[8] Remarkably, little attention has been given to the differences between those ventricular tachyarrhythmias provoked by single extrastimuli, and those requiring fast drive-trains and multiple extrastimuli.

Is it acceptable to test only once? The reproducibility of electrophysiological tests is not absolute[9]; with repeated procedures apparent, drug efficacy is progressively reduced.[10] Another and very important problem of electrophysiological testing is its failure to adequately reflect the actions of two of the most powerful antiarrhythmic drugs: the beta-blockers and amiodarone. It is well-recognized that if a ventricular tachyarrhythmia is rendered noninducible by the administration of amiodarone, this is likely to foretell a good clinical situation. The patients in whom the drug fails, however, do not do as badly as expected. In approximately half, there are no further arrhythmic events.[11,12] The electrophysiology result is therefore misleading. A consequence has been the suspicion of electrophysiological testing and a vogue for empiric amiodarone therapy. A similar problem arises with beta-blockers which may act through autonomic modulation. This cannot be adequately assessed or reproduced in electrophysiological studies. The majority of affected post-MI patients are potential candidates for routine beta-blockade for general prognostic reasons, although concerns regarding left ventricular performance may dictate that this therapy is used less frequently than is appropriate.

Ventricular Ectopic Beat Suppression

Invasive electrophysiological testing is invasive. It requires trained personnel and specialized equipment. Several less demanding assessment strategies have been examined. In the majority of patients affected by sustained monomorphic VT, there are occasional ventricular ectopic beats. In the ESVEM study,[13] the utility of titrating drug therapy to suppress ventricular ectopic beats (performed through Holter monitoring investigations) was compared directly with drug management based on electrophysiological testing. This controversial study suggested that it was "easier" to find a "successful" antiarrhythmic drug based on ectopic beat suppression than it was on the noninducibility of a ventricular tachyarrhythmia by programmed stimulation. Perhaps surprisingly, however, this study suggested that in neither case did it really matter as the outlook for patients was not particularly well-correlated with arrhythmia suppression measured by either technique. The ESVEM study has been widely discussed. It enrolled an unusual group of patients. They had to be evaluated by both Holter and programmed stimulation techniques. Thus, they had to have an electrically inducible ventricular tachyarrhythmia and high levels of ambient ventricular ectopic activity. It is not clear whether the results of the ESVEM study can be applied to more general VT patients. Intuitively, and on the basis of other studies,[14,15] it would seem that programmed electrical stimulation assessment of sustained monomorphic VT is the most direct and most relevant evaluation of the drug arrhythmia interaction.

Signal-Averaged Late Potentials

Patients subjected to sustained monomorphic VT often have signal-averaged late potentials. These represent the delayed ventricular activation of myocardial cells lying within an infarct territory. It had been hoped that antiarrhythmic drug therapy which would prove successful in the long-term might be identified by consistent changes on the signal-averaged electrocardiogram. This has not proved the case, and currently, there is no role for signal averaging in assessing antiarrhythmic drug utility.

Heart Rate Variability

Heart rate variability (HRV) correlates with prognosis postmyocardial infarction, but it is not specifically linked to sustained monomorphic VT.

There are suggestions that drug modification of HRV might be useful in tracking a prognostically beneficial intervention but this may relate more to total cardiac events than to a specific single arrhythmia.

QT Dispersion

QT dispersion which is emerging as a very important marker of inhomogeneity of recovery of excitability, has been linked with post-MI prognosis and also with sustained monomorphic VT.[16,17] This is consistent with evidence of arrhythmia-related myocardial dispersion of refractoriness.[18] Drug-provoked abnormalities of QT dispersion may identify disadvantageous clinical situations and it may be in the future that QT dispersion will offer some help in antiarrhythmic drug evaluation.

The Utility of Antiarrhythmic Drugs

The fact that there are several nonpharmacological interventions for sustained monomorphic VT, including map-directed cardiac surgery, revascularization, radiofrequency, and DC ablation, suggests that all cannot be well with antiarrhythmic drug therapy for this indication. It is difficult to establish levels of efficacy for individual agents, as protocols that are followed vary so widely. Overall, it is unlikely that antiarrhythmic drug efficacy is better than 40% (Figure 1). The class I antiarrhythmic drugs including propafenone,

VENTRICULAR ARRHYTHMIAS
The 'benefit' of drugs

	arrhythmia control	mortality
Class I	~ 50%	= or ↑
II	~ 20%	↓
III	~ 60%	= or slight ↓
IV	1%	= or ↑

Figure 1. Overall utility of the four classes of Vaughan Williams antiarrhythmic drugs in respect of arrhythmia control and mortality impact.

AMIODARONE
Ventricular Tachycardia

83 patients, inducible VT. 23 months follow up.
19 with 'no' VEBs; 64 with VEBs

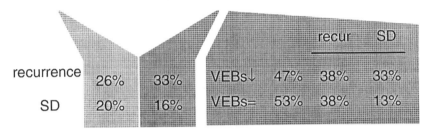

Nasir et al, AJC, 1994

Figure 2. Amiodarone's effect on ventricular tachycardia. Despite the drug, arrhythmia recurrence and sudden death (SD) rates are high. In those patients whose ventricular ectopic beats (VEBs) are reduced by amiodarone, there is no evidence of a particular benefit in the reduction of sudden death or arrhythmia recurrence. (Data adapted from Nasir et al.[21])

flecainide, and mexiletine are undoubtably effective.[19,20] Quinidine and procainamide may also have a limited role.

Empiric amiodarone therapy is widely used[21,22] and has the attraction that therapy is prescribed without formal testing. No large studies of amiodarone use for sustained VT have been reported, whether against placebo or in direct comparison with other antiarrhythmic agents. In a recent study of patients with inducible monomorphic VT,[21] amiodarone's impact on arrhythmia recurrences and sudden death was correlated with the drug's effect on ventricular ectopic beats. Despite amiodarone, VT recurrence rates were high (up to 32%) as was the rate of sudden death (up to 20%) (Figure 2).

Amiodarone has been tested against the cardioverter defibrillator. In that circumstance, amiodarone's efficacy in terms of sudden death and total mortality was poorer than that of the implantable cardioverter defibrillator.[23] Nonetheless, if amiodarone's results are compared to historical controls, then a reasonable efficacy can be inferred. Drugs other than antiarrhythmic agents may become important.

Modest attempts have been made to determine the usefulness or otherwise of combination antiarrhythmic therapy[24] but no study has yet been large enough to produce other than interesting anecdotal descriptions.

Other Drug Interventions

Most of the emphasis in control of VT postinfarction has been directed to electrical modification of the surviving myocardium. As often as there is coexisting left ventricular impairment, the negative inotropic impact of many antiarrhythmic drugs seriously limits their usefulness. Ideally, arrhythmia control might come from a modification of the architecture of the infarct, or better, by the prevention of the circumstances which create an arrhythmogenic scar.

The angiotensin-converting enzyme (ACE) inhibitors are known to influence the remodeling process after infarction. They also may regress left ventricular hypertrophy, perhaps by altering wall tension. There are some indications that these agents may also influence VT.[25] The V-Heft II study[25] was conducted in heart failure patients but many of them were postinfarction. Holter monitoring revealed on follow-up that those who received an ACE inhibitor had reduced rates of VT compared to those who received a nitrate hydralazine combination. Admittedly, the vast majority of these VT incidents were nonsustained, but there is a persuasive logic that links wall tension abnormalities, not just with triggered automatic arrhythmias, but also with inhomogeneity of recovery of refractoriness. It may emerge that ACE inhibitors will be a useful adjunctive agent in the drug management of postinfarction VT.

Successful thrombolysis with useful myocardial reperfusion has many immediate and late benefits. From an electrophysiological point of view, infarct size is smaller and late potentials are less likely to be found. Programmed stimulation has also showed that electrically inducible VT is less common in successfully thrombolyzed infarct patients. No reliable registers of post-MI VT exist, but anecdotally, there appears to be fewer patients presenting with this arrhythmia in the thrombolytic era.

Conclusions

Antiarrhythmic drug management of sustained monomorphic VT postinfarction is a troubled clinical area. The concept of electrophysiological testing to show the utility of administered drugs was established almost 20 years ago. There has been surprisingly little development in the procedure and the concept since then. Perhaps the lack of enthusiasm derives from the relatively poor performance of antiarrhythmic drug therapy for this indication. Nonetheless, for those patients in whom drugs work, this is an excellent option. More should be done to identify such responding patients, sparing them consideration of surgery or an implantable device. It seems unlikely that many new antiarrhythmic drugs will be developed. The pure potassium channel blockers have not so far lived up to their promise, but it may be that older and traditional agents have more to offer than is currently recognized. New electrical assessment techniques including QT dispersion and HRV could prove to be valuable, both in risk assessment and for drug evaluation.

References

1. Leclercq JF, Coumel P, Denjoy I, et al. Long-term follow-up after sustained monomorphic ventricular tachycardia: causes, pump failure, and empiric antiarrhythmic therapy that modify survival. *Am Heart J* 1991;121(6 Pt 1):1685–1692.
2. Wellens HJ, Duren DR, Lie KI. Observations on mechanisms of ventricular tachycardia in man. *Circulation* 1976;54(2):237–244.
3. de Bakker JM, van Capelle FJ, Janse MJ, et al. Macroreentry in the infarcted human heart: the mechanism of ventricular tachycardias with a "focal" activation pattern. *J Am Coll Cardiol* 1991;18(4):1005–1014.
4. Bourke JP, Richards DA, Ross DL, et al. Routine programmed electrical stimulation in survivors of acute myocardial infarction for prediction of spontaneous ventricular tachyarrhythmias during follow-up: results, optimal stimulation protocol and cost-effective screening. *J Am Coll Cardiol* 1991;18(3):780–788.
5. Wolfe CL, Nibley C, Bhandari A, et al. Polymorphous ventricular tachycardia associated with acute myocardial infarction. *Circulation* 1991;84:1543–1551.
6. Ostermeyer J, Kirklin JK, Borggrefe M, et al. Anti-tachycardia surgery in ventricular arrhythmia. *Herz* 1990;15(2):126–138.
7. Waller TJ, Kay HR, Spielman SR, et al. Reduction in sudden death and total mortality by antiarrhythmic therapy evaluated by electrophysiologic drug testing: criteria of efficacy in patients with sustained ventricular tachyarrhythmia. *J Am Coll Cardiol* 1987;10(1):83–89.
8. Hummel JD, Strickberger SA, Daoud E, et al. Results and efficiency of programmed ventricular stimulation with four extrastimuli compared with one, two, and three extrastimuli. *Circulation* 1994;90(6):2827–2832.
9. Rosenbaum MS, Wilber DJ, Finkelstein D, et al. Immediate reproducibility of electrically induced sustained monomorphic ventricular tachycardia before and during antiarrhythmic therapy. *J Am Coll Cardiol* 1991;17(1):133–138.
10. Fogoros RN, Elson JJ, Bonnet CA, et al. Reproducibility of successful drug trials in patients with inducible sustained ventricular tachycardia. *PACE* 1992;15(3):295–303.
11. Hamer AW, Finerman WB Jr, Peter T, et al. Disparity between the clinical and electrophysiologic effects of amiodarone in the treatment of recurrent ventricular tachyarrhythmias. *Am Heart J* 1981;102(6 Pt 1):992–1000.
12. Manolis AS, Uricchio F, Estes NAD. Prognostic value of early electrophysiologic studies for ventricular tachycardia recurrence in patients with coronary artery disease treated with amiodarone. *Am J Cardiol* 1989;63(15):1052–1057.
13. Mason J, for the ESVEM Investigators. A comparison of electrophysiologic testing with Holter monitoring to predict antiarrhythmic drug efficacy for ventricular tachyarrhythmias. *N Engl J Med* 1993;329:445–451.
14. Kim SG, Felder SD, Figura I, et al. Comparison of programmed stimulation and Holter monitoring for predicting long-term efficacy and inefficacy of amiodarone used alone or in combination with a class 1A antiarrhythmic agent in patients with ventricular tachyarrhythmia. *J Am Coll Cardiol* 1987;9(2):398–404.
15. Mitchell LB, Duff HJ, Manyari DE, et al. A randomized clinical trial of the

noninvasive and invasive approaches to drug therapy of ventricular tachycardia. *N Engl J Med* 1987;317(27):1681–1687.

16. Pye M, Quinn A, Cobbe S. QT interval dispersion: a non-invasive marker of susceptibility to arrhythmia in patients with sustained ventricular arrhythmias? *Br Heart J* 1994;71(6):511-n514.

17. Perkiomaki J, Koistinen M, Yli-Mayry S, et al. Dispersion of QT interval in patients with and without susceptibility to ventricular tachyarrhythmias after previous myocardial infarction. J *Am Coll Cardiol* 1995;26(1):174–179.

18. Misier AR, Opthof T, van Hemel NM, et al. Dispersion of 'refractoriness' in noninfarcted myocardium of patients with ventricular tachycardia or ventricular fibrillation after myocardial infarction. *Circulation* 1995;91(10):2566–2572.

19. Anonymous. A multicentre, randomized trial on the benefit/risk profile of amiodarone, flecainide and propafenone in patients with cardiac disease and complex ventricular arrhythmias. Antiarrhythmic Drug Evaluation Group (A.D.E.G.). *Eur Heart J* 1992;13(9):1251–1258.

20. Haissaguerre M, Warin JF, Benchimol D, et al. Oral flecainide in the treatment of refractory arrhythmias. Long-term follow-up of 98 patients. *Arch Mal Coeur Vaiss* 1987;80(3):357–363.

21. Nasir N Jr, Doyle TK, Wheeler SH, et al. Usefulness of Holter monitoring in predicting efficacy of amiodarone therapy for sustained ventricular tachycardia associated with coronary artery disease. *Am J Cardiol* 1994;73(8):554–558.

22. Olson PJ, Woelfel A, Simpson RJ Jr, et al. Stratification of sudden death risk in patients receiving long-term amiodarone treatment for sustained ventricular tachycardia or ventricular fibrillation. *Am J Cardiol* 1993;71(10):823–826.

23. O'Brien BJ, Buxton MJ, Rushby JA. Cost effectiveness of the implantable cardioverter defibrillator: a preliminary analysis. *Br Heart J* 1992;68(2):241–245.

24. Marchlinski FE, Buxton AE, Kindwall KE, et al. Comparison of individual and combined effects of procainamide and amiodarone in patients with sustained ventricular tachyarrhythmias. *Circulation* 1988;78(3):583–591.

25. Fletcher R, Cintron G, Johnson G, et al. for the V-Heft II VA Cooperative Studies Group. Enalapril decreases prevalence of ventricular tachycardia in patients with chronic congestive heart failure. *Circulation* 1993;87(Suppl VI):49–55.

Chapter 6

The Identification and Management of Patients with Hypertrophic Cardiomyopathy at High Risk of Sudden Cardiac Death

Alistair K.B. Slade, MA, MRCP,
A. John Camm, MD, FRCP

Introduction

Hypertrophic cardiomyopathy has fascinated clinicians since its first description over 30 years ago by Teare.[1] While initially, studies focused on the classic variant of hypertrophic cardiomyopathy with asymmetrical septal hypertrophy, it has become clear from extensive family studies and routine health screening that the condition exists in a spectrum of morphological forms.

Currently, the condition is defined by the presence of a hypertrophied and nondilated left and/or right ventricle in the absence of a cardiac or systemic cause.[2,3] Patients may be profoundly disabled due to abnormalities of diastolic function, systolic left ventricular outflow tract gradients, ischemia, and arrhythmias, or they may be completely asymptomatic. Presentation may be in early infancy or may occur in old age. While this broad spectrum of morphological and symptomatic presentations has modified the initial belief that hypertrophic cardiomyopathy carries a uniformly poor prognosis, the identification of the patient at risk of sudden cardiac death remains paramount.

The condition carries an increased risk of sudden cardiac death, classically thought to be arrhythmogenic in origin. In a typical referral center population, there is a mortality from sudden cardiac death of 2% to 3%.[4,5] In

From *Practical Management of Cardiac Arrhythmias* edited by Nabil El-Sherif, and Jean Lekieffre. Futura Publishing Co., Armonk, NY, © 1997.

children and adolescents, where sudden death may be the presenting feature of the disease, this figure rises to 5% to 6%. It is the most common cause of sudden cardiac death in patients under the age of 30.[6-8]

Genetics

Shortly after the initial reports of the disease, it rapidly became evident that certain families have a malignant pedigree with a high incidence of sudden cardiac death.[10] With the explosion of interest in mapping the human genome, a number of mutations were shown to be linked with hypertrophic cardiomyopathy. Initially, mutations affecting beta myosin heavy chains were described on chromosome 14, but other chromosomes have now been implicated.[12,13] More recently, mutations affecting other contractile proteins such as alpha-tropomyosin and troponin T have been identified.[14] Attempts have been made to correlate particular mutations with an adverse outcome,[15-17] but it has been long established that phenotypic expression is not wholly dictated by the underlying genetic abnormality.[18] It is well documented that premature sudden cardiac death can coexist with end-stage systolic heart failure within the same kindred.[19] It would seem premature to base therapeutic intervention, particularly, prophylactic defibrillator implantation on a genetic basis alone, although it seems likely that certain mutations carry an increased risk of sudden cardiac death.

Myocardial Disarray

Gross anatomical morphology and symptomatic status do not predict future sudden cardiac death. The central importance of the characteristic histologic feature of hypertrophic cardiomyopathy, myocardial disarray would seem to be established.[20] Myocyte disarray associated with an excess of loose connective tissue is quantitatively different in hypertrophic cardiomyopathy from the appearances seen in other forms of hypertrophy. The disorganized muscle bundles have a characteristic whorled pattern on light microscopy. Ultrastructural examination by electron microscopy has demonstrated that there is also disorganization of the myofibrils within individual cells (Figure 1). The clinical consequences of myocyte disarray are electrical instability of the heart, which must be relevant in the pathogenesis of sudden death. In addition, the cellular disorganization may contribute to the abnormalities of ventricular diastolic function. It is uncertain whether the development of myocardial disarray and of myocardial hypertrophy are unrelated responses to a molecular or a developmental abnormality or are contingent upon each other.[21] The recognition of patients who have severe left ventricular hypertrophy and minimal disarray and those who have severe disarray and minimal

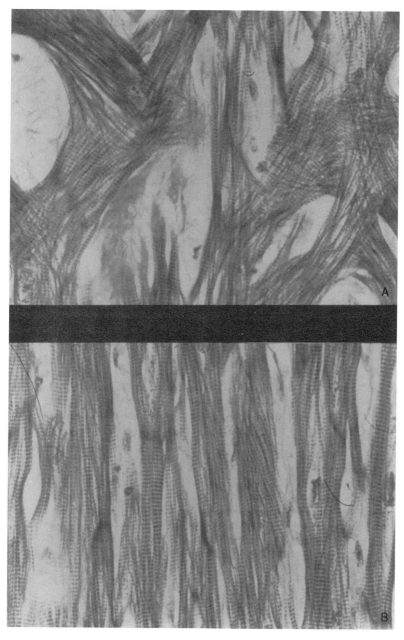

Figure 1. (A): Normal myocardial cellular architecture **(B):** Disordered myocardial architecture demonstrating myocardial disarray—the histologic hallmark of hypertrophic cardiomyopathy.

hypertrophy is consistent with the former hypothesis.[22] The extent of disarray would seem to be associated with the risk of sudden cardiac death. There is greater cellular disarray in the hearts of adolescents who die suddenly than in adults who die suddenly. Disarray is least in adults who die from other causes.[4,23] Until recently, no quantitation of myocardial disarray or its effect on electrophysiological parameters of conduction has been available.

Abnormalities of Peripheral Vasomotor Control

Exertional syncope is an important symptom and carries an increased risk of sudden cardiac death.[5] Classically exertional syncope in hypertrophic cardiomyopathy was thought to be due to true obstruction to left ventricular outflow in a manner akin to aortic stenosis. The occurrence of exertional syncope in patients without left ventricular outflow tract gradients even with pharmacological provocation, and the finding of exercise hypotension despite a normal increase in cardiac output has forced a revision of opinion; although it is likely that in a proportion of patients true obstruction does exist. A significant proportion of sudden deaths in hypertrophic cardiomyopathy occur in association with exertion.[24] Such sudden deaths may not always be associated with arrhythmias.

Frenneaux et al, studied 129 consecutive patients with hypertrophic cardiomyopathy to evaluate the response of blood pressure to exercise.[25] Distinctly differing patterns of response were observed. The normal response to exercise with a steady rise in blood pressure on exercise and a steady fall on recovery was seen in 64 patients. Of the remaining patients, five showed a continuous fall in blood pressure from the commencement of exercise, and 38 showed a dramatic fall from peak values while exercising. A subgroup of 14 patients with exercise hypotension were further studied with invasive hemodynamic measurements. At peak exercise, they showed similar cardiac index as compared to 14 controls with a normal blood pressure response but had a significantly lower systemic vascular resistance.

Patients with exercise hypotension had smaller left ventricular end-diastolic dimensions as assessed by echocardiography, and had a significantly higher incidence of known risk factors such as a young age and an adverse family history suggesting the possible importance of hemodynamic instability as a factor in initiating sudden cardiac death. Interestingly, the older patients described symptoms of fatigue, light-headedness, and presyncope causing them to discontinue exercise while younger patients who have a higher incidence of syncope did not experience such warning symptoms. The failure of this early warning system in the young may be an important determinant of exertional syncope and sudden death. It is postulated that activation of the ventricular baroreceptor reflex occurs, leading to withdrawal of peripheral sympathetic tone, and that this is explained by abnormally high left ventricular wall stress consequent on increased wall thickness, reduced cavity size, and increased sympathetic drive. Such abnormalities would be magnified in patients with the smallest left ventricular cavity dimensions.

The abnormal drop in systemic vascular resistance during erect exercise is strongly associated with an inappropriate increase in forearm blood flow during supine leg exercise. Counihan et al studied 103 consecutive patients with hypertrophic cardiomyopathy during symptom-limited supine bicycle exercise with forearm blood flow measurement by plethysmography.[26] The normal response of reduction in forearm blood flow was seen in 64 patients as blood was preferentially transmitted to the exercising musculature. No change or an increase in forearm blood flow suggesting inappropriate peripheral vasomotor control was observed in 39 patients. Again, the abnormal population had echocardiographic evidence of smaller left ventricular end-diastolic dimensions. This latter group also showed an association with factors suggesting an adverse prognosis, providing further evidence of the possible importance of hemodynamic instability as a risk factor for sudden cardiac death.

Prospective evaluation of the abnormalities of blood pressure response on exercise reveal it to be an important risk factor. In 167 patients evaluated prospectively between January 1988 and February 1994, 67 had abnormal blood pressure responses on exercise. After a mean follow-up, of nearly 3 years, sudden cardiac death occurred in 13 patients, 10 of whom had abnormal exercise blood pressure responses. This suggests that evaluation of the blood pressure response should become incorporated into current noninvasive risk stratification.[27]

Risk Stratification Techniques

One of the main aims in assessing patients with hypertrophic cardiomyopathy is the identification of individual risk for sudden death. In young patients (who have the highest incidence of sudden cardiac death) syncope and a family history of hypertrophic cardiomyopathy and sudden premature death are specific, but relatively insensitive, predictors of sudden death.[9,10] In older patients, the presence of nonsustained ventricular tachycardia on Holter monitoring adds to risk stratification but is still only weakly predictive of sudden cardiac death.[11] The current status of these conventional risk factors for sudden cardiac death will be reviewed together with newer and more contentious approaches to risk stratification: signal-averaged electrocardiography; measurement of indices of heart rate variability; abnormalities of exercise hemodynamics; electrophysiological study with programmed ventricular stimulation; and a novel electrophysiological approach designed to quantify the electrical effects of myocardial disarray.

Holter Monitoring

Nonsustained ventricular tachycardia is seen on Holter monitoring in approximately 25% of patients with hypertrophic cardiomyopathy and the presence of such episodes on Holter monitoring carries a sevenfold increased risk of sudden cardiac death.[11,28] Such arrhythmias appear to be clinically benign. Attacks are almost invariably asymptomatic, occurring at night or during periods of predominant vagal tone. The ventricular rate is usually relatively slow (mean heart rate at 140 beats per minute in one series of 400 episodes in 52 patients). Analysis of different episodes in the same patient show multiple morphologies suggesting multiple origins in keeping with the diffuse histopathological nature of the disease. The presence of such arrhythmias is the best readily available marker of increased risk of sudden cardiac death in the adult patient. The negative predictive accuracy is high (97%), but the positive predictive accuracy is low (23%), reflecting the fact that the majority of patients with nonsustained ventricular tachycardia on Holter do not die during short-term follow-up.

Signal-Averaged Electrocardiogram

The signal-averaged electrocardiogram is a useful technique in identifying patients at risk of developing sustained monomorphic ventricular tachycardia and sudden cardiac death after myocardial infarction. Refinements to the technique such as frequency-domain analysis and spectral temporal mapping improve the predictive accuracy. Its application in hypertrophic cardiomyopathy is less useful. In a study of 121 patients, free from antiarrhythmic medication, Kulakowski et al looked at the predictive value of conventional criteria for abnormalities of the signal-averaged electrocardiogram.[29] Nonsustained ventricular tachycardia was seen in 27 of the patients. Abnormal time-domain signal-averaged electrocardiograms were seen in three of the population of patients with nonsustained ventricular tachycardia and three of the remainder. The most useful criterion for identifying patients with nonsustained ventricular tachycardia was a reduced (less than 40 μVolts) voltage of the initial 40 msecs of the signal-averaged complex. Nine patients in this study had catastrophic cardiac events (three sudden cardiac deaths and six patients who had been resuscitated from out-of-hospital ventricular fibrillation), but all had a normal time domain signal-averaged electrocardiogram.

The failure of the signal-averaged electrocardiogram was thought to be due to several factors: (1) late potentials are a marker for the development of sustained monomorphic ventricular tachycardia which is rare in hypertrophic cardiomyopathy; (2) the arrhythmogenic substrate in hypertrophic cardiomyopathy is more diffusely located in the myocardium than the scar which, is the basis for postmyocardial infarction ventricular tachycardia; and (3) the hypertrophic process interferes with the measurement of late potentials.

Heart Rate Variability

Abnormalities of autonomic function such as heart rate variability and baroreflex activity have been shown to be important predictors of future arrhythmic events including sudden cardiac death after myocardial infarction. The application of the technique of heart rate variability to patients with hypertrophic cardiomyopathy might be of theoretical benefit in risk stratification in a population with documented abnormalities of autonomic function, and in whom abnormalities of autonomic function have been thought by some, to be central to the development of the condition.

Counihan et al looked at time-domain and spectral-domain parameters of heart rate variability in a referral population of 104 patients in sinus rhythm, free from antiarrhythmic medication.[30] Although abnormalities of heart rate variability were found in certain subgroups the technique did not add to the predictive accuracy of conventional risk stratification techniques.

Arrhythmias in Hypertrophic Cardiomyopathy

Evidence for an Arrhythmic Cause of Sudden Cardiac Death

The majority of cases of sudden cardiac death in hypertrophic cardiomyopathy are thought to be due to ventricular fibrillation,[31] although individual case reports have documented complete heart block, asystole, myocardial infarction, and supraventricular tachycardia, especially atrial fibrillation, conducted rapidly to the ventricles via the atrioventricular node or by an accessory pathway, as antecedent events.[4,6,7,32] The triggering factors may also include the hemodynamic abnormalities described above (Figure 2). The importance of hemodynamic factors is shown in the case of a 52-year-old woman with hypertrophic cardiomyopathy, syncope, and frequent nonsustained ventricular tachycardia which occurred during Holter monitoring.[33] After complaining of palpitation and breathlessness, the patient rested but symptoms persisted with the disappearance of her left ventricular outflow tract murmur and loss of consciousness. During this syncopal episode, peripheral pulses were absent and signs of anoxia developed. Spontaneous recovery occurred. Analysis of the Holter revealed that loss of consciousness developed during sinus tachycardia (130 beats per minute) in the absence of arrhythmias and evidence of syncope.

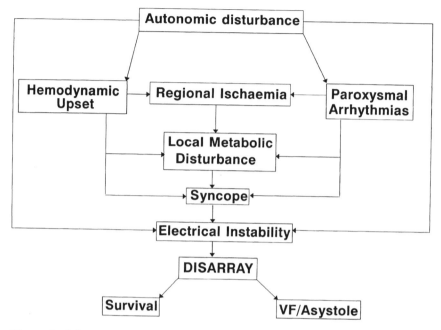

Figure 2. Schematic diagram illustrating the interrelationship between autonomic dysfunction, hemodynamic upset, paroxysmal arrhythmias and the arrhythmogenic substrate in the pathogenesis of sudden death in hypertrophic cardiomyopathy.

Atrial Fibrillation

Atrial fibrillation is the most commonly sustained arrhythmia seen with a prevalence in most series of 15% to 20%.[11,34,35] The establishment of atrial fibrillation was classically held to represent an important stage in the disease process with universal functional deterioration and the risk of systemic emboli. The lack of worsened outcome of a cohort of patients with hypertrophic cardiomyopathy with atrial fibrillation is reported in a retrospective study of 52 patients from 1960 to 1985.[36] The acute onset of atrial fibrillation led to symptomatic deterioration in 89%, but restoration of sinus rhythm (63%), or control of ventricular rate with appropriate medical therapy (30%), led to restoration of original NYHA functional class. Survival in the group with atrial fibrillation was compared to that of 122 patients, matched for age, sex, known risk factors, and year of diagnosis, who remained in sinus rhythm during the same time period. There were 19 deaths in the group with atrial fibrillation (6 sudden, 6 from cardiac failure, 2 following myocardial infarction, 2 from stroke, and 3 from noncardiac causes); 5-year mortality was 14%.

Overall survival was similar in the patients who remained in sinus rhythm during the study period. Interestingly, none of the six patients with atrial fibrillation who were aged < 21 years at diagnosis died, compared to 11 (31%) of 35 patients of a similar age at diagnosis, who did not develop atrial fibrillation. In those aged > 21 years at diagnosis, 22 of 46 (48%) patients with atrial fibrillation died, compared to 17 of 87 (20%) patients with sinus rhythm. This difference was not statistically different.

Thus, symptomatic deterioration associated with the acute onset of atrial fibrillation may be seen in patients who have impaired left ventricular function, but the majority of such patients can be restored to their previous functional class by treatment, even if they remain in atrial fibrillation. Furthermore, the development of atrial fibrillation was not shown to have an adverse effect on prognosis. A short duration of atrial fibrillation and amiodarone therapy were the most powerful predictors of a successful return to sinus rhythm. Patients with paroxysmal or established atrial fibrillation are at risk of emboli and should be anticoagulated.[11]

These observations should be tempered by the fact that paroxysmal atrial fibrillation may initiate hemodynamic deterioration and sudden cardiac death before presentation to hospital.[32] This possible triggering factor for sudden cardiac death was vividly demonstrated in a 45-year-old female who underwent evaluation of DDD pacing with the insertion of temporary pacing wires. Passage of a guide-wire into the right atrium, induced atrial fibrillation with a ventricular rate of 170 to 190 beats per minute, resulting in hypotension and myocardial ischemia that rapidly deteriorated within 15 seconds to ventricular fibrillation (Figure 3).

The Role for Programmed Ventricular Stimulation

The role of programmed electrical stimulation in hypertrophic cardiomyopathy is controversial. Programmed ventricular stimulation was evolved primarily to induce clinically relevant ventricular arrhythmias in the context of ischemic heart disease. When considering whether the technique is appropriate when applied to hypertrophic cardiomyopathy, several points need to be considered. The first issue is, whether the commonly stimulated arrhythmias, ventricular fibrillation, polymorphic ventricular tachycardia, or ventricular flutter in any way mimic the clinical arrhythmias that cause death in hypertrophic cardiomyopathy, and therefore increase understanding of the mechanism of arrhythmogenesis. The second issue is the specificity of programmed stimulation in identifying high-risk patients. It is likely that, *as a group*, patients with hypertrophic cardiomyopathy are more likely to develop arrhythmias with programmed stimulation than patients with normal ventri-

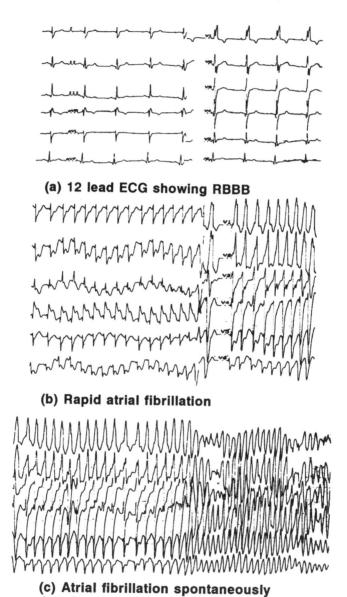

(a) 12 lead ECG showing RBBB

(b) Rapid atrial fibrillation

**(c) Atrial fibrillation spontaneously
deteriorating to ventricular fibrillation
after 20 seconds**

Figure 3. Sequential ECG tracings showing rapid transition from sinus rhythm to rapid atrial fibrillation with marked ST segment depression with subsequent spontaneous deterioration to ventricular fibrillation.

cles and that high-risk patients, *as a group*, are more fragile than low-risk patients. Aggressive stimulation may be required to produce an arrhythmia in patients who have survived ventricular fibrillation. However, the same protocol will induce an arrhythmia in a large number of low-risk patients and controls who will not die suddenly. This lack of discrimination makes programmed stimulation unhelpful in the management of patients, unless other stratification methods are employed to refine the high-risk group. The literature remains controversial.

In Fananapazir's et al series of 155 patients with hypertrophic cardiomyopathy undergoing electrophysiological study, a variety of responses to programmed ventricular stimulation were observed.[37] Nonsustained ventricular tachycardia was induced in 22 (14%) patients, sustained arrhythmias (defined in this study as 3 to 30 consecutive ventricular beats at 120 or greater beats per minute terminating spontaneously, or requiring termination due to hemodynamic embarrassment) were induced in 66 (43%) of which monomorphic ventricular tachycardia was seen in 16, polymorphic ventricular tachycardia in 48, and ventricular fibrillation in 2. Induction of sustained arrhythmias required two extrastimuli in 19 patients and three extrastimuli in 47. A left ventricular site for extrastimulation was required in 15 patients. 16 out of 17 survivors of out-of-hospital ventricular fibrillation required 3 extrastimuli to produce sustained arrhythmia. It was claimed that the induction of sustained ventricular arrhythmia (polymorphic ventricular tachycardia in the majority of the patients that were studied) is an abnormal finding in hypertrophic cardiomyopathy that may provide a useful guide to therapy; although the study also concluded that programmed ventricular stimulation using less than 3 extrastimuli, induced ventricular tachycardia in only a small percentage of patients with hypertrophic cardiomyopathy. Further follow-up data from this group is available. An aggressive stimulation protocol involving right and left ventricular sites with up to three extrastimuli, induced ventricular fibrillation in 70% of survivors of out-of-hospital cardiac arrest. What is of concern is that 68 patients out of 230 (32%) had a positive result with programmed ventricular stimulation, yet remained free from a cardiac event during follow-up, rendering the use of programmed ventricular stimulation poorly specific for identifying high-risk patients.[38] This lack of specificity makes the technique inappropriate in guiding therapy, particularly if that therapy is an implantable cardioverter defibrillator.

The experience with programmed ventricular stimulation at St. George's Hospital has been less helpful.[39] A total of 52 patients have undergone programmed stimulation up to stage 8 of the Wellens protocol. Twelve of the series developed ventricular fibrillation or polymorphic ventricular tachycardia requiring defibrillation (a positive response), whereas, 40 did not. Only two of the six patients with documented ventricular fibrillation were inducible.

The other ten were nonventricular fibrillation patients who were inducible and have remained free from arrhythmic events and were also patients with a follow-up of between 2 and 4 years. The absence of use of a third extrastimulus in this experience is a possible criticism. The incidence of polymorphic ventricular tachycardia, usually thought to be a nonspecific response, rises steeply with the use of a third stimulus.[40] Rendering, in our opinion, the use of a third extrastimulus unhelpful in targeting appropriate therapy.

The combined European experience of programmed ventricular stimulation is in general agreement with the National Institute of Health (NIH). Induction of ventricular arrhythmias require very aggressive stimulation protocols. What is different, is that, the patients with inducible polymorphic ventricular tachycardia have not experienced the adverse outcome that the NIH studies would have predicted for them.[41,42]

A Novel Electrophysiological Technique

An alternative electrophysiological approach to risk stratification aims to record electrophysiological measurements which reflect the underlying myocardial disarray.[20] It is based on the hypothesis that increased myocardial disarray leads to an increased number of possible conduction paths due to variations in fiber length and tortuosity. These different pathways would be expected to conduct with variable velocity on the basis of their physical properties.[43] Thus, inhomogeneous conduction may occur with pathways recruited or blocked, depending on the refractory state of the ventricle. Such dispersion of conduction may form one component of the substrate for reentry and hence ventricular fibrillation.

The method is based on the analysis of the separate components of paced right ventricular electrograms recorded at multiple right ventricular sites. Such electrograms may contain components due to the individual conduction paths close to the electrodes. The electrograms are recorderd during a computer-controlled pacing sequence with an extrastimulus every third beat, which has a gradually decreased coupling interval down to ventricular effective refractory period. With decreasing extrastimulus coupling, interval individual pathways may be blocked or recruited and the presence of such pathways may be inferred by studying the number of components within the recorded electrograms.

Thirty-seven consecutive patients with hypertrophic cardiomyopathy were initially studied, including 4 patients who had sustained out-of-hospital cardiac arrest and were assumed or documented as having sustained ventricular fibrillation, 5 patients with nonsustained ventricular tachycardia on Holter, 15 patients with sudden death in a first-degree relative and 13 patients considered to be at low risk.[44]

The analysis of the conduction curves that were generated focused on two variables: (1) the point at which latency began to increase; and (2) the width of the electrogram at ventricular effective refractory period. The different appearances of normal and abnormal conduction curves is illustrated (Figure 4). Normal controls showed an increase in electrogram width and increased latency at short coupling intervals. In contrast, patients who had sustained prior ventricular fibrillation showed early increase in latency, a markedly increased electrogram width and increased numbers of transitions. A scatter plot of change of electrogram duration against S1S2 coupling interval, at which latency increases produced highly significant discrimination between the patients who had sustained cardiac arrest and who showed a marked increase in electrogram width, early increase in latency and controls, and low-risk patients who demonstrated a late increase in latency and only a small increase in electrogram width. Patients with familial sudden death and nonsustained ventricular tachycardia formed an intermediate group (Figure 5).

The technique has now been prospectively evaluated in a further cohort of 64 patients.[39] Of this new cohort, three had documented ventricular fibrillation, with a further patient having sustained sudden cardiac death assumed to be due to ventricular fibrillation, 25 had nonsustained ventricular tachycardia on Holter, 21 had a family history of premature sudden cardiac death, 19 had syncope, and 14 had no conventional risk factors. All patients underwent the same pacing protocol as the original cohort. Three of the ventricular fibrillation group lay within the original VF group while only 6 out of 60 nonventricular fibrillation patients were within this group. Interestingly, the patients with nonsustained ventricular tachycardia and a family history of sudden cardiac death lay spread across the spectrum of abnormalities from normal to the ventricular fibrillation group (Figure 6). This result gives possible insight into the well-established fact that only a proportion of patients identified as being at increased risk after the detection of nonsustained ventricular tachycardia, go on to sustain an adverse cardiac event.

This technique is now to be evaluated further. In a multicenter trial, patients identified as being at high risk on the basis of conventional risk stratification, together with the electrogram fractionation technique, will be implanted with an ICD and then randomized to either placebo or amiodarone therapy. Such an approach will allow an evaluation of the various techniques of risk stratification, an assessment of the ICD in the treatment of high-risk hypertrophic cardiomyopathy patients, and finally, a prospective evaluation of amiodarone in the prevention of sudden cardiac death.

Therapy to Prevent Sudden Cardiac Death

Conventional risk factor stratification identifies a cohort of patients who are at an increased risk of sudden cardiac death. In approximately 30% of

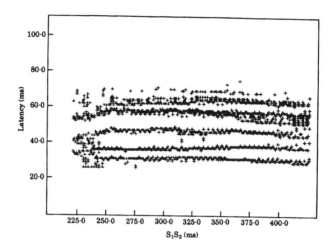

Control

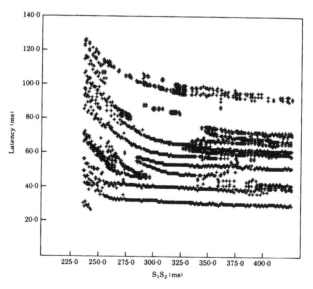

VF Patient

Figure 4. Conduction curve from a control subject and a patient with ventricular fibrillation. The short duration and nonfractionated appearance of the electrogram in the control patient contrasts with the increased number of transitions, increase in electrogram width and early increase in latency in the patient with ventricular fibrillation.

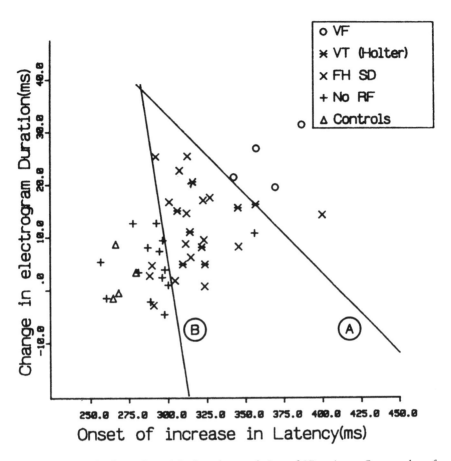

Figure 5. Results from the original study population of 37 patients. Scatter plot of change in electrogram duration against S1S2 at which latency starts to increase. The discriminant line A separates the patients with ventricular fibrillation (VF) from the remainder (p<0.0001) and the line B separates the VF, nonsustained ventricular tachycardia on Holter (NSVT) and family history of sudden cardiac death patients (FHSD) from low-risk patients (No RF) and controls (p<10^{-6}).

this group, a probable initiating mechanism which is amenable to specific therapy can be identified. Paroxysmal atrial fibrillation can be effectively prevented with amiodarone. Sustained monomorphic ventricular tachycardia, although very rare, can be treated with: drugs and/or an ICD; conduction disease with a pacemaker; rapid atrioventricular conduction via an accessory pathway by radiofrequency catheter ablation; ischemia with high-dose verapamil; and left ventricular outflow tract obstruction by dual-chamber pac-

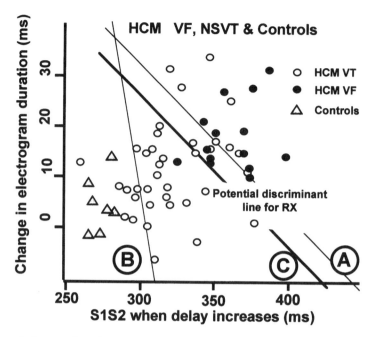

Figure 6. Scatter plot of patients with VF, NSVT and FHSD. Lines A and B are as above in figure 6. Line C is the discriminant line that separates the VF group from the rest of the population. Eight of 30 patients with NSVT and 3 of 31 patients with FHSD fall to the right of this line and are potential recipients of the implantable cardioverter defibrillator. VF = ventricular fibrillation; NSVT = Nonsustained ventricular tachycardia; FHSD = family history of sudden cardiac death.

ing[45–47] or myectomy.[48] In the remainder (approximately 70%), the patient is recognized to be at an increased risk, but there are either multiple potential triggers or no identifiable triggers which can be targeted. Such patients include those who have been resuscitated from out-of-hospital ventricular fibrillation, those with syncopal episodes, adults with nonsustained ventricular tachycardia on Holter, and those with multiple sudden deaths in young first degree relatives.

There are a number of therapeutic approaches to this group of patients at high risk, centered on pharmacotherapy, surgery, dual-chamber pacing, or implantation of the ICD.

Drugs

Although *beta-blocking agents and calcium antagonists* have been shown to provide symptomatic benefit, there is no evidence to suggest improved survival.[5,49] Indeed, the use of verapamil can be associated with serious complications.[50] It can suppress impulse formation in the sinus node and adversely affect conduction through the atrioventricular node. It has been associated with the development of complete heart block in patients with preexisting, but unsuspected conduction disease. The combination of conduction disturbance, negative inotropism, and vasodilator properties has caused pulmonary edema and death in some patients.[50]

In adults with nonsustained ventricular tachycardia, suppression can be achieved and the risk of sudden cardiac death diminished with low-dose *amiodarone*, maintaining plasma levels less than 1.5 mg/ml. In a nonrandomized but well-controlled study, there was 7% annual mortality in those treated with conventional agents versus zero mortality at 3 years in those who received amiodarone.[51] The mode of action of amiodarone at this low dose, particularly in the absence of sustained spontaneous arrhythmias, is speculative. Prevention of primary arrhythmias, raising the threshold of ventricular fibrillation, attenuating the ventricular response during atrial fibrillation and an effect on the control of peripheral blood flow may all be relevant.

Other studies have not shown such a beneficial effect with amiodarone. The NIH experience reports a significant incidence of sudden death in patients with hypertrophic cardiomyopathy taking amiodarone. Seven of fifty patients taking amiodarone at doses of 400 mg daily, died suddenly during follow-up, six of these deaths occurring the loading period.[52] Electrophysiological evaluation of patients on amiodarone showed a variety of effects, including production of important conduction abnormalities in about 20% of patients, and facilitation of ventricular tachycardia induction in about half of the studied population.[53]

There are major differences between the two apparently contradictory experiences. The NIH study used amiodarone in a higher dosage with concomitant medication in a group of patients with refractory symptoms, amiodarone being used primarily for symptomatic relief. McKenna et al,[51] used amiodarone in low dose (mean plasma concentration less than 1.5 mg/ml) for prevention of sudden cardiac death in high-risk adults identified by Holter ECG monitoring.

Newer class III agents are being developed and may prove useful in this field. Dofetilide has been evaluated in a small group of high-risk patients and appears to have a beneficial effect on inducibility, both acutely and after 3 days of oral therapy.[54] No long-term data are yet available.

The Implantable Cardioverter Defibrillator

The use of the automatic ICD remains controversial in patients with hypertrophic cardiomyopathy. Its use is rational in those rare patients with documented, sustained tachyarrhythmias whose arrhythmia fails to be suppressed after electrophysiologically guided drug testing, and those who have recurrent episodes of ventricular tachycardia/ventricular fibrillation, or episodes of collapse due to sustained tachycardia, despite medical therapy. Its use in other high-risk patients, even those with recurrent syncope, is not justified. In most cases, the initiating mechanism of syncope is not clear (myocardial ischemia, peripheral vasodilatation, or acute obstruction of the left ventricular outflow tract are all potential mechanisms in an individual), and the rationale for defibrillation is uncertain. The device might restore sinus rhythm (if this were not the rhythm anyway), without restoring cardiac output.

Even in patients with one episode of out-of-hospital ventricular fibrillation, the use of the automatic ICD is controversial. A series of 33 survivors of cardiac arrest was reported recently.[55] The 18 patients with a resting or provocable left ventricular outflow tract gradient, underwent surgery (septal myotomyectomy in 17, and mitral valve replacement in 1), and all but 2 received antiarrhythmic therapy with a class I agent postoperatively; the remaining 17 received medical therapy alone (a class I agent in 11, and amiodarone in 4). Five patients survived more than one cardiac arrest, four of whom were in the medical group, and there were 11 deaths (eight disease related) during follow-up for a mean of 7 years. Four patients, two in each group, died suddenly, and four, all in the surgical group, died of progressive heart failure. Actuarial survival for the whole group was 97% at 1 year, 74% at 5 years, and 61% at 10 years, which is not significantly different from the survival for a group of patients with hypertrophic cardiomyopathy who have not experienced cardiac arrest. Thus, in hypertrophic cardiomyopathy, aborted episodes of sudden death do not carry the same ominous prognosis with which they are associated in coronary artery disease. Such patients do however, represent a difficult management problem, and more information about them is needed. The availability of the ICD with improved logging of arrhythmic events and the rhythm immediately preceding arrhythmia detection, may provide the follow-up data in this group, which would help to decide which patients should have an implantable cardioverter defibrillator implanted. The more precise identification of those patients at the greatest risk of sudden death, coupled with the improved peri-implant mortality/morbidity of newer transvenous lead systems, may make the ICD implantation a logical and cost-effective form of therapy.[56,57]

Surgery

The experience of surgical treatment in this group of patients is limited in most centers, although over 1000 cases have been reported worldwide. The majority of patients have had symptoms refractory to medical therapy, and usually, an outflow tract gradient. The most common procedure is the removal of a segment of the upper anterior septum (myectomy), usually via a transaortic approach, although a transventricular approach has also been employed. There is no doubt that myectomy can significantly improve symptoms in these difficult patients, but abolition of the outflow tract gradient is not necessarily the explanation of its success.[48,58]

The operation has been associated with improved symptoms, improved objective measures of exercise capacity[59] and myocardial perfusion,[60] but an initial surgical series showed mortality up to 15%, together with complications such as complete heart block, aortic regurgitation, and ventricular septal defect. More recent series show improved survival with no mortality in a series of 43 children and young adults,[61] and 1 death from 83 patients less than 65-years old.[62] The use of intraoperative echocardiography to direct surgery may improve perioperative mortality and can also be reduced by the use of this technique.[63] Mitral valve replacement has also been advocated in some patients.[64] Good results have been obtained in the relatively small number of patients whose condition is complicated by severe mitral regurgitation.

Although there have been no reported controlled trials of the effect of myectomy on survival, the surgical experience of workers at Düsseldorf is of interest. After successful myotomy/myectomy, their results have shown a greatly reduced incidence of syncope and sudden death.[65]

Dual-chamber pacing with a short atrioventricular delay has recently been rediscovered with enthusiasm as an alternative to surgery after sporadic description over the last 25 years.[45,66–70] Claims have been made that chronic pacing produces regression of left ventricular hypertrophy and that the prognosis of paced patients appears to be significantly better than the background prognosis of a typical referral population.[46] Such claims have yet to be substantiated. DDD pacing seems capable of producing a reduction in left ventricular outflow tract gradient of only approximately 50%. This compares unfavorably with one surgical cohort in whom a gradient reduction of 87% has been observed,[71] and in which a residual gradient of more than 15 mm Hg was an independent predictor of mortality after myectomy. Whether the larger residual gradient seen after DDD pacing is important remains unanswered. In the meantime it would be unwise to assume that DDD pacing has any impact on sudden cardiac death.

Conclusions

Current noninvasive risk stratification techniques provide a reassuringly high negative predictive accuracy, but precise identification of high-risk patients remains elusive. Conventional invasive electrophysiology adds to noninvasive risk stratification but still lacks high, positive predictive accuracy. A novel electrophysiological approach which attempts to individually quantify the electrophysiological effects of myofibrillar disarray has produced promising results. It appears more discriminating and may offer for the first time a specific indication of risk of sudden death. Further multicenter prospective studies, now in the process of being set up, will help to establish the true role of electrogram fractionation as a technique to more precisely identify the individual at greatest risk of sudden cardiac death, and thus, potentially guide therapy.

The pathogenesis of sudden death in hypertrophic cardiomyopathy is complex. There is clearly a distinct myocardial structural abnormality which contains the substrate for lethal ventricular arrhythmias. A variety of triggers may initiate the episode leading to ventricular fibrillation. These may be physiological or pathological in the form of paroxysmal supraventricular or ventricular arrhythmias (Figure 2). Susceptible individuals with abnormal exercise hemodynamics and autonomic function may be highly intolerant of such arrhythmias and such patients might be suitable targets for appropriate antiarrhythmic therapy.

The precise identification of individuals at risk remains elusive. Nevertheless, continued advances in our understanding of mechanisms of sudden death in hypertrophic cardiomyopathy, and closer links between electrophysiological and structural abnormalities may yet allow specific individual targeting of optimal therapy.

References

1. Teare RD. Asymetrical hypertrophy of the heart in young adults. *Br Heart J* 1958; 20:1–8.
2. Maron BJ, Epstein SE. Hypertrophic cardiomyopathy: a discussion of nomenclature. *Am J Cardiol* 1979;43:1242–1244.
3. Goodwin JF. The frontiers of cardiomyopathy. *Br Heart J* 1982;48:1–18.
4. McKenna WJ, Goodwin JF. The natural history of hypertrophic cardiomyopathy. *Curr Probl Cardiol* 1981;6:1–26.
5. McKenna W, Deanfield J, Faruqui A, England D, Oakley C, Goodwin J. Prognosis in hypertrophic cardiomyopathy: role of age and clinical, electrocardiographic and hemodynamic features. *Am J Cardiol* 1981;47:532–538.
6. Maron BJ, Bonow RO, Cannon RO, Leon MB, Epstein SE. Hypertrophic cardiomyopathy. Interrelations of clinical manifestations, pathophysiology, and therapy (1). *N Engl J Med* 1987;316:780–789.
7. Maron BJ, Bonow RO, Cannon RO, Leon MB, Epstein SE. Hypertrophic cardiomyopathy. Interrelations of clinical manifestations, pathophysiology, and therapy (2). *N Engl J Med* 1987;316:844–852.
8. Maron BJ, Roberts WC, McAllister HA, Rosing DR, Epstein SE. Sudden death in young athletes. *Circulation* 1980;62:218–229.
9. Fiddler GI, Tajik AJ, Weidman W, McGoon DC, Ritter DG, Giuliani ER. Idiopathic hypertrophic subaortic stenosis in the young. *Am J Cardiol* 1978;42: 793–799.

10. Maron BJ, Lipson LC, Roberts WC, Savage DD, Epstein SE. "Malignant" hypertrophic cardiomyopathy: identification of a subgroup of families with unusually frequent premature death. *Am J Cardiol* 1978;41:1133–1140.
11. McKenna WJ, England D, Doi YL, Deanfield JE, Oakley C, Goodwin JF. Arrhythmia in hypertrophic cardiomyopathy. I: Influence on prognosis. *Br Heart J* 1981;46:168–172.
12. Jarcho JA, McKenna W, Pare JA, et al. Mapping a gene for familial hypertrophic cardiomyopathy to chromosome 14q1. *N Engl J Med* 1989;21:1372–1378.
13. Watkins H, MacRae C, Thierfelder L, et al. A disease locus for familial hypertrophic cardiomyopathy maps to chromosome 1q3. *Nature Genetics* 1993;3:333–337.
14. Watkins H, McKenna WJ, Thierfelder L, et al. Mutations in the genes for cardiac troponin T and alpha-tropomyosin in hypertrophic cardiomyopathy. *N Engl J Med* 1995;332:1058–1064.
15. Watkins H, Rosenzweig A, Hwang DS, et al. Characteristics and prognostic implications of myosin missense mutations in familial hypertrophic cardiomyopathy. *N Engl J Med* 1992;326:1108–1114.
16. Marian AJ, Mares A Jr, Kelly DP, et al. Sudden cardiac death in hypertrophic cardiomyopathy. Variability in phenotypic expression of beta-myosin heavy chain mutations. *Eur Heart J* 1995;16:368–376.
17. Fananapazir L, Epstein ND. Genotype-phenotype correlations in hypertrophic cardiomyopathy: insights provided by comparisons of kindreds with distinct and identical beta-myosin heavy chain mutations. *Circulation* 1994;89:22–32.
18. Solomon SD, Wolff S, Watkins H, et al. Left ventricular hypertrophy and morphology in familial hypertrophic cardiomyopathy associated with mutations of the beta-myosin heavy chain gene. *J Am Coll Cardiol* 1993;22:498–505.
19. Hecht GM, Klues KG, Roberts WC, Maron BJ. Co-existence of sudden cardiac death and end-stage heart failure in familial hypertrophic cardiomyopathy. *J Am Coll Cardiol* 1993;22:489–497.
20. Davies MJ. The current status of myocardial disarray in hypertrophic cardiomyopathy. *Br Heart J* 1984;51:361–363.
21. Perloff JK. Pathogenesis of hypertrophic cardiomyopathy: hypotheses and speculations. *Am Heart J* 1981;101:219–226.
22. McKenna WJ, Stewart JT, Nihoyannopoulos P, McGinty F, Davies MJ. Hypertrophic cardiomyopathy without hypertrophy: two families with myocardial disarray in the absence of increased myocardial mass. *Br Heart J* 1990;63:287–290.
23. McKenna WJ, Alfonso F. Arrhythmias in the cardiomyopathies and mitral valve prolapse. In: Zipes D, Rowlands D (eds.): *Progress in Cardiology.* Philadelphia: Lea and Febiger, 1988, pp 59–75.
24. Maron BJ, Roberts WC, Epstein SE. Sudden death in hypertrophic cardiomyopathy: a profile of 78 patients. *Circulation* 1982;65:1388–1394.
25. Frenneaux MP, Counihan PJ, Caforio AL, Chikamori T, McKenna WJ. Abnormal blood pressure response during exercise in hypertrophic cardiomyopathy. *Circulation* 1990;82:1995–2002.
26. Counihan PJ, Frenneaux MP, Webb DJ, McKenna WJ. Abnormal vascular responses to supine exercise in hypertrophic cardiomyopathy. *Circulation* 1991;84:686–696.
27. Sadoul N, Prasad K, Slade AKB, et al. Abnormal blood presure response during exercise is a marker of risk of sudden death in young patients with hypertrophic cardiomyopathy. *Eur Heart J* 1995;16 (Suppl):504(Abstract).
28. Maron BJ, Savage DD, Wolfson JK, Epstein SE. Prognostic significance of 24

hour ambulatory electrocardiographic monitoring in patients with hypertrophic cardiomyopathy: a prospective study. *Am J Cardiol* 1981;48:252–257.
29. Kulakowski P, Counihan PJ, Camm AJ, McKenna WJ. The value of time and frequency domain, and spectral temporal mapping analysis of the signal-averaged electrocardiogram in identification of patients with hypertrophic cardiomyopathy at increased risk of sudden death. *Eur Heart J* 1993;14:941–950.
30. Counihan PJ, Fei L, Bashir Y, Farrell TG, Haywood GA, McKenna WJ. Assessment of heart rate variability in hypertrophic cardiomyopathy. Association with clinical and prognostic features. *Circulation* 1993;88:1682–1690.
31. Nicod P, Polikar R, Peterson KL. Hypertrophic cardiomyopathy and sudden death. *N Engl J Med* 1988;318:1255–1257.
32. Stafford WJ, Trohman RG, Bilsker M, Zaman L, Castellanos A, Myerburg RJ. Cardiac arrest in an adolescent with atrial fibrillation and hypertrophic cardiomyopathy. *J Am Coll Cardiol* 1986;7:701–704.
33. McKenna W, Harris L, Deanfield J. Syncope in hypertrophic cardiomyopathy. *Br Heart J* 1982;47:177–179.
34. McKenna WJ, Franklin RC, Nihoyannopoulos P, Robinson KC, Deanfield JE. Arrhythmia and prognosis in infants, children and adolescents with hypertrophic cardiomyopathy. *J Am Coll Cardiol* 1988;11:147–153.
35. Savage DD, Seides SF, Maron BJ, Myers DJ, Epstein SE. Prevalence of arrhythmias during 24-hour electrocardiographic monitoring and exercise testing in patients with obstructive and nonobstructive hypertrophic cardiomyopathy. *Circulation* 1979;59:866–875.
36. Robinson K, Frenneaux MP, Stockins B, Karatasakis G, Poloniecki JD, McKenna WJ. Atrial fibrillation in hypertrophic cardiomyopathy: a longitudinal study. *J Am Coll Cardiol* 1990;15:1279–1285.
37. Fananapazir L, Tracy CM, Leon MB, et al. Electrophysiologic abnormalities in patients with hypertrophic cardiomyopathy. A consecutive analysis in 155 patients. *Circulation* 1989;80:1259–1268.
38. Fananapazir L, Chang AC, Epstein SE, McAreavey D. Prognostic determinants in hypertrophic cardiomyopathy. Prospective evaluation of a therapeutic strategy based on clinical, Holter, hemodynamic, and electrophysiological findings. *Circulation* 1992;86:730–740.
39. Saumarez RC, Slade AKB, Grace AA, Sadoul N, Camm AJ, McKenna WJ. The significance of paced electrograms in hypertrophic cardiomyopathy: a prospective study. *Circulation* 1995;91:2762–2768.
40. Wellens HJ, Brugada P, Stevenson WG. Programmed electrical stimulation of the heart in patients with life-threatening ventricular arrhythmias: what is the significance of induced arrhythmias and what is the correct stimulation protocol? *Circulation* 1985;72:1–7.
41. Kuck KH, Kunze KP, Schluter M, Nienaber CA, Costard A. Programmed electrical stimulation in hypertrophic cardiomyopathy. Results in patients with and without cardiac arrest or syncope. *Eur Heart J* 1988;9:177–185.
42. Borgreffe M, Podczeck A, Breithardt G. Electrophysiological studies in hypertrophic cardiomyopathy. *Circulation* 1986;74 (Suppl II):1922(Abstract).
43. Noble D. *The Initiation of the Heartbeat*. Oxford: Oxford University Press, 1979.
44. Saumarez RC, Camm AJ, Panagos A, et al. Ventricular fibrillation in hypertrophic cardiomyopathy is associated with increased fractionation of paced right ventricular electrograms. *Circulation* 1992;86:467–474.

45. Jeanrenaud X, Goy JJ, Kappenberger L. Effects of dual-chamber pacing in hypertrophic obstructive cardiomyopathy. *Lancet* 1992;339:1318–1323.
46. Fananapazir L, Epstein ND, Curiel RV, Panza JA, Tripodi D, McAreavey D. Long term results of dual chamber pacing in obstructive hypertrophic cardiomyopathy. Evidence for progressive symptomatic and hemodynamic improvement and reduction of left ventricular hypertrophy. *Circulation* 1994;90:2731–2742.
47. Slade AKB, Sadoul N, Shapiro L, et al. DDD pacing in hypertrophic cardiomyopathy: a multicentre clinical experience. *Heart* 1996;75:44–49.
48. McIntosh CL, Maron BJ. Current operative treatment of obstructive hypertrophic cardiomyopathy. *Circulation* 1988;78:487–495.
49. Bonow RO, Rosing DR, Bacharach SL, et al. Effects of verapamil on left ventricular systolic function and diastolic filling in patients with hypertrophic cardiomyopathy. *Circulation* 1981;64:787–796.
50. Epstein SE, Rosing DR. Verapamil: its potential for causing serious complications in patients with hypertrophic cardiomyopathy. *Circulation* 1981;64:437–441.
51. McKenna WJ, Oakley CM, Krikler DM, Goodwin JF. Improved survival with amiodarone in patients with hypertrophic cardiomyopathy and ventricular tachycardia. *Br Heart J* 1985;53:412–416.
52. Fananapazir L, Leon MB, Bonow RO, Tracy CM, Cannon RO, Epstein SE. Sudden death during empiric amiodarone therapy in symptomatic hypertrophic cardiomyopathy. *Am J Cardiol* 1991;67:169–174.
53. Fananapazir L, Epstein SE. Value of electrophysiologic studies in hypertrophic cardiomyopathy treated with amiodarone. *Am J Cardiol* 1991;67:175–182.
54. Fananapazir L, Cropp A. Dofetilide (UK 68,798) prevents ventricular tachycardia in patients with hypertrophic cardiomyopathy. *J Am Coll Cardiol* 1992;19:224A (Abstract).
55. Cecchi F, Maron BJ, Epstein SE. Long-term outcome of patients with hypertrophic cardiomyopathy successfully resuscitated after cardiac arrest. *J Am Coll Cardiol* 1989;13:1283–1288.
56. Anderson MH, Camm AJ. Implications for present and future applications of the implantable cardioverter-defibrillator resulting from the use of a simple model of cost efficacy. *Br Heart J* 1993;69:83–92.
57. Zipes DP, Roberts D. Results of the international study of the implantable pacemaker cardioverter-defibrillator. A comparison of epicardial and endocardial lead systems. The Pacemaker-Cardioverter-Defibrillator Investigators. *Circulation* 1995;92:59–65.
58. Maron BJ, Merrill WH, Freier PA, Kent KM, Epstein SE, Morrow AG. Long-term clinical course and symptomatic status of patients after operation for hypertrophic subaortic stenosis. *Circulation* 1978;57:1205–1213.
59. Redwood DR, Goldstein RE, Hirshfeld J, et al. Exercise performance after septal myotomy and myectomy in patients with obstructive hypertrophic cardiomyopathy. *Am J Cardiol* 1979;44:215–220.
60. Cannon RO, Dilsizian V, O'Gara PT, et al. Impact of surgical relief of outflow obstruction on thallium perfusion abnormalities in hypertrophic cardiomyopathy. *Circulation* 1992;85:1039–1045.
61. Mohr R, Schaff HV, Puga FJ, Danielson GK. Results of operation for hypertrophic obstructive cardiomyopathy in children and adults less than 40 years of age. *Circulation* 1989;80:I191–I196.
62. Mohr R, Schaff HV, Danielson GK, Puga FJ, Pluth JR, Tajik AJ. The outcome

of surgical treatment of hypertrophic obstructive cardiomyopathy. Experience over 15 years. *J Thorac Cardiovasc Surg* 1989;97:666–674.

63. Marwick TH, Stewart WJ, Lever HM, Lytle BW, Rosenkranz ER, Duffy CI. Benefits of intraoperative echocardiography in the surgical management of hypertrophic cardiomyopathy. *J Am Coll Cardiol* 1992;20:1066–1072.

64. Krajcer Z, Leachman RD, Cooley DA, Ostojic M, Coronado R. Mitral valve replacement and septal myomectomy in hypertrophic cardiomyopathy. Ten-year follow-up in 80 patients. *Circulation* 1988;78:I35-I43.

65. Schulte HD, Bircks WH, Loesse B, Godehardt EA, Schwartzkopff B. Prognosis of patients with hypertrophic obstructive cardiomyopathy after transaortic myectomy. Late results up to twenty-five years. *J Thorac Cardiovasc Surg* 1993;106: 709–717.

66. Gilgenkrantz J, Cherrier F, Petitier H, Dodinot B, Houplon M, Legoux J. Cardiomyopathie obstructive du ventricle gauche avec bloc auriculo-ventriculaire complet. Considerations therapeutiques. *Arch Mal Coeur* 1968;61:439–453.

67. Hassenstein P, Storch HH, Schmitz W. Results of electrical pacing in patients with hypertrophic obstruction cardiomyopathy. *Thoraxchir Vask Chir* 1975;23: 496–498.

68. Duck HJ, Hutschenreiter W, Pankau H, Trenckmann H. Atrial synchronous ventricular stimulation with reduced AV delay time as a therapeutic principle in hypertrophic obstructive cardiomyopathy. *Z Gesamte Inn Med* 1984;39:437–447.

69. McDonald K, McWilliams E, O'Keeffe B, Maurer B. Functional assessment of patients treated with permanent dual chamber pacing as a primary treatment for hypertrophic cardiomyopathy. *Eur Heart J* 1988;9:893–898.

70. Fananapazir L, Cannon RO, Tripodi D, Panza JA. Impact of dual-chamber permanent pacing in patients with obstructive hypertrophic cardiomyopathy with symptoms refractory to verapamil and beta-adrenergic blocker therapy. *Circulation* 1992;85:2149–2161.

71. Mohr R, Schaff HV, Danielson GK, Puga FJ, Pluth JR, Tajik AJ. The outcome of surgical treatment of hypertrophic obstructive cardiomyopathy. Experience over 15 years. *J Thorac Cardiovasc Surg* 1989;97:666–674.

Chapter 7

Mechanisms and Management of Congenital and Acquired Long QT Syndromes

Ralph Lazzara, MD

Congenital Long QT Syndromes

The congenital long QT syndromes (LQTSs) are most commonly inherited in an autosomal dominant mode (the Romano-Ward syndrome)[1,2] and very rarely in an autosomal recessive pattern (the Jervell and Lange-Nielsen syndrome).[3] Recent discoveries have revealed that the Romano-Ward syndrome can result from multiple genetic defects that express abnormal sarcolemmal ion channel proteins.[4–11] These dysfunctional ion channels transmit abnormal currents that prolong repolarization, and by mechanisms not fully clarified, generate arrhythmias.

The acquired LQTSs are caused by various drugs and conditions that have in common the alteration of transsarcolemmal currents in such a manner that repolarization is prolonged.[12] Investigation of the ever-increasing list of drugs that may cause this syndrome has virtually always disclosed actions to block K^+ channels that conduct K^+ currents mediating repolarization.[13] Most commonly, the composite current designated I_k is affected in one or more of its components, and a frequent victim is the current I_{kr}, the same current implicated in one form of the LQTS.[8,9]

Observations of an association between prolonged repolarization and oscillations during repolarization have been made by various investigators for many years.[14–16] Oscillations during repolarization have been defined as early afterdepolarizations (EADs), a definition which includes transient delays in repolarization without frank depolarization (Figure 1). A role for EADs in the LQTS was proposed when it was observed that electrocardiographic changes resembling the clinical syndrome and torsades de pointes could be induced in intact dogs following reduction of repolarizing K^+ currents by intravenous

From *Practical Management of Cardiac Arrhythmias* edited by Nabil El-Sherif, and Jean Lekieffre. Futura Publishing Co., Armonk, NY, © 1997.

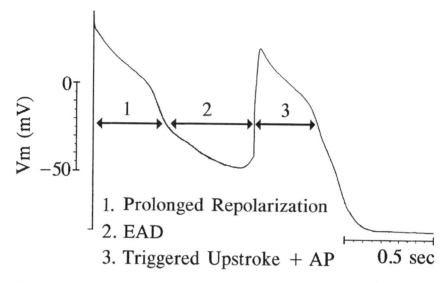

Figure 1. Illustration of the three phases in which abnormal current mechanisms operate to lead to triggered arrhythmias due to early afterdepolarization(EAD). The first phase: involves the various mechanisms that can effect currents during repolarization and induce prolonged repolarization. The second phase: reflects the disturbances that cause the deviation from the course of repolarization that is the EAD proper. The third phase: includes currents that generate the triggered upstroke and action potential (AP) that induce the arrhythmia.

CsCl.[17] These changes were accompanied by EADs' generation. A number of experimental models for investigating prolonged repolarization have been developed including the inhibition of various repolarizing outward K^+ currents, or the enhancement of inward currents during repolarization including Na^+ current (I_{Na}) or the L-type Ca^{2+} current (I_{CaL}).[18] EADs have been observed in the various models when repolarization is sufficiently prolonged though the levels of repolarization at which they occur and their characteristics have differed.[18] In addition, there have been numerous demonstrations of EADs in patients with LQTS with the technique of monophasic action potential recording.[19–22] The earliest such demonstrations were made with suction electrodes in the late 1970s.[19] Though it is generally agreed that EADs are the trigger mechanisms for arrhythmogenesis in the LQTS and contribute to the electrocardiographic abnormalities reflected in the abnormal T-U waves, other electrophysiological mechanisms, notably reentry, may contribute importantly to arrhythmogenesis. The marked dispersion of refractoriness observed in LQTS provides a plausible basis for the involvement of reentrant mechanisms in arrhythmogenesis.[23] A role has been postulated for the recently discovered M cells, those cells in the mid-myocardium that display longer action potentials, in arrhythmogenesis by virtue of EADs' generation and participation in macroreentrant circuits.[24]

For the purpose of elucidating the ionic currents that generate EADs, various models have been developed ex vivo in isolated tissues or myocytes including inhibition of K^+ currents by Cs^+ [25-27], enhancement of Ca^{2+} current by BAY K-8644,[28,29] enhancement of Na^+ current by sea anemone toxins anthopleuran and ATX II,[30,31] and intense β-adrenergic stimulation.[32-34] The diversity of EADs observed in various settings makes it clear that multiple ionic mechanisms for EAD development must exist, depending on the conditions and the level of membrane potential at which the EADs are generated.

Consideration of the ionic mechanisms for EAD generation necessitates a distinction between the abnormalities of currents that prolong repolarization; those currents that produce the initial deviation of repolarization from its expected time course (i.e., the EAD proper[26]) and those currents that produce the more intense depolarization that may follow, termed the triggered upstroke (Figure 1). In some cases, especially at depolarized levels of membrane potential, the membrane potential may oscillate without an obvious differentiation of an EAD and a triggered upstroke. The EADs could result from the introduction or intensification of an inward current or a reduction of one of the outward currents mediating repolarization. So far, two hypotheses have received the most attention, both involving surges of inward currents during repolarization. One hypothesis proposed by January and coworkers,[28,29] is that a fraction of L-type Ca^{2+} channels reopen when repolarization is prolonged within a voltage range in which voltage-dependent activation and inactivation curves overlap (i.e., a range in which both activation and inactivation gates are open in some of the channels). For the L-type Ca^{2+} channel, this "window" range would be near the level of the plateau of the action potential. It has been demonstrated that prolonged residence of the membrane potential in the window range can lead to an increase in L-type Ca^{2+} current. In addition, Zeng and Rudy[35] have pointed out that the dual mechanisms for inactivation of L-type Ca^{2+} channels with differing time courses also provide a possible means for reopening of channels during repolarization. Ca^{2+}-dependent inactivation is rapid in onset, tracing the course of cytosolic Ca^{2+} which rises rapidly from release of Ca^{2+} by the sarcoplasmic reticulum, and declines more slowly with reuptake by the sarcoplasmic reticulum and extrusion by Na:Ca exchange. Voltage-dependent inactivation may have a relatively slow onset. If Ca^{2+}-dependent inactivation is rapidly removed during repolarization, as with adrenergic enhancement of sarcoplasmic reticulum uptake, and voltage-dependent inactivation is not fully developed, a substantial proportion of L-type Ca^{2+} channels might reopen.

Another hypothesis, introduced by Szabo and coworkers, is that inward

Na:Ca exchange current could be enhanced by secondary spontaneous release of Ca^{2+} from the sarcoplasmic reticulum during repolarization, as has been demonstrated in diastole in relation to delayed afterdepolarizations that occur in states of Ca^{2+} loading.[26,27] This hypothesis is predicated on the occurrence of Ca^{2+} loading with prolonged repolarization because of continued inflow of I_{CaL} during the prolonged plateau and the reduced efficiency of Ca^{2+} extrusion by Na:Ca exchange at depolarized levels of membrane potential. Spontaneous release of Ca^{2+} by the scarcoplasmic reticulum in states of Ca^{2+} loading is a well-demonstrated but not fully understood phenomenon. The spontaneous release of Ca^{2+} is postulated to activate an inward current via Na:Ca exchange and perhaps other Ca^{2+} activated inward currents such as that conducted by nonselective cationic channels. This mechanism could operate at later stages of repolarization and more repolarized levels of membrane potential at which I_{CaL} is not activated. It is possible that either or both mechanisms may be operative in certain of the LQTS.

These complex arrhythmogenic mechanisms involving I_{CaL} or spontaneous release of Ca^{2+}, set into motion by prolonged repolarization, may be termed arrhythmogenic cascades. In theory, the arrhythmic end result could be aborted or suppressed by interventions aimed at various stages in the process. For example, the arrhythmogenic cascade involving Ca^{2+} loading and the spontaneous release of Ca^{2+} could be suppressed by reducing Ca^{2+} loading by various means including inhibition of I_{CaL}, or by affecting the storage, transport or release properties of the sarcoplasmic reticulum (if spontaneous release were well enough understood), or by inhibiting the currents activated by cytosolic Ca^{2+} such as Na:Ca exchange current.

In the condition of prolongation of repolarization due to enhancement of long-lasting Na^+ current, either or both of the previously described mechanisms could be active. The prolonged plateaus observed could lead to the reopening of Ca^{2+} channels; Ca^{2+} loading is likely to occur because of the long repolarization and the effect of Na^+ loading to reduce Ca^{2+} extrusion via Na:Ca exchange. On the other hand, other mechanisms for a depolarizing current surge may be called into play when Na^+ channels function abnormally in this manner.[31]

Since the first description of the electrocardiographic abnormalities of the LQTS by Jervell and Lange-Nielsen,[36] the powerful effect of adrenergic stimulation to provoke sudden death was appreciated. This striking provocative effect became the basis for hypotheses of pathophysiology[37] and for effective treatment by agents that block β-adrenergic receptors. Data from the international registry indicate that prevention of arrhythmic death can be achieved for prolonged periods in about 80% of patients, though success rates of such therapy over a long life-span remain to be determined.[38] In the minority that fail pharmacological therapy, removal of cardiac stimulation from the left side (left cardiac sympathectomy), an approach based on experimental observation indicating a dominance of the left sympathetic innervation in the syndrome, also is protective over 5 years in more than 90% of cases.[38]

The important role of adrenergic stimulation in the congenital LQTS does not appear to have a parallel in the acquired LQTS in which β-adrenergic stimulation has been used to ameliorate the syndrome presumably by speeding the heart rate. In the acquired LQTS, the more important and immediate provocative factor appears to be the lengthening of the diastolic interval intermittently by pauses or continuously in bradycardia.[12] One approach to therapy in the acquired LQTS has been the elimination of long diastolic intervals by β-adrenergic stimulation, atropine or temporary pacing. There are indications that this factor may also operate in the congenital LQTS, despite the attention that has been devoted to adrenergic stimulation. Some patients appear to benefit from pacing in addition to reduction of adrenergic influence.[39]

The action of long diastolic intervals to accentuate prolonged repolarization is well-established and extensively clarified, but the influence of adrenergic stimulation on EADs is not clear. A number of investigators have demonstrated that EADs can be induced with intense adrenergic stimulation in myocytes, but it is debated whether the ionic mechanism is due to a reactivation of I_{CaL} during repolarization, or Ca^{2+} loading and spontaneous release of Ca^{2+} from the sarcoplasmic reticulum or both.[32-35] The relative contributions of α- and β-stimulation to EAD generation have scarcely been explored. EAD generated by block of K^+ currents can be accentuated by combined β- and α-adrenergic stimulation[40] or by alpha adrenergic stimulation alone.[41] Similarly, EAD in patients with the congenital LQTS have been shown to be accentuated by combined beta and alpha adrenergic stimulation.[12,21] A therapeutic role for alpha, as well as beta blockade has been suggested.[42] Finally, the gathering evidence for the importance of Ca^{2+} transport suggests that block of I_{CaL} or reduction of cellular Ca^{2+} by other means could have therapeutic benefit in either the congenital or acquired LQTS. There are isolated reports of benefit of Ca^{2+} blockers in both the congenital and acquired long QT syndromes,[20,21] as illustrated in Figure 2, and the evidence that magnesium, a physiological Ca^{2+} blocker, is beneficial in the acquired LQTS is substantial.[43]

Very recently, there have been breath-taking discoveries concerning specific genetic abnormalities that may produce the LQTS and each has been shown to express an abnormal sarcolemmal ion channel. Mutations in the gene that express the Na^+ channel, SCN5A, have been shown to express a channel that fails to inactivate normally, leading to a greater than normal steady flow of Na^+ current during repolarization.[7,10] Mutations in a gene, HERG, that encodes a K^+ channel shown to transmit I_{kr}, expresses an abnormal channel that transmits reduced I_{kr}.[8,9] Most recently, the gene on chromo-

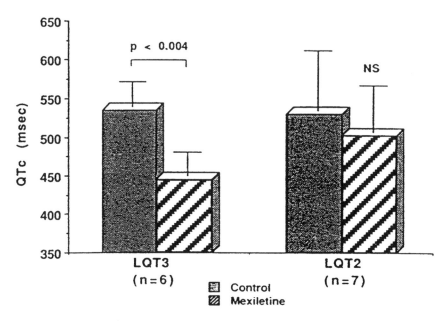

Figure 2. Effects of verapamil on early afterdepolarization (EAD) amplitude and nonsustained ventricular tachycardia in a 64-year-old man with nonfamilial LQTS. **Panels A and B** were recorded shortly before verapamil administration and **Panel C** was recorded approximately 5 minutes after the onset of the 2-minute verapamil infusion. **Panels A and B**: Ventricular pacing at cycle length 400 msec and pauses of 1200 msec and 1240 msec resulted in large post-pause EADs, which were associated with a 6-beat and a 5-beat episode of ventricular tachycardia. **Panel C**: Following verapamil, 5 mg IV, ventricular pacing at cycle length 400 msec and a longer pause of 1290 msec failed to elicit a post-pause (triggered) ventricular extrasystole. The post-pause EAD persists (arrow), although diminished in amplitude. (Reprinted by permission from *J Cardiovasc Electrophysiol* 1990;1(2):170–195).

some 11, the first chromosome linked to the LQTS, has been identified and has the amino acid sequence associated with the expression of a K^+ channel but the specific K^+ current involved has not been identified.[11] These gene defects account for most of the families with this syndrome that have been subjected to linkage analysis. There appears to be a gene on chromosome 4 which has not yet been identified.[6]

These discoveries already have led to attempts to distinguish phenotypes and to specific therapeutic strategies. It has been reported that patients with the Na^+ channel defect respond to the Na^+ channel blocker mexiletine, with striking shortening, almost normalization, of the long QT interval, whereas patients with the mutations in HERG resulting in reduced I_{Kr} do not show a significant response (Figure 3).[44] Also, for reasons not fully clear, defects

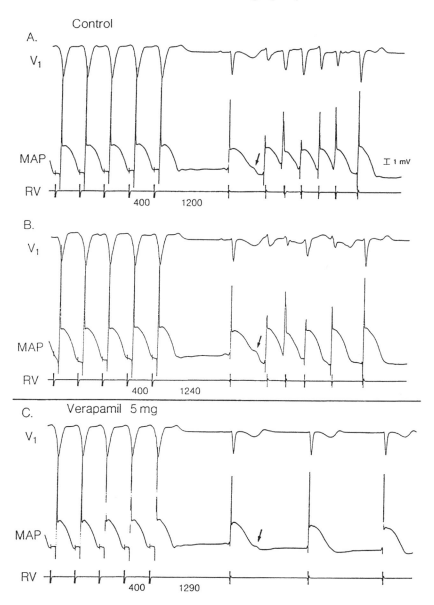

Figure 3. The effects of mexiletine on the corrected QT intervals (QT_c) of patients with the long QT syndrome(LQTS) caused by defects in the Na^+ channel gene SCN5A (LQT3) and of patients with the LQTS caused by defects in HERG encoding the K^+ channel for I_{Kr} (LQT2). The QT_c in patients with LQT3 was significantly reduced almost to normal, whereas that in patients with LQT2 was not significantly altered. (Reproduced by permission from *Circulation* 1995:3381–3386).

Table 1
Therapeutic Targets

Congenital LQTS
—The Defective Gene
—The Abnormal Expressed Protein
—The Functional Abnormality of the Expressed Protein
—The Arrhythmogenic Cascade
Acquired LQTS
—The Factor Affecting Repolarization Currents
—The Arrhythmogenic Cascade

in SCN5A, the Na^+ channel gene, may be associated with a relatively normal response of the QT interval to increasing rate and relatively less adrenergic sensitivity but the small number of patients so far studied make these conclusions tenuous. Another study preliminarily reported has indicated that patients with defects in HERG resulting in reduced I_{Kr} demonstrate marked shortening of the QT interval with modest elevations of extracellular K^+.[45] It has been shown that I_{Kr} is augmented by increases in extracellular K^+.[9]

Two of the three experimental approaches to models for EAD generation, those involving reduction of K^+ currents and those involving enhancement of Na^+ currents now have counterparts in the naturally occurring congenital LQTS. A third model, the enhancement of Ca^{2+} current, does not have a counterpart; no abnormalities of genes encoding Ca^{2+} channels have yet to be uncovered. Nevertheless, it has been noted that Ca^{2+} transport may be involved in arrhythmogenesis when repolarization is prolonged either by reduction of K^+ currents or enhancement of Na^+ current. Established and potential therapeutic approaches to the LQTS are listed in Tables 1 and 2.

The acquired LQTS induced by antiarrhythmic agents present a special

Table 2
Therapy of Long QT Syndrome

Congenital (Adrenergic Dependent)	*Acquired (Pause Dependent)*
Beta Receptor Blockers	Remove Inciting Factor
Calcium Channel Blockers	Mg^{2+} Infusion
Na Channel Blockers?	Calcium Channel Blockers
Alpha Receptor Blockers?	Heart Rate Increase
K^+ Supplement?	—Isoproterenol
Left Cardiac Sympathectomy	—Atropine
Permanent Pacing	—Temporary Pacing
Implantable Defibrillator	

dilemma. Recent clinical trials have indicated a superiority of the class III action (i.e., prolongation of repolarization and refractoriness over Na^+ channel blockade as represented by approved and commonly used agents in the primary and secondary prevention of ventricular tachycardia and ventricular fibrillation).[46] The risk of torsades de pointes deters the use of agents that prolong repolarization in low-risk populations such as those with supraventricular arrhythmias and those that may be targeted for primary prevention of ventricular tachycardia and ventricular fibrillation. To fully realize the powerful antiarrhythmic action of prolongation of repolarization and refractoriness, the generation of EADs must be averted. A more complete understanding of the ionic mechanisms for EAD generation could point the way to achieving greatly prolonged repolarization without EADs generation. So far, the evidence suggests that investigation of the alterations of Ca^{2+} transport when repolarization is prolonged, might be a promising direction and could lead to drugs that incorporate actions that mitigate the arrhythmogenic alterations in Ca^{2+} transport, or that prolong repolarization in such a manner that the arrhythmogenic alterations in Ca^{2+} transport might not be induced.

References

1. Romano C, Gemme G, Pongiglione R. Aritmie cardiache rare in eta pediatrica. *Clin Pediatr* 1963;45:656–683.
2. Ward OC. A new familial cardiac syndrome in children. *J Irish Med Assoc* 1964; 54:103–106.
3. Fraser GR, Froggatt P, Murphy T. Genetical aspects of the cardio-auditory syndrome of Jervell and Lange-Nielsen (congenital deafness and electrocardiographic abnormalities). Ann Hum Genet 1964;28:133–156.
4. Keating M, Atkinson D, Dunn C, Timothy K, Vincent GM, Lepert M. Linkage of a cardiac arrhythmia, the long QT syndrome, and the Harvey ras-1 gene. *Science* 1991;252:704–706.
5. Jiang C, Atkinson D, Towbin JA, et al. Two long QT syndrome loci map to chromosomes 3 and 7 with evidence for further heterogeneity. *Nature Genet* 1994; 8:141–147.
6. Schott JJ, Carpentier F, Peltier S, et al. Mapping of a gene for long QT syndrome to chromosome 4q25–27. *Am J of Human Genet* 1995;57(5):1114–1122.
7. Wang Q, Shen J, Splawski I, et al. SCN5A mutations associated with an inherited cardiac arrhythmia, long QT syndrome. *Cell* 1995;80:805–811.
8. Curran ME, Splawski I, Timothy KW, Vincent GM, Green ED, Keating MT. A molecular basis for cardiac arrhythmia: HERG mutations cause long QT syndrome. *Cell* 1995;80:795–803.
9. Sanguinetti MC, Jiang C, Curran ME, Keating MT. A mechanistic link between an inherited and an acquired cardiac arrhythmia: HERG encodes the I_{kr} potassium channel. *Cell* 1995;81:299–307.
10. Bennett PB, Yazawa K, Makita N, George AL Jr. Molecular mechanism for an inherited cardiac arrhythmia. *Nature* 1995;376:683–685.
11. Wang Q, Curran ME, Splawski I, et al. Positional cloning of a novel potassium

channel gene: KVLQT1 mutations cause cardiac arrhythmias. *Nature Genet* 1996; 12(1):17–23.

12. Hohnloser SH, Singh BH. Proarrhythmia with class III antiarrhythmic drugs: definition, electrophysiologic mechanisms, incidence, predisposing factors, and clinical implications. *J Cardiovasc Electrophysiol* 1995;6(pt II):920–936.

13. Jackman WM, Friday KJ, Anderson JL, Aliot EM, Clark M, Lazzara R. The long QT syndromes: a critical review, new clinical observations and a unifying hypothesis. *Prog Cardiovasc Dis* 1988;31:115–172.

14. Goldenberg M, Rothberger CJ. Uber die Wirkung von Veratrin auf den Purkinjefaden. *Pflügers Arch* 1936;328:137–152.

15. Schmidt RE. Versuche mit aconitin zum problem der spontanen erregungabildung im herzen. *Pflügers Arch* 1960;217:526–536.

16. Matsuda K, Hoshi T, Kameyama S. Effects of aconitine on the cardiac membrane potential of the dog. *Jpn J Physiol* 1959;9:419–429.

17. Brachmann J, Scherlag BJ, Rosenshtraukh LV, Lazzara R. Bradycardia-dependent triggered activity: relevance to drug-induced multiform ventricular tachycardia. *Circulation* 1983;68:846–856.

18. El-Sherif N, Craelius W, Boutjdir M, Gough WB. Early afterdepolarizations and arrhythmogenesis. *J Cardiovasc Electrophysiol* 1990;1(2):145–160.

19. Bonatti V, Rolli A, Botti G. Recording of monophasic potentials of the right ventricle in long QT syndrome complicated by severe ventricular arrhythmias. *Eur Heart J* 1983;4:168–179.

20. Jackman WM, Szabo B, Friday KJ, et al. Ventricular tachyarrhythmias related to early afterdepolarizations and triggered firing: relationship to QT interval prolongation and potential therapeutic role for calcium channel blocking agents. *J Cardiovasc Electrophysiol* 1990;1(2):170–195.

21. Shimizu W, Ohe T, Kurita T, Tokuda T, Shimomura K. Epinephrine-induced ventricular premature complexes due to early afterdepolarizations and effects of verapamil and propranolol in a patient with congenital long QT syndrome. *J Cardiovasc Electrophysiol* 1994;5:438–444.

22. El-Sherif N, Bekheit SS, Henkin R. Quinidine-induced long QTU interval and torsade de pointes: role of bradycardia-dependent early afterdepolarizations. *J Am Coll Cardiol* 1989;14:242–257.

23. Priori SG, Napolitano C, Diehl, Schwartz PJ. Dispersion of the QT interval. A marker of therapeutic efficacy in the idiopathic long QT syndrome. *Circulation* 1994;89:1681–1689.

24. Antzelevitch C, Sicouri S. Clinical relevance of cardiac arrhythmias generated by afterdepolarizations role of M cells in the generation of U waves, triggered activation and torsade de pointes. *JACC* 1994;23(1):259–277.

25. Marban E, Robinson SW, Wier WG. Mechanisms of arrhythmogenic delayed and early afterdepolarizations in ferret ventricular muscle. *J Clin Invest* 1986;78: 1185–1192.

26. Szabo B, Sweidan R, Rajagopalan CV, et al. Role of $Na^+:Ca^+$ exchange current in Cs^+ induced early afterdepolarizations in Purkinje fibers. *J Cardiovasc Electrophysiol* 1994;5:933–944.

27. Szabo B, Kovacs T, Lazzara R. Role of calcium loading in early afterdepolarizations generated by Cs^+ in canine and guinea pig Purkinje fibers. *J Cardiovasc Electrophysiol* 1995;6(10):796–812.

28. January CT, Riddle JM, Salata JJ. A model for early afterdepolarizations: induction with the Ca^{2+} channel agonist Bay K 8644. *Circ Res* 1988;62:563–571.

29. January CT, Riddle JM. Early afterdepolarizations: mechanisms of induction and block: a role for L-type Ca^{2+} current. *Circ Res* 1989;64:977–989.
30. El-Sherif N, Zeller RH, Craelius W, Gough WB, Henkin R. QTU prolongation and polymorphic ventricular tachyarrhythmias due to bradycardia-dependent early afterdepolarizations. Afterdepolarizations and ventricular arrhythmias. *Circ Res* 1988;63:286–305.
31. Boutjdir M, Restivo M, Wei Y, Stergiopoulos K, El-Sherif N. Early afterdepolarization formation in cardiac myocytes: analysis of phase plane patterns, action potential, and membrane currents. *J Cardiovasc Electrophysiol* 1994;5:609–620.
32. Priori SG, Corr PB. Mechanisms underlying early and delayed afterdepolarizations induced by catecholamines. *Am J Physiol* 1990;258:H1796–H1805.
33. Yamada K, Corr PB. Effects of β-adrenergic receptor activation on intracellular calcium and membrane potential in adult cardiac myocytes. *J Cardiovasc Electrophysiol* 1991;3:209–224.
34. De Ferrari GM, Viola M, D'Mato E, Antolini R, Fort I. Distinct patterns of calcium transients during early and delayed afterdepolarizations induced by isoproterenol in ventricular myocytes. *Circulation* 1995;91(10):2510–2515.
35. Zeng J, Rudy Y. Early afterdepolarizations in cardiac myocytes: mechanism and rate dependence. *Biophys J* 1995;68:949–964.
36. Jervell A, Lange-Nielsen F. Congenital deaf-mutism; functional heart disease with prolongation of the QT interval and sudden death. *Am Heart J* 1957;54:59–68.
37. Schwartz PJ, Malliani A. Electrical alternation of the T-wave: clinical and experimental evidence of its relationship with the sympathetic nervous system and with the long QT syndrome. *Am Heart J* 1975;89:45–50.
38. Schwartz PJ, Locati EH, Moss AJ, Crampton RS, Trazzi R, Ruberti U. Left cardiac sympathetic denervation in the therapy of congenital long QT syndrome: a worldwide report. *Circulation* 1991;84:503–511.
39. Eldar M, Griffin JC, Abbott JA, et al. Permanent cardiac pacing in patients with the long QT syndrome. *J Am Coll Cardiol* 1987;10:600–607.
40. Ben-David J, Zipes DP. Differential response to right and left ansae subclaviae stimulation of early afterdepolarizations and ventricular tachycardia induced by cesium in dogs. *Circulation* 1988;78:1241–1250.
41. Ben-David J, Zipes DP. α-adrenoceptor stimulation and blockade modulates cesium-induced early afterdepolarizations and ventricular tachyarrhythmias in dogs. *Circulation* 1990;82:225–233.
42. Grubb BP. The use of oral labetalol in the treatment of arrhythmias associated with the long QT syndrome. *Chest* 1991;100(6):1224–1225.
43. Banai S, Tzivoni D. Drug therapy for torsade de pointes. *J Cardiovasc Electrophysiol* 1993;4:206–210.
44. Schwartz PJ, Priori SG, Locati EH, et al. Long QT syndrome patients with mutations of the SCN5A and HERG genes have differential responses to Na^+ channel blockade and to increases in heart rate. Implications for gene-specific therapy. *Circulation* 1995;92:3381–3386.
45. Compton SJ, Lux RL, Ramsey MR, et al. Gene-derived therapy in inherited long QT syndrome: correction of abnormal repolarization by potassium. *PACE* 1996; 19(4 Part II):642.
46. Lazzara R. From first class to third class: recent upheaval in antiarrhythmic therapy—lessons from clinical trials. *Am J Cardiol* 1996 (In Press).

PART II

Catheter Ablation Techniques

Chapter 8

Radiofrequency Ablation:
Physical Basis and Principles

Thomas Lavergne, MD, Xavier Copie, MD,
Claude Sebag, MD, Jacky Ollitrault, MD,
Jean Yves Le Heuzey, MD, Louis Guize, MD

Introduction

The potential therapeutic benefit of radiofrequency (RF) energy has been suggested by d'Arsonval at the end of the eighteenth century. He reported that when this type of current flows through a subject, it induces a slight warmth at the contact point between skin and electrical wire.[1] The electrosurgical knife was the direct clinical application of this observation and was well-developed by Cushing and Bovie.[2] The effects of RF current application on biological tissues are dependent on the characteristics of the energy used and of the delivering electrodes. Thus, RF currents may lead to tissue electrocoagulation, or tissue section with simultaneous hemostasis.[3]

The interruption of atrioventricular conduction using RF energy was studied as early as 1978, by Mitsui et al.[4] However, its extensive experimental evaluation occurred[5] after fulguration demonstrated for the first time that suppression of an arrhythmogenic myocardial site could be achieved by using a transcatheter approach.[6] Since its first clinical application,[7] RF current has been recognized as the best energy for the treatment of various arrhythmias, and especially supraventricular arrhythmias.[8] Technical improvements should lead to the extension of indications such as ventricular tachycardias complicating organic heart disease, or certain types of atrial fibrillation.[9]

Radiofrequency Currents Characteristics

Radiofrequency energy is an electromagnetic sine wave with a frequency ranging from 100 to 3000 kHz (cycles per second). The power can be calculated according to the formula:

From *Practical Management of Cardiac Arrhythmias* edited by Nabil El-Sherif, and Jean Lekieffre. Futura Publishing Co., Armonk, NY, © 1997.

$$P = U \times I \times \cos\phi$$

where P (W) is the power, U (V) the voltage, I (A) the current, and ϕ the phase angle between current and voltage curves.

Maximum power is obtained when there is no phase shift ($\phi = 0°$, cos $\phi = 1$). Phase displacement results in lower power to be delivered, and can even result in no power at all, if $\phi = 90°$.[10] Modifications of impedance is a common cause of phase shift. Other factors that affect the efficiency of energy delivery are a mismatch between generator, internal impedance, and the circuit impedance, or energy losses along connecting wires, caused by inductive and capacitive coupling.[11,12]

Radiofrequency currents can be applied according to different modes: continuous or pulsed. In the pulsed mode, current delivery is periodically interrupted in order to limit the heating process. Using the high energy delivered by electrosurgical units, these two modes result in different histologic lesions: continuous mode achieving tissue section, and pulsed mode coagulation lesion.[13] For transcatheter myocardial ablation, the power used is six times lower than the power used in electrosurgical units, and pulsed mode does not show any advantages as compared to continuous mode,[14] which is currently used (Figure 1).

Radiofrequency energy is delivered to the tissue between two electrodes. According to the position and characteristics of these electrodes, one can consider unipolar or bipolar configuration:

(1) In unipolar configuration, which is the standard mode, the current is delivered between two electrodes with very different

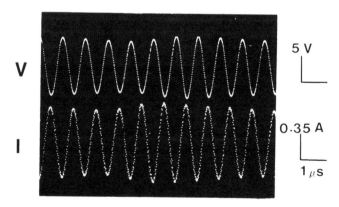

Figure 1. Radiofrequency waveform used for percutaneous ablation of arrhythmogenic myocardial areas. Energy is delivered by a continuous pulse of a 750 MHz frequency sine wave. I = current; V = voltage.

areas. The electrode catheter (or "active" electrode) is small and is positioned close to the endocardium at the target site. The other electrode (dispersive electrode) is large (area above 150 cm^2) and applied on the skin surface. The location of this dispersive electrode on the body does not substantially alter the electric field within the first millimeter of active electrode, and for myocardial ablation it is usually placed below the left scapula of the patient.[15]

(2) In the bipolar configuration, the current is delivered between two small electrode catheters. These electrodes can be located on the same catheter, and being so, are adjacent,[16] or are positioned on two different catheters on either side of the target tissue, usually the septum.[17]

For the same energy, unipolar delivery results in larger lesions than bipolar delivery.[16] However, using a high power, bipolar delivery with electrodes positioned on either side of the target tissue, may achieve transseptal lesions.[17]

Physical Properties of Radiofrequency Currents

Owing to their high frequency ($>$ 100 kHz), RF currents do not induce neuromuscular cell depolarization and do not result in painful muscular contraction.[13] Hence, RF ablation does not require general anesthesia during the procedure.

From a theoretical point of view, biological effects of RF energy can result in three distinct physical phenomenons: (1) thermic; (2) faradic; and (3) electrolytic injury. Although the last two phenomenons are probably of minor importance compared to tissue heating for myocardial tissue injury, direct electrical effect may explain part of the early electrophysiological effects occurring immediately during RF application, such as conduction blocks or spontaneous automaticity.[18] In fact, the main mechanism by which RF current induces tissue injury, is the conversion of electrical energy into heat. Tissue heating involves an active (or resistive) heating and passive components (Figure 2).[19]

Active, or resistive heating, is the result of increased molecular vibrations in the tissue submitted to an electromagnetic field. Energy dissipation is proportional to impedance, current density squared, and the duration of application. Within an RF current circuit, maximal heating occurs at the point where the current density is high and electrical conductivity is low, that is at the electrode-tissue interface.[15] Tissue heating in one site is inversely proportional to the fourth power of the distance from the active electrode.[3] Thus

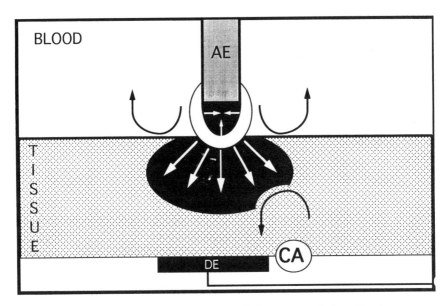

Figure 2. Schematic representation of thermal phenomenon induced in the myocardial tissue by radiofrequency (RF) energy. RF currents are delivered between the active electrode (AE) and the dispersive electrode (DE). The active electrode, applied against the endocardium, is continuously washed by blood flow. Radiofrequency current flow creates a localized area of resistive heating at the electrode—tissue interface **(white rim)**. Heating of the active electrode and myocardium is the consequence of thermal conduction from the electrode-tissue interface **(white arrows)**. Thermic losses are due to convection related to blood flow, primarily at the endocardium **(black arrows)**, but also next to the coronary artery (CA).

resistive heating decreases rapidly with increased distance from the active electrode.

Passive heating results from heat conduction from the active heated volume. Heat is transmitted retrogradely to the active electrode and antegradely to the surrounding myocardium. Thermal losses result from convection due to blood flow during exchanges with bloodstream.[19] Convective losses are maximum where blood flow is high (i.e., subendocardial layers, myocardium close to large arterial or venous coronary vessels), but seem to be minimal in the myocardium itself, and especially in the heated tissue area because blood flow is reduced.[20]

According to the characteristics of heating process (mechanism, kinetic, magnitude), three regions can be distinguished[21]:

(1) The active electrode which is heated indirectly, by conduction from the active heated rim. Thus the temperature measured on

the inner side of this electrode is lower than that of the electrode-tissue interface.[22]

(2) The electrode-tissue interface which is directly heated by the resistive process. The heating kinetic fits with a mono-exponential curve and its half-life is short, the plateau being obtained after only a few seconds.[23,24]

(3) The myocardium which is heated passively according to the thermodynamic laws.[19] Its curve fits also with a more complex mono-exponential function. Heating is slower and maximal heat is not obtained before 60 seconds, whatever the type of electrode.[19,25,26] Thermic increase is not uniform in the myocardium, but is distributed in the depth of the myocardium with a gradient.[27] Values of isothermic curves are dependent on the energy delivered.[27]

Thermic increase must be over 45°C, but less than 100°C to provide an adequate tissue lesion. Ideal temperature is between 70° and 90°C.[15] For temperatures above 100°C, deleterious effects such as bubbles and coagulum formation at the catheter tip, catheter sticking, and char formation can occur. Bubbles and coagulum are a consequence of protein alteration. They isolate the active electrode and induce a rise in impedance. Therefore any rise in impedance is a consequence of these phenomenons and interruption of current application is then mandatory.

Tissue Lesion

Tissue lesions induced by RF current application are dependent on the intensity, kinetic, and duration of tissue heating. Irreversible cellular modifications are obtained for temperatures above 50°C. These cellular modifications are the result of alterations of the phospholipidic membrane, protein coagulation, and enzyme inactivation, as well as mitochondrial lesions.[28] Such lesions involve common and specialized myocardial cells, but also microvascular endothelial cells.[20,28]

Hence, tissue lesion is the consequence of two mechanisms with different time periods. The first one is the result of the direct effect of heating on cellular structure and metabolism. The second is delayed, and is the consequence of ischemic and inflammatory phenomenons related to microvascular injury. This phenomenon can explain parts of the evolution of electrophysiological modifications which are seen in some patients, such as delayed completion of the effect, or, on the contrary, recovery of baseline electrophysiological properties.[29,30]

Anatomical Aspects

Anatomical lesion morphology is dependent on the magnitude of temperature elevation:

(1) Below 100°C, lesions are a homogenous desiccation, without alteration of myocardial architecture.[28]

(2) Above 100°C, lesions are more complex and include tissue vaporization (See color Figure 3 following p. 110) and char formation.[15,31] Such lesions promote myocardial wall fragilization, especially in thin structure such as the atrial free walls[32] or coronary venous vessels, and thrombus formation[33] as a consequence of endocardium alteration.

Gross examination reveals ovoid lesions (See color Figure 4A following p. 110), with a main axis parallel to the endocardium and 1 or 2 mm below.[25,34] Histologic aspects of acute lesions include a central area with coagulation necrosis, surrounded by a moderate inflammatory and hemorrhagic infiltrate. A peripheral zone shows normal myocardial tissue but with altered microvasculature.[34] These lesions will lead to cicatricial fibrosis with clear cut limits and without disruption of tissular architecture (See color Figure 4B following p. 110).[32]

Lesions Size

During in vitro studies in controlled conditions, lesion size depends on the power delivered,[5] duration of RF current delivery,[5,11] the pressure of electrode catheter on the endocardium,[11,35] the length and radius of the active electrode[36] and its position against the endocardium.[37]

However, in vivo, all these parameters cannot be controlled adequately, and tissue-electrode interface temperature is the parameter most closely related to lesion size.[19,23] In animal studies, lesions can vary in length from 0.5 to 9.50 mm, and from 0.1 to 7.55 mm in depth, according to the protocol and type of electrode used[11,16,23,34,37,38] (See color Figure 5 following p. 110). Thus lesion volumes range from 78 to 388 mm³. As compared to lesions produced by DC shock, those induced by RF energy are smaller,[39] but are more homogenous and better limited.

Kinetic of Lesion Formation

In vivo, the lesion size fits well with a mono-exponential curve as well as in vitro.[5,38] The time constant is close to 3 seconds for depth, and 6 seconds for diameter, when contact is stable.[38] This kinetic is not dependent on the size of the active electrode.[26,38] Therefore, 90% of lesion size is reached before 20 seconds, but stationarity is not reached before 40 seconds.[38]

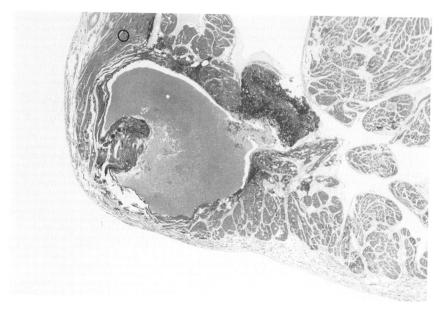

Figure 3. Histologic aspect of an experimental radiofrequency (RF) lesion secondary to an RF current application in atrium (15 W × 30 sec). The atrial wall has been vaporized and replaced by a large hemorrhagic vacuole. This vacuole is separated from the epicardium by only a thin layer of atrial tissue and thus makes the atrial wall fragile with the risk of perforation.

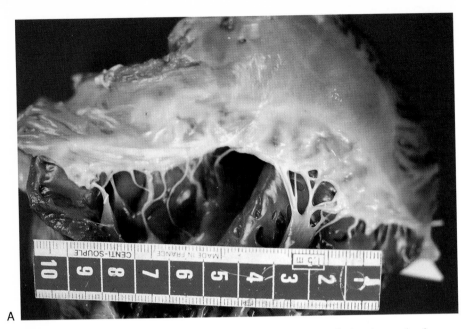

A

Figure 4. (A): Macroscopical aspect of a radiofrequency (RF) lesion 1 month after atrioventicular (AV) nodal ablation for chronic atrial fibrillation with fast ventricular response in patient with dilated cardiomyopathy. This represents part of the piece of cardiectomy obtained at transplantation. There is an oval lesion at the top of Koch triangle. The lesion is opalescent with clear cut edges and a few hemorrhagic areas.

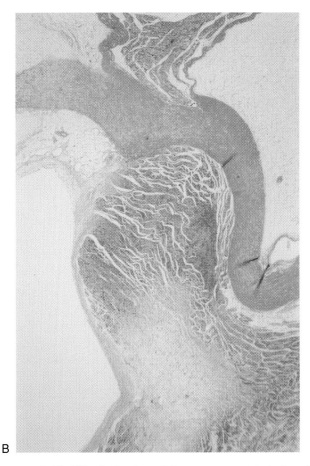

B

Figure 4. *(continued)* **(B)**: Histologic view of the same anatomical piece. There is a large fibrotic area replacing AV node on the right side of the atrial septum, but the interventricular septum did not show lesion (Masson trichrome).

110C

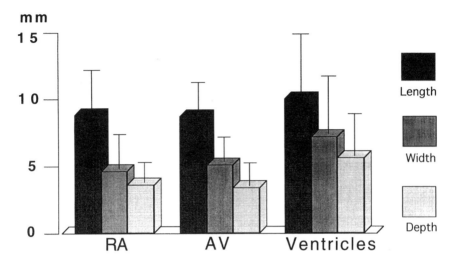

Figure 5. Histogram of the mean lesion size obtained experimentally in vivo in different cardiac structures. RA = right atrium; AV = AV junction.

Optimization of RF Ablation

In order to extend the clinical indications of RF ablation, some improvement of the method is mandatory, such as the increase of the lesion's effect, decrease of its adverse effect, and the monitoring of lesion formation.

Increase in Lesional Effect

The clinical development of RF ablation results mainly from catheter technology improvement which occurred at the beginning of the 1990s. A specific catheter has been designed with a larger active electrode than the classical electrophysiological electrode [40,41] and a steerable tip. However, the extent of tissue lesion may not be always sufficient, especially when the target substrate is large or deeply located in the myocardium, as it is the case with ischemic ventricular tachycardia. Several approaches have been advocated to increase lesion volume. The aims of these approaches were to increase the power delivered to the tissue but also to prevent the occurrence of overheating. This goal can be partly achieved by different options:

(1) Keeping the active electrode temperature below 90°, using a power self-adjusted generator. [42]

(2) Increasing the size of the active electrode. Compared to conventional electrophysiological electrodes, a length of 4 mm in-

creases lesion size to more than twice the volume.[40] Longer electrodes (e.g., 8 mm) would result in a larger lesion but requires a higher energy and may lead to more complications, especially rhythmic.[43]

(3) Cooling the active electrode with internal or external liquid perfusion.[26, 44] Active electrode with external liquid perfusion can increase lesion volume (700 vs 275 mm³), and lesion depth (9.9 vs 2.6 mm) compared to conventional electrodes.[26] However, lesions that are too large can lead to dangerous complications.

Preventing Adverse Effects

To prevent adverse effects such as tissue vaporization and carbonization, temperature should remain below 100°C. The monitoring of electrical and thermic parameters can detect and even prevent harmful overheating.[15,45]

In Vivo Monitoring of Lesion Size

Theoretically, monitoring the lesion formation could provide information on acute effects of the method, explaining some of the electrophysiological failures could predict long-term results, and even detect potentially harmful lesions (tissue vacuolization or endocardial thrombus). Electrode temperature is the best physical parameter related to the size of the lesion, but constitutes an indirect approach.[19,23] Echocardiographic and angioscopic imaging should provide in the future, the tool for direct imaging of the lesion.[46,47]

Monitored Parameters

Several parameters can be monitored during RF application in order to optimize its results.

Electrical Impedance

The measurement of this parameter is of particular importance:

(1) The quality of the electrode tissue contact: the impedance measured before RF application with a low RF energy pulse reflects a good contact between the electrode and the myocardium when it exceeds 135 Ω.[48]

(2) The formation of the lesion, which determines a decrease of the impedance during pulse application.[49]

(3) The detection of overheating, which is associated with bubbles and coagulum formation, resulting in an abrupt impedance increase. Impedance rise is unlikely if electrode temperature remains below 100°C[34] and can be predicted by the value of the impedance measured prior to or during RF application. Thus the incidence of the impedance rise during RF pulse is low when pre-RF impedance is ≤ 120 Ω,[50] and greater when the impedance decrease at the beginning of the RF pulse exceeds 15 Ω.[51]

Active Electrode Temperature

Three general types of thermometry probes have been used for the measurement of electrode temperature during RF application: thermocouples; thermistors; and fiberoptic thermometers.[45] In order to obtain a good assessment of electrode-tissue temperature, the thermometry probe should be in direct contact with the endocardium[22] and positioned perpendicular to the endocardium.[45]

Measuring electrode temperature has several advantages:

(1) It reflects the quality of electrode tissue contact. In fact, this contact seems to be at best, assessed by the radio between power and electrode temperature, a ratio lower than 1:5, reflecting a good contact (Figure 6).[52]

(2) It provides an indirect assessment of the size of the lesion. In vivo, the size of the lesion correlates best with the electrode temperature than with the power or the duration of RF application.[19,23] In clinical settings, Langberg et al have shown that persistent electrophysiological effects are associated with a higher mean electrode temperature value than transient effects.[24] Nevertheless, this parameter is not well-correlated with long-term clinical efficacy.[53]

(3) It allows the prevention of impedance rise, due to tissue overheating. Haines and Verow have well shown that maintaining a temperature below 90° lowers the risk of impedance rise.[34] However, this risk is not totally eliminated as intramyocardial temperature can be higher than that of the active electrode.

In clinical practice, monitoring temperature of the active electrode is more useful to assess tissue-electrode contact and prevent impedance rises, than for the assessment of the size of the lesion.

Other Potentially Useful Techniques for RF Ablation

Transesophageal echocardiography allows catheter positioning, decreasing fluoroscopy time.[54] It can also detect bubbles which occur during

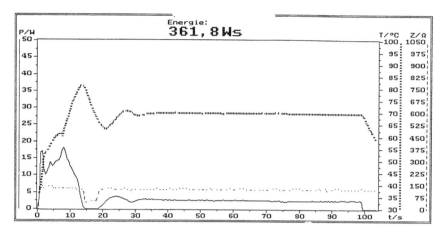

Figure 6. Panel A. Impedance (I), power (P), and temperature (T) curves recorded during radiofrequency (RF) current application. The generator used a closed loop system to control the electrode temperature. The evolution of the three parameters provides information on the quality of the contact between the electrode and the tissue. **Panel A.** At the beginning of RF current application, there is a steep rise in power, which secondly decreases as temperature increases. Power is adapted to maintain the temperature close to 70° C. Simultaneously, there is an initial decrease in impedance, related to tissue lesion. Such evolution is seen when the electrode-tissue contact is stable, achieving tissue lesion.

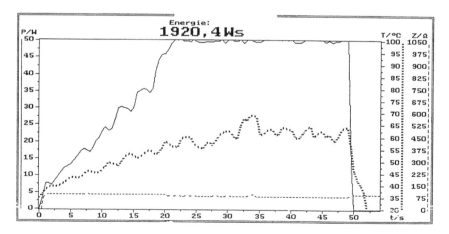

Figure 6. *(continued)* **Panel B.** Power increases rapidly to reach the maximum value of 50 W, but the electrode temperature remains below 40° C, and impedance did not change. This evolution is seen when contact between the electrode and the tissue is poor, and no lesion has occurred.

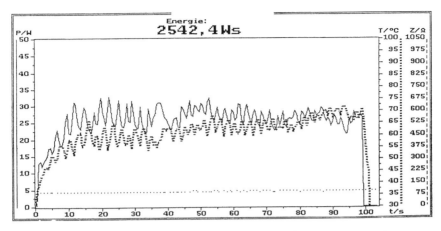

Figure 6. *(continued)* **Panel C.** Variations in power and temperature are important during RF application, which is the witness of an unstable electrode-tissue contact.

30% of RF pulse, preceding impedance rise. The bubbles' occurrence are usually associated with thrombus formation.[55]

The intravascular echocardiography seems to provide more accurate information than the transesophageal approach, and is more comfortable for the patient and the physician.[46] Moreover, this method could allow assessment of the size of the lesion, since modifications in tissue echogenicity following RF current application have been reported.[56] Angioscopy has also been proposed to help the positioning of the ablation catheter in the coronary sinus and to assess the lesion formation.[47]

Equipment

Radiofrequency catheter ablation should be performed in highly trained centers, with extensive knowledge in invasive electrophysiology, and high quality electrophysiological and fluoroscopy equipments.[57] These conditions are required to increase success rates, as well as diminish procedure duration, fluoroscopy time, and the incidence of complications. Specific equipment is constituted by a generator and two electrodes.

Generators

Monitored parameters have been progressively improved, whereas waveforms have remained the same, because within the range of frequencies used, there are no significant differences with respect to tissue effects. A generator should allow the monitoring of electrical parameters (power or voltage, and impedance), but also temperature. It should provide automatic systems that can cut energy delivery in case of excessive rise of temperature or impedance. Some of them can adapt to the power delivered to electrode temperature in order to prevent undesirable overheating.

Catheters

Catheters currently used in ablation procedure have a steerable distal part and an active electrode of large area (27 mm2).[40,41] Current development of catheters for RF ablation are under way. One aim is to provide catheters allowing greater lesions. This aim could be reached by increasing the size of the active electrode,[43] or by cooling the active electrode with internal or external liquid perfusion.[26,44] Moreover, other shapes of catheters are under development, to allow the creation of linear lesions that could be useful for the treatment of arrhythmias with a large anatomical substrate such as atrial fibrillation.

Conclusion

During the last decade, RF ablation has been recognized as the first-line ablative method. Its clinical efficacy and safety has been well-established. However, the technical principles of the method should not be overlooked, as well as the utilization of specific equipment, to improve results and to decrease the incidence of adverse effects. The ability of performing more extensive lesions and linear lesions could extend its indication to arrhythmias, specially to these which are not yet treated with this method.

References

1. D'Arsonval M. Action physiologique des courants alternatifs. *C R Soc Biol Paris* 1891;43:283–287.
2. Cushing H, Bovie WT. Electrosurgery as an aid to the removal of intracranial tumors. *Surg Gynecol Obstet* 1928;47:751–758.
3. Organ LW. Electrophysiologic principles of radiofrequency lesion making. *Appl Neurophysiol* 1976/77;39:69–76.
4. Mitsui I, Tima H, Okamura K, et al. Transvenous electrocautery of the atrioventricular connection guided by the His electrogram. *Jpn Circ J* 1978;42:313–318.
5. Hoyt RH, Huang SK, Marcus FI, et al. Factors influencing trans-catheter radiofrequency ablation of the myocardium. *J Appl Cardiol* 1986;1:469–486.
6. Scheinman MM, Morady F, Hess DS, et al. Catheter-induced ablation of the atrioventricular junction to control refractory supraventricular arrhythmias. *JAMA* 1982;248:851–855.

7. Laver ;ne T, Guize L, Le Heuzey JY, et al. Closed-chest AV junction ablation by high frequency energy transcatheter dessication. Lancet 1986;ii:858–859.
8. Scheinman MM. North American Society of Pacing and Electrophysiology (NASPE) survey on radiofrequency catheter ablation: implications for clinicians, third party insurers, and government regulatory agencies. *PACE* 1992;15: 2228–2231.
9. Haissaguerre M, Gencel L, Fischer B, et al. Successful catheter ablation of atrial fibrillation. *J Cardiovasc Electrophysiol* 1994;5:1045–1052.
10. Hoffmann E. Biophysical parameters of radiofrequency catheter ablation. *Int J Cardiol* 1992;37:213–222.
11. Haverkamp W, Hindricks G, Gulker H, et al. Coagulation of ventricular myocardium using radiofrequency alternating current: biophysical aspects and experimental findings. *PACE* 1989;12(Pt II):187–195.
12. Mackey S, Lampe L, Marcus FI. Power losses in the energy delivery system during ablation. *Circulation* 1993;88 (Pt 2):I-400 (Abstract).
13. Marcus FI. The use of radiofrequency energy for intracardiac ablation: historical perspectives and results of experiments in animals. In: Breithardt G, Borggrefe M, Zipes DP (eds): *Nonpharmacological Therapy of Tachyarrhythmias*. Mount Kisco, NY: Futura Publishing Co., 1987, pp 213–223.
14. An H, Saksena S, Janssen M, et al. Radiofrequency ablation of ventricular myocardium using active fixation and passive contact catheter delivery systems. *Am Heart J* 1989;118:69–77.
15. Hindricks G, Haverkamp W. Determinants of radiofrequency induced lesion size: what are the important parameters to monitor during energy application? In: Huang SKS (ed): *Radiofrequency Catheter Ablation of Cardiac-Arrhythmias: Basic Concepts and Clinical Applications*. Armonk, NY: Futura Publishing Co., 1994, pp 97–112.
16. Huang SR, Bharati S, Graham A, et al. Closed chest catheter dessication of the atrio-ventricular junction using radiofrequency energy: a new method of catheter ablation. *J Am Coll Cardiol* 1987;9:349–358.
17. Ring ME, Huang SKS, Graham A, et al. Catheter ablation of the ventricular septum with radiofrequency energy. *Am Heart J* 1989;117:1233–1240.
18. Nath S, Lyach C, Whayne JG, et al. Cellular electrophysiological effects of hyperthermia on isolated guinea pig papillary muscle—implications for catheter ablation. *Circulation* 1993;88:1826–1831.
19. Haines DE, Watson DD. Tissue heating during radiofrequency catheter ablation: a thermodynamic model and observations in isolated perfused and superfused canine right ventricular free wall. *PACE* 1989;12:962–977.
20. Nath S, Whayne JC, Kaul S, et al. Effects of radiofrequency catheter ablation on regional myocardial blood flow. *Circulation* 1994;89:2667–2672.
21. Wittkampf FHM. Temperature response in radiofrequency catheter ablation. *Circulation* 1992;86:1648–1650.
22. Blouin LT, Marcus F, Lampe L. Assessment of effects of a radiofrequency energy field and thermistor location in an electrode catheter on the accuracy of temperature measurement. *PACE* 1991;14:807–813.
23. Hindricks G, Haverkamp W, Gülker H, et al. Radiofrequency coagulation of ventricular myocardium: improved prediction of lesion size by monitoring catheter tip temperature. *Eur Heart J* 1989;10:972–984.
24. Langberg JJ, Calkins H, El-Atassi R, et al. Temperature monitoring during radio-

frequency catheter ablation of accessory pathways. *Circulation* 1992;86: 1469–1474.

25. Wittkampf FHM, Simmers TA, Hauer RNW, et al. Myocardial temperature response during radiofrequency catheter ablation. *PACE* 1995;18:307–317.

26. Nakagawa H, Yamanashi WS, Pitha JV, et al. Comparison of in vivo tissue temperature profile and lesion geometry for radiofrequency ablation with a saline-irrigated electrode versus temperature control in a canine thigh muscle preparation. *Circulation* 1995;91:2264–2273.

27. Cosman ER, Rittman WJ. Physical aspects of radiofrequency energy applications. In: Huang SKS (ed): *Radiofrequency Catheter Ablation of Cardiac-Arrhythmias: Basic Concepts and Clinical Applications.* Armonk, NY: Futura Publishing Co., 1994, pp 13–23.

28. Nath S, Haines DE. Pathophysiology of lesion formation by transcatheter radiofrequency ablation. In: Huang SKS (ed): *Radiofrequency Catheter Ablation of Cardiac-Arrhythmias: Basic Concepts and Clinical Applications.* Armonk, NY: Futura Publishing Co., 1994, pp 25–39.

29. Langberg JJ, Borganelli SM, Kalbfleisch SJ, et al. Delayed effects of radiofrequency energy on accessory atrioventricular connections. *PACE* 1993;16(Pt I): 1001–1005.

30. Langberg JJ, Calkins H, Kim YN, et al. Recurrence of conduction in accessory atrioventricular connections after initially successful radiofrequency catheter ablation. *J Am Coll Cardiol* 1989;13:468–482.

31. Avitall B, Morgan M, Hare J, et al. Intracardiac explosions during radiofrequency ablation: histopathology in the acute and chronic dog model. *Circulation* 1992; 86(Pt I): I-191.

32. Lavergne T, Prunier L, Guize L, et al. Transcatheter radiofrequency ablation of atrial tissue using a suction catheter. *PACE* 1988;11:906–915.

33. Haines DE, Verow A. Observations on electrode-tissue interface temperature and effect on electrical impedance during radiofrequency ablation of ventricular myocardium. *Circulation* 1990;82:1034–1038.

34. Huang SKS, Graham AR, Wharton K. Radiofrequency ablation of the left and right ventricles: anatomic and electrophysiologic observations. *PACE* 1988;11: 449–459.

35. Haines DE. Determinants of lesion size during radiofrequency catheter ablation: the role of electrode-tissue contact pressure and duration of energy delivery. *J Cardiovasc Electrophysiol* 1991;2:509–515.

36. Haines DE, Watson DD, Verow AF. Electrode radius predicts lesion radius during radiofrequency energy heating. Validation of a proposed thermodynamic model. *Circulation* 1990;67:124–129.

37. Chan R, Johnson S, Seward J, et al. Effect of ablation catheter tip/endocardial surface orientation on radiofrequency lesion size in canine ventricle. *Eur J of Cardiac Pacing and Electrophysiol* 1994;4(Suppl 4):185 (Abstract).

38. Simmers TA, Wittkampf FHM, Hauer RNW, et al. In vivo ventricular lesion growth in radiofrequency catheter ablation. *PACE* 1994;17(II):523–531.

39. Lavergne T, Le Heuzey JY, Bruneval P, et al. Comparative effects of electrical catheter ablation and radiofrequency dessication in the canine right ventricle. *Circulation* 1986;74(Suppl II):II-186.

40. Langberg JJ, Lee MA, Chin MC, et al. Radiofrequency catheter ablation: the effect of electrode size on lesion volume in vivo. *PACE* 1990;13:1242–1248.

41. Jackman WM, Wang XZ, Friday KJ, et al. Catheter ablation of atrioventricular

junction using radiofrequency current in 17 patients. Comparison of standard and large tip catheter electrodes. *Circulation* 1991;83:1562–1576.

42. Pires LA, Huang SKS, Wagshal AR. Temperature-guided radiofrequency catheter ablation of closed-chest ventricular myocardium with a novel thermistor tipped catheter. *Am Heart J* 1994;127:1614–1618.

43. Langberg JJ, Gallagher M, Strickberger SA, et al. Temperature-guided radiofrequency catheter ablation with very large distal electrode. *Circulation* 1993;88: 245–249.

44. Wharton J, Nibley C, Sykes CM, et al. Establishment of a dose response relationship for high power chilled-tip radiofrequency current ablation in sheep. *J Am Coll Cardiol* 1995;1A:293A (Abstract).

45. Haines DE. Temperature monitoring in radiofrequency catheter ablation. In: Huang SKS (ed): *Radiofrequency Catheter Ablation of Cardiac-Arrhythmias: Basic Concepts and Clinical Applications.* Armonk, NY: Futura Publishing Co., 1994, pp 83–95.

46. Jue J, Lesm MD, Ossipo V, et al. Real time quantification of radiofrequency ablation injury using a 15N MHz intracardiac imaging catheter. *Circulation* 1992; 86:I-784 (Abstract).

47. Fujimura O, Lawton A, Koch CA. Direct in vivo visualization of right cardiac anatomy by fiberoptic endoscopy: observation of radiofrequency-induced acute lesions around the ostium of the coronary sinus. *Eur Heart J* 1994;15:534–540.

48. Strickberger SA, Vorperian VR, Man KC, et al. Relation between impedance and endocardial contact during radiofrequency catheter ablation. *Am Heart J* 1994: 128:226–229.

49. Ring ME, Huang SKS, Gorman C, et al. Determinants of impedance rise during catheter ablation of bovine myocardium with radiofrequency energy. *PACE* 1989; 12:170–176.

50. Hoffmann E , Remp T, Gerth A, et al. Does pre-ablation impedance measurement improve the safety of radiofrequency catheter ablation? *Eur Heart J* 1993;13:34 (Abstract).

51. Remp T, Hoffmann E, Gerth A, et al. Drop in impedance and safety during catheter ablation: validation of a predictive marker for impedance rise. *Eur Heart J* 1994;15:286.

52. Stellbrink C, Haltern G, Ziegert K, et al. Different temperature curves observed during temperature guided ablation of accessory pathway correlate with application sequence. *PACE* 1994;17:II-788 (Abstract).

53. Calkins H, Prystowsky E, Carlson M, et al. Temperature monitoring during radiofrequency catheter ablation procedures using closed loop control. *Circulation* 1994;90:1279–1286.

54. Lai W, Al-Khatib Y, Klitzner TS, et al. Biplanar transesophageal echocardiographic direction of radiofrequency catheter ablation adolescents with the Wolff-Parkinson-White syndrome. *Am J Cardiol* 1993;71:872–874.

55. Gallais Y, Lascault G, Tonet J, et al. Transesophageal echocardiographic assessment of radiofrequency beating a accurate method to detect thrombus formation during catheter ablation. Eur Heart J 1994;15:38.

56. Chu E, Kalman JM, Kwasman MA, et al. Intracardiac echocardiography during radiofrequency catheter ablation of arrhythmias in humans. *J Am Coll Cardiol* 1994;24:1351–1357.

57. Daubert JC, Levy S, Medvedowsky JL. Recommandations sur les bonnes pratiques dans les techniques intracavitaires de diagnostic et de traitement des arythmies cardiaques. *Arch Mal Coeur* 1994;87:1213–1224.

Chapter 9_____

Catheter Ablation and Modulation of the Atrioventricular Junction:
Current Issues

Jacques Clémenty, MD, Frank Robert, MD, Laurent Gencel, MD, Michel Haïssaguerre, MD, Philippe Le Métayer, MD, Philippe Gosse, MD, Pierre Jaïs, MD

The catheter ablation of the atrioventricular (AV) junction for the treatment of uncontrollable atrial arrhythmia was first proposed in 1982 by two different groups, led by Scheinman[1] and Gallagher.[2] However, since symptom relief is the sole purpose of the method, and since neither mandatory antithrombotic treatment nor the requirement for implantation of a definitive pacing device, which in itself can have lethal complications, can be eliminated, the method has been somewhat neglected despite the deleterious effects of antiarrhythmic drugs,[3-4] basically because the ablation method provides complete cure of junctional, ventricular and atrial arrhythmias.[5,6,7]

In order to overcome these drawbacks, techniques which modulate without completely interrupting AV conduction have been proposed. An objective evaluation of this special method which transforms tachycardias into bradycardias is now possible, 15 years after its introduction.

Ablation of the Atrioventricular Junction

Technical Data

There has been a considerable amount of technical advancement since the method was initially introduced.

Thermal energy delivery by radiofrequency (RF) electrical currents has replaced high-energy endocavitary shock (fulguration). The electrical arc created by an endocavitary shock produces a high temperature (1700°C) and

121

high pressure (140 atm) bubble at the tip of the catheter.[8,9] The lesion produced lacks precision and is arrhythmogenic.[10] With RF, temperature rise is minimal resulting in homogeneous, and weakly arrhythmogenic lesions.[11]

The result is a dessication of the conduction structures. The importance of controlling temperature is well established. Above 100°C, tissue at the tip of the catheter coagulates, resulting in an abrupt rise in impedance and a microblock which prevents penetration of the thermal energy leading to ablation failure.[12]

General anesthesia is required for fulguration while RF is generally unpainful.

Two studies[13,17] have compared the results of the two techniques. An equivalent AV block is created (complete AV block achieved in 81% and 85% of the cases) but fewer sessions are required for RF (1.05 versus 1.21). The rate of early complications is the same (8% and 9%) and there are fewer major complications with RF (2.3% versus 6.8%). The improvement in patient comfort makes RF preferable in all cases. The smaller elevation in CPK levels indicates the lesions produced are smaller.

The use of wide-tipped ablation electrodes has totally changed the effectiveness of RF. The requirement for a perfect electrode-myocardium contact can now be met with stereo-manipulated catheters which also facilitate access to the target site. Wide-tipped electrodes (4 to 8 mm) increase the surface area and the depth of the lesions.[15,16]

Radiofrequency delivery can be standardized to optimize results (fewer failures, fewer complications). Current protocols use an energy level from 10 to 50 Watts, 30 to 120 second salves, temperature control at 75°C, catheter cleansing whenever impedance rises, routine anticoagulation at the end of each procedure because of the risk of thrombus formation in the right atrium,[17,18] minimal analgesia during the procedure, hospital surveillance for 5 to 7 days, and careful clinical follow-up for one year.[19]

The direct route is still preferred for ablation of the AV junction. In case of failure, the intra-aortic left sided approach can be used effectively without supplementary complications.[20] We used this route in 8 out of 81 consecutive patients (10%). Because of the economic implications related to single-use catheters, when several attempts via the right route have failed, the left route with the same catheter may be recommended before changing the catheter.

The electrophysiological target for ablation has also changed.

Fulguration is aimed at the trunk of the His bundle, and consequently, the rate of pacemaker dependence is high, due to lack of an escape rhythm (Figure 1).

In order to preserve underlying automatism, RF is aimed at the proximal part of the HIS bundle and the compact AV node. The ideal site has a charac-

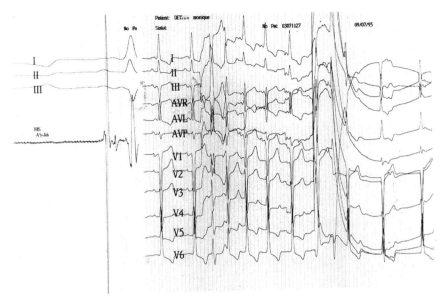

Figure 1. Ablation of the AV junction. Left: The electrophysiological target A/H > 1. Right: Radiofrequency firing creating an AV block. Junction escape.

teristic ample atrial deflection (A) and a weak His deflection (4) (A/H ratio >1). In patients with atrial fibrillation, cardioversion may be attempted before ablation, or alternatively, the target is the point where the His activity disappears under the F waves, when the catheter is drawn from the ventricular cavity into the atrium.[21] Alison, et al[22] thus achieved an escape rhythm in 98% of his cases.

The mean escape cycle is 1,500 ms; the origin would be situated at the junction between the AV node and the His trunk, although all authors do not fully agree on this point. In any case, long-term escape rhythm is observed in only 40% of the fulguration patients.

Technological progress has provided a wider choice of pacemakers adapted for implantation after ablation. The established presence of major chronotropic incompetence after ablation[24] imposes rate-responsiveness. In addition, a retrospective study[25] also established that 4 years after ablation of the AV junction, 30% of the patients have an intermittent sinus rhythm without any antiarrhythmic drug. Currently available dual-chamber pacemakers with a rate-responsive captor can be proposed for many patients after ablation of the AV junction (Figure 2).

124   •   Practical Management of Cardiac Arrhythmias

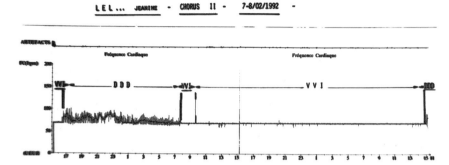

Figure 2. DDD fallback pacing after ablation of the AV junction. **Left:** Sinus rhythm: normal circadian cycle. **Right:** Atrial fibrillation. VVI fallback pacing at 70 bpm. Note the total chronotropic incompetence (rate-responsiveness is required).

Results

Outcome after ablation of the atrioventricular junction should be evaluated according to criteria, considering both electrocardiographic data and symptom relief, assessed in terms of quality of life. This evaluation should include all early and late complications.

Our personal experience[27] with two consecutive series is summarized in Table 1.

Electrocardiographic data obtained after RF show that high degree AV block is achieved in 98% of the cases, in 96% after one session. A mean 6 firings with a average energy of 28 ± 17 watts is applied for 51 ± 25 sec. These figures are slightly higher than those for fulguration. Long-term criteria for success after fulguration have been defined as the persistence of AV block 24 hours after the procedure.[28] For RF, long-term results are acquired immediately, but a few cases of late recovery,[29] or inversely late success,[30] have been reported.

The escape rhythm raises several problems. Patient survival depends on its presence in case of defective pacemaker function.

Data in the literature are rather sparse. The pacemaker has to be inhibited to determine whether an escape rhythm is present. Of course, the pacemaker cannot be inhibited too long and reproducibility over several days, which depends on the adrenergic status and the circadian cycle, remains unknown. In our study, we inhibited pulse delivery for 6 seconds. Although it may take more than 6 seconds for some escape rhythms to appear, once triggered, the rate is >10 bpm.

Most studies report that 25% to 30% of the patients never develop an escape rhythm after RF.

Table 1
Two Populations Undergoing Ablation of the AV Junction by Fulguration
and by Radiofrequency (personal data)

Parameter	Fulguration	Radiofrequency
Number	317	81
Study period	1982–1992	1993–1995
Sex (M/F) %	52/47	58/42
Mean age (years)	67 ± 10	70 ± 11
Atrial fibrillation (% of patients)	61	80
Number of antiarrhythmic drugs	2.8 ± 1.2	3.5 ± 1.1
Failure rate of medical antiarrhythmic treatment	70%	66%
Number of firings	2.0 ± 0.8	5.9 ± 4.0
Energy level	645 ± 260 joules	30 (51 ± 25) Watts
Left-sided approach (%)	0	10
More than one session (%)	18	4
Final 3rd degree AV block (%)	90.7	98
Escape rhythm (%)	20	50
VVI (%)	25	1
VVIR (%)	68	66
DDDR (%)	7	33

In our experience, the escape cycle has a monomorphic configuration over time, though the rate tends to decelerate (35 ± 7.8 bpm versus 37 ± 5 bpm).

Presence of an escape rhythm after ablation is a positive predictive factor for long-term escape. It must be remembered, however, that most patients are given antiarrhythmic drugs at the time of ablation. These inhibitory drugs are later discontinued, favoring the development of an escape rhythm.

Early complications occur only in 8% to 10% of the cases. Most are benign: vagal malaise; hematoma at the point of insertion, phlebitis of the lower limbs; hematoma or ecchymosis over the pacemaker. Severe complications such as pericardial fremitus or sustained ventricular rhythm disorders are unusual (1% to 3% of the cases)[31,32] (Table 2).

Mortality is the major late complication. In our series of 317 patients who underwent fulguration, mortality was 17% after a mean 48-month follow-up, comparable to results reported by Rosenqvist,[33] after 41 months.

Death may be caused by a noncardiac condition (intercurrent disease) or be of cardiac origin. The natural history of the underlying heart disease is the cause of death in most cases. Sudden death however remains problematic. We observed 13 cases in our fulguration series and 1 case in our radiofrequency series (Table 3).

Table 2
Results After Ablation of the AV Junction by Fulguration
and by Radiofrequency (personal data)

Parameter	Fulguration	Radiofrequency
Number of patients	317	81
Mean follow-up (months)	48 ± 29	18 ± 7
Complications	8%	9%
Quality of life		
Improvement	91%	88%
Unchanged	15%	10%
Worse	4%	2%
Deaths	18%	10%
Hospitalized	1%	0%
Cardiac cause	8%	7%
Noncardiac cause	5%	1.5%
Sudden death	4%	1.5%

Table 3
Sudden Death After Ablation of the AV Junction (14 personal cases)

Patient	Ablation Method	Age (years)	Delay (months)	Cardiopathy	LV Function (% EF)	Rhythm Disorder	Sessions	Number of Firings	Post-ablation ECG
1	Fulg.	66	76	hypertension	30%	chronic AF	4	8	Failure
2	Fulg.	52	19	hypertension	normal	paroxysmal AF	1	2	3^d AV Block
3	Fulg.	75	60	hypertension	23%	paroxysmal AF	1	2	3^d AV Block
4	Fulg.	61	16	myocardial infarction	?	paroxysmal AF	1	1	3^d AV Block
5	Fulg.	70	34	congestive heart disease	15%	paroxysmal AF	1	1	3^d AV Block
6	Fulg.	66	30	valvulopathy	20%	paroxysmal AF inter-atrial	1	2	3^d AV Block
7	Fulg.	95	25	valvulopathy	43%	conduction disorder	1	2	Failure
8	Fulg.	80	37	hypertension	?	paroxysmal AF	1	2	Failure
9	Fulg.	67	21	congestive heart disease	17%	paroxysmal AF	1	1	3^d AV Block
10	Fulg.	74	19	ischemia	LV aneurysm	paroxysmal AF	1	2	3^d AV Block
11	Fulg.	57	26	ischemia	20%	flutter paroxysmal	3	6	3^d AV Block
12	Fulg.	79	28	idiopathic	normal	junctional TC	1	1	3^d AV Block
13	Fulg.	67	16	valvulopathy	26%	paroxysmal AF	1	1	3^d AV Block
14	RadioF	46	16	congestive heart disease ischemia	40%	paroxysmal AF	1	2	3^d AV Block

Fulg. = fulguration; RadioF = radiofrequency; AF = atrial fibrillation; EF = ejection fraction

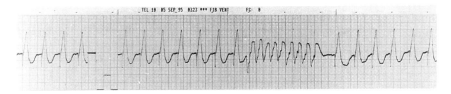

Figure 3. Torasades de pointes and ventricular tachycardia after ablation of the AV junction.

The underlying heart disease obviously plays a role. Eight out of the 14 patients had an ejection fraction under 30%. These patients also had a high incidence of ventricular arrhythmias and sudden death, even without ablation.

There is debate over the effect of the technique itself. The advent of RF has not totally eliminated sudden death, but it is difficult to compare series due to the lack of common selection criteria and variable length of follow-up. Nevertheless, late development of a ventricular rhythm disorder cannot be totally excluded.[34]

Dependence on the pacemaker is a problem in case of defective or totally interrupted pulse delivery. It can be noted that in 12 out of 14 cases the interval to death was 16 to 37 months, meaning that early pacemaker dysfunction due to a secondary rise in the stimulation threshold can be excluded because this phenomenon usually occurs within the first 3 months after implantation. In 3 patients, ablation was not caused by high degree AV block, indicating that this mechanism of dependency cannot always be incriminated. None of the pacing units in this series had to be recalled for premature wear.

In a few documented cases, defective pacemaker response to exercise can be incriminated in the sudden death (Figure 3).

The overall actuarial survival curves (Figure 4) show that prognosis is excellent in patients free of heart disease, because their life expectancy is comparable with that of patients given medical treatment for their atrial fibrillation. The question to be addressed then becomes the patient's quality of life during this survival period.

The remarkable effect of ablating the AV junction on symptoms was recognized from the very first series of fulguration. Our personal experience is summarized in Table 4.

It can be noted that dyspnea persists in a large number of patients. It happens that this particular series included a large number of patients paced in VVI mode (25%) which, due to the inherent chronic chronotropic incompetence, would explain a large part of the residual dyspnea.

The hemodynamic benefit of ablating the AV junction has been emphasized by several authors. Left ventricular dysfunction is improved by ablation

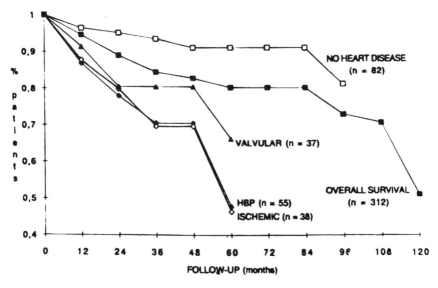

Figure 4. Actuarial survival curve after fulguration of the His network. Prognosis depends on the underlying heart disease.

Table 4
Symptoms in 317 Patients Before and After Radiofrequency
Ablation of the AV Junction

Symptom	Before Ablation	After Ablation
Palpitations	143	8
Dyspnea	88	54
Malaise	40	3
Asthenia	26	6
Syncope	21	0
Dizziness	12	3
Chest pain	11	2
Anxiety	8	0
Total	349	76

as is particularly evident in patients with prior dysfunction. Improvement is less obvious when left ventricular function is only slightly impaired.[33,35,36]

In our series of 81 patients treated with RF, an analysis of left ventricular function was possible in 20 cases and showed that 3 of them had severe dysfunction. In 17 patients with a normal left ventricle, there was no change. Early alterations in left ventricle function seen after fulguration are not observed with RF.

Results of quality of life studies have been quite encouraging. Drug consumption is decreased. Olgin and Scheinman[37] found that the number of hospitalizations decreased from 4 ± 3 admissions annually to 0.7 ± 1.4 admissions annually after ablation. This drop off is similar to that found for fulguration in the series reported by Rosenqvist (2.4 ± 2 to 0.3 ± 0.5).[33]

We evaluated quality of life in our series of 81 patients treated with RF using a quantified questionnaire. Interpretable data could be obtained for 52 of the patients but data were unreliable for 29. Quality of life was judged better in 46 patients (88%), unchanged in 5 (10%) and worse in 1 (2%). This study demonstrates the excellent capacity of AV junction ablation to improve quality of life, but also underlines how difficult it is to obtain reliable measurements which can be generalized for larger populations.[38]

The risk of cerebral vascular events or transient cerebral ischemia remains unchanged after ablation of the AV junction. The risk reaches 14% in patients given no antithrombotic treatment and is much lower in anticoagulated patients.[13] The main problem is patient compliance and the quality of the anticoagulation achieved. In our own series of patients treated with RF, we had 4 cerebral vascular events during the 18-month follow-up in elderly patients that were given aspirin. The preventive effect of aspirin might therefore be insufficient. The rule has been to continue anticoagulation after ablation of the AV junction for atrial fibrillation.

Ablation of the AV junction is thus a simple technique to apply. It is principally indicated in all patients with refractory atrial arrhythmia, unresponsive to medical therapy and inaccessible to other specific action.

Major early complications are rare. It has been established that symptom relief improves quality of life, reduces the need for anticoagulant therapy thus decreasing the need for drugs, and improves left ventricle performance.

The risks are mainly those related to definitive pacing. The exact proportion of the risk related to the proarrhythmogenic effect of the underlying heart disease, the ablation itself and the pacemaker remains to be fully established (2% to 4% sudden deaths) especially when there is a severe structural cardiopathy involved (with the exclusion of the tachymyocardiopathy).[39]

Further extension of the indication to other categories of patients must be evaluated case by case. It is of the utmost importance to rapidly organize randomized prospective studies comparing this technique with medical therapy.

Modulation of Nodal Conduction

The limitations of complete ablation of the AV junction, especially definitive pacing, have led to the search for another technique which could slow down AV conduction enough to provide symptom relief without requiring definitive pacing.

Modulation of the Rapid Pathway

Occasional observations of first degree AV block after fulguration of the HIS bundle clearly demonstrate that the electric results of modulation of the compact node are not identical in all patients.[40,41]

In certain patients, the PR interval adapts normally to exercise, while inversely in others, the degree of the AV block progresses leading to a fall in the ventricular rate (Figure 5).

The first systematic evaluation of modulation was presented by Duckeck, et al[42] who showed that modulation with RF increases the AH interval by 50% or raises the Wenckebach cycle above 400 msec. These results were very discouraging. Modulation was only technically possible in 35% of the cases. There was little effect on symptom relief (32% improvement, 37% complete AV block).

Modulation of the Slow Pathway

Work on AV conduction after selective ablation of the AV node for the treatment of paroxysmal nodal tachycardia led to work on modulation of the slow pathway. Briefly summarized, modulating the rapid pathway situated in the compact node lengthens the AH interval without significantly affecting the anterograde refractory period of the AV node and the Wenckebach cycle. There is also a slow pathway and its ablation has no effect on the AH interval but lengthens the refractory period and the Wenckebach cycle.[43]

There have been three studies in the literature confirming the usefulness of this method.

Feld, et al[44] used the method in 10 patients and had successful results in 7 with reduction of the atrial fibrillation rate (128 to 83 bpm at rest), reduction of the maximal rate recorded on the Holter or at exercise (164 to 123 bpm), and no AV block after 17 applications per patient and a 14-month follow-up.

Della Bella, et al[45] applied the method in 17 patients and found that the

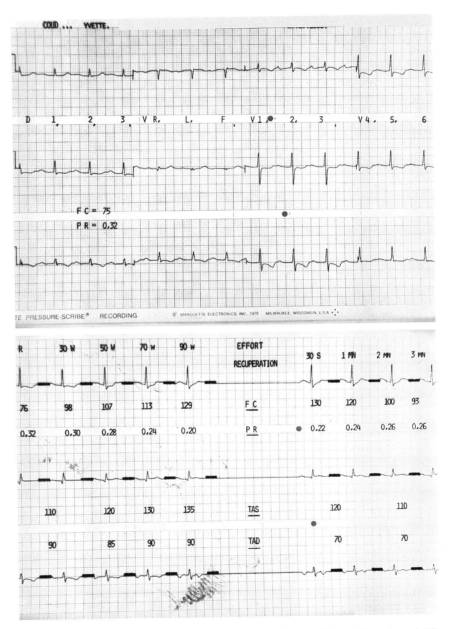

Figure 5. "Successful" modulation of the rapid pathway. **Above:** Lengthened PR interval. **Below:** Normal adaptation of the PR interval to exercise.

PR interval was lengthened from 270 to 390 msec, the Wenckebach cycle from 346 to 450 msec, and the mean atrial fibrillation rate reduced from 165 to 95 bpm. After 5 to 15 applications per patient and a 5-month follow-up, there were 2 AV blocks and 3 residual palpitations.

For Williamson, et al[46] the method was successful in 14 out of 17 patients with 5 AV blocks (21%). Atrial fibrillation rate fell from 180 to 126 bpm after an 8-month follow-up. There were 3 recurrences and one sudden death.

Modulation of the slow pathway is possible in a large number of patients as supported by data reported by Haïssaguerre, et al[47,48] who found that 80% of normal subjects have a recordable slow pathway potential (Figure 6).

Certain difficulties should be emphasized. The first problem is to localize the slow pathway. Electrophysiological mapping is possible in patients with

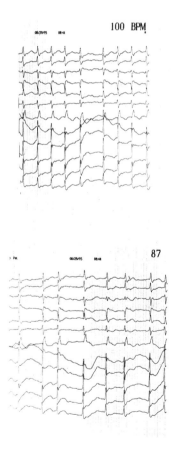

Figure 6. Modulation of the slow pathway. Clear reduction in heart rate and mean atrial fibrillation.

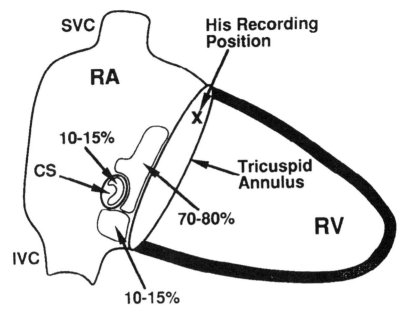

Figure 7. Topography of the slow pathway (in Zipes and Jalife).

a sinus rhythm[47] but anatomic localization is the only possibility in patients with a permanent fibrillation.[49,50] Wide topographic variations have been observed for the slow pathway leading to the need for successive firings (Figure 7).

Another difficulty results from the preceding (i.e., to obtain an effect on ventricular rate) the firings must come close to the compact AV node, increasing the risk of creating an AV block by inadvertently destroying the rapid pathway.

These limitations related to methodology are further complicated by electrophysiological limitations. It has been established that after ablation of the slow pathway, AV conduction in atrial fibrillation no longer depends on the refractory period of the rapid pathway. This period may be short, allowing rapid ventricular rate to persist.

The real effects of modulation on symptoms of atrial fibrillation have not yet been established. In paroxysmal forms, even if the ventricular rate is reduced, an irregular rate can be perceived by the patients (two of the three symptomatic patients in Della Bella's series were in sinus rhythm which would suggest that complete ablation would be useful). The exact role of irregular RR cycles in the genesis of atrial fibrillation-related rhythmic cardiopathy is also an unknown factor.

Conclusions

Modulation of the AV conduction can be proposed in candidates for complete ablation due to the risk of non sinus AV block. The technique consists of successive firings starting in the medioseptal area and working towards the compact node. Ablation should be started by applying 15 to 30 Watts for 60 seconds then gradually lowering the energy level as firings approach the compact AV node. When the rate suddenly changes, firings are stopped. The mean frequency should be lowered below 100 bpm and above 120 bpm with atropine.

This technique is a first step before complete ablation. It can be easily applied in permanent atrial fibrillation. If ablation is done in sinus rhythm, potential recordings serve as a guide for controlling reduction of the Wenckebach point above 120 bpm.

References

1. Scheinman MM, Morady F, Hess DS, et al. Catheter ablation induced of atrial ventricular junction to control refractory supraventricular arrhythmias. *JAMA* 1982;248:851–855.
2. Gallagher JJ, Svenson RH, Kasell JH, et al. Catheter technique for closed chest ablation of ventricular conduction system: a therapeutic alternative for the treatment of refractory supraventricular tachycardia. *N Engl J Med* 1982;306:194–200.
3. Coplen SE, Antman EM, Berlin JM. Efficacy and safety of quinidine therapy for maintenance of sinus rhythm after cardioversion. A meta-analysis of randomized control trials. *Circulation* 1990;82:1106–1116.
4. Flaker GC, Blackshear JL, McBride R, et al. Antiarrhythmic therapy and cardiac mortality in atrial fibrillation. *J Am Coll Cardiol* 1992;20:527–532.
5. Haïssaguerre M, Warin JF, Le Metayer Ph., et al. Closed-chest ablation of retrograde conduction in patients with atrioventricular nodal reentrant tachycardia. *N Engl J Med* 1989;320:426–433.
6. Fontaine G, Frank R, Gallais Y, et al. Fulguration et radiofrequence dans la tachycardie ventriculaire. *Arch Mal Coeur* 1994;87:1589–1607.
7. Touboul P, Kirkorian C, Moncada E. Traitement intracardiaque du flutter auriculaire par courant de radiofréquence. *Arch Mal Coeur* 1994;87:1555–1561.
8. Holt PM, Boyd EG-CA. Hematologic effects of high energy endocardial ablation technique. *Circulation* 1986;75:1029–1036
9. Bardy GH, Goltorti F, Stewart RB, et al. Catheter mediated electrical ablation, the relation between current and pulse width on voltage break down and shock wave generation. *Circ Res* 1988;63:409–414.
10. Hauer RNW, Robles de Medina EO, Borpst C, et al. Proarrhythmic effects of ventricular electrical catheter ablation in dogs. *Am Coll Cardiol* 1987;10:1350–1356.
11. Witkampf FHM, Hauer RNW, Robles de Medina EO. Control of radiofrequency lesion size by power regulation. *Circulation* 1989;80:962–968.
12. Haines DE. The biophysics of radiofrequency catheter ablation in the heart. The importance of temperature monitoring. *PACE* 1993;16(II):586–591
13. Olcin JE, Scheinman MM. Comparison of high energy direct current and radio-

frequency catheter ablation of the ventricular junction. *J Am Coll Cardiol* 1993; 21:557–564.

14. Morady F, Calkins H, Langberg JJ, et al. A prospecive randomized comparison of direct current and radiofrequency ablation of the ventricular junction. *J Am Coll Cardiol* 1993;21:102–109.

15. Jackman WW, Wang X, Friday KJ, et al. Catheter ablation of ventricular junction listing radiofrequency current in 17 patients comparison of standard and large type catheter electrodes. *Circulation* 1991;83:1562–1576.

16. Yeung-Lai-Wah JA, Alison JF, Conergan L, et al. High success rate of atrioventricular mode ablation with radiofrequency energy. *J Am Coll Cardiol* 1991;18: 1753–1758.

17. Kunze KP, Schuter M, Costard A, et al. Right atrial thrombus formation after transvenous catheter ablation of the atrioventricular node. *J Am Coll Cardiol* 1985; 6:1428–1430.

18. Moro C, Aragoncillo P, Jorge P. Thrombus apposition on catheter ablation injuries. *Europ Heart J* 1989;10:853–857.

19. Lavergne T, Sebag C, Alitrant J. Ablation par courants de radiofrequence; aspects théoriques et techniques. *Arch Mal Coeur* 1994;87:1547–1553.

20. Sousa J, Elatassi R, Rosenhelk S. Radiofrequency catheter ablation of atrioventricular junction from the left ventricle. *Circulation* 1991;84:567–571.

21. Touboul P, Canu C, Claudel P, et al. His bundle ablation for atrial fibrillation: Indications and results In: Olsson SB, Allessie M, Campbell RWF, (ed.). *Atrial Fibrillation Mechanisms and Therapeutic Strategies.* Futura Publishing Co: Armonk, 1994, p. 307–323.

22. Alison JF, Yeung JA, Schulzer M, et al. Characterization of junctional rhythm after atrioventricular node ablation. *Circulation* 1995;91:84–90.

23. Vijgen J, Ector H, de Geest H. Underlying heart rhythm after catheter ablation of atrio-ventricular conduction system. *J Cardiovasc Electrophysiol* 1990;1:209–213.

24. Clementy J, Coste P, Bricaud H. Functional evaluation of patients 6 to 60 months after transvenous ablation of atrioventricular conduction. *Europ Heart J* 1977; 8(Supp II):65 (Abstract).

25. Bernard V, Clementy J, Gencel L, et al. Choix du mode de stimulation après ablation du faisceau de HIS. Expérience tirée d'une enquête rétrospecive portant sur 192 malades. *Arch Mal Coeur* 1994;87, (S. 11):1581–1589.

26. Mond HG, Barold S. Dual chamber rate adaptive pacing in patients with paroxysmal supra-ventricular tachyarrhythmias. *PACE* 1993;16:2168–2185.

27. Poquet F, Gencel L, Le Métayer Ph., et al. Long term survival after closed chest his bundle ablation with DC SHOCK for supra ventricular arrhythmias. *PACE* 1994;17 (P.E. II):2150–2155.

28. Lemery R, Brugada P, Della Bella P, et al. Predictors of long term success during closed chest catheter ablation of atrioventricular junction. *European Heart J* 1989; 10:826–832.

29. Huang SKS, Bharati S, Graham AR, et al. Chronic incomplete atrioventricular block induced by radiofrequency catheter ablation. *Circulation* 1989;80:951–961.

30. Stein KM, Lerman BB. Delayed success following radiofrequency catheter ablation. *PACE* 1993;16 (Part I):698–701.

31. Sadoul N, de Chillou C, Lamouri F, et al. Resultats, complications, et suivi au long cours de l'ablation percutanée de la conduction auriculo-ventriculaire. *Arch Mal Coeur* 1994;87:1453–1458.

32. Canu G, Moncada E, Claudel JP, et al. Evolution à long terme après ablation électrique du faisceau de HIS dans le traitement des tachycardies supraventriculaire. *Arch Mal Coeur* 1994;87:1447–1451.

33. Rosenqvist M, Lee MA, Moulinier G, et al. Long-term follow-up of patients after transcatheter direct current ablation of the atrioventricular junction. *J Am Coll Cardiol* 1990;16:1467–1474.

34. Perry JC, Kearney DL, Friedman RA, et al. Late ventricular arrhythmia and sudden death following direct current catheter ablation of the atrioventricular junction. *Am J Cardiol* 1992;70:765–768.

35. Huang S. Advances in application of radiofrequency current to ablation therapy. *PACE* 1991;14:28–42.

36. Lemery R, Brugada P, Cheriex E, et al. Reversibility of tachycardia induced left ventricular dysfunction after closed chest catheter ablation of the atrioventricular junction for intractable atrial fibrillation. *Am J Cardiol* 1987;60:1406–1408.

37. Olgin J, Scheianman M. Catheter ablation of atrioventricular mode for the treatment of supraventricular tachyarrhythmias. In: Zipes D and Jalife J. *Cardiol Electrophysiol P* 1453–1460. W.B. Saunders, Philadelphia 1995.

38. Kay GN, Bubien RS, Epstein AE, et al. Effect of catheter ablation of the atrioventricular junction on quality of life and exercise tolerance of paroxysmal atrial fibrillation. *Am J Cardiol* 1988;62:741–744.

39. Denes P. Radiofrequency catheter ablation of the A.V. node. *J Am Coll Cardiol* 1991;18:1759–1760.

40. Kunze KP, Schluter M, Geiger M, et al. Modulation of atrioventricular nodal conduction using radiofrequency current. *Am J Cardiol* 1988;61:657–658.

41. Avitall B, Khan M, Krum D, et al. Repeated use of ablation catheters: a prospective study. *J Am Coll Cardiol* 1993;22:1367–1377.

42. Duckeck W, Engelstein ED, Kuck KH. Radiofrequency current therapy in atrial tachyarrhythmias modulation versus ablation of atrioventricular nodal conduction. *PACE* 1993;16:629–636.

43. Jazayeri MR, Sra JS, Deshpande SS. Electrophysiologic spectrum of atrioventricular nodal behavior in patients with atrioventricular nodal reentrant tachycardia undergoing selective fast or slow pathway ablation. *J Cardiovasc Electrop* 1993;4:99–111.

44. Feld GK, Fleck RP, Fujimura OS, et al. Control of rapid ventricular response by radiofrequency catheter modification of the atrioventricular node in patients with medically refractory atrial fibrillation. *Circulation* 1994;90:2299–2307.

45. Della Bella P, Carbucicchio C, Tondo C, et al. Modulation of atrioventricular conduction by ablation of the slow atrioventricular node pathway in patients with dry refractory atrial fibrillation or flutter. *J Am Coll Cardiol* 1995;25:39–46.

46. Williamson BD, Man KC, Daoud E. Radiofrequency catheter modification of atrioventricular conduction to control ventricular rate during atrial fibrillation. *N Engl J Med* 1994;331:910–917.

47. Haïssaguerre M, Gaita F, Fischer B, et al. Elimination of atrioventricular nodal reentrant tachycardia using discrete slow potentials to guide application of radiofrequency. *Circulation* 1992;85:2162–2175.

48. Jackman NM, Beckman KJ, McLelland JH, et al. Treatment of supraventricular tachycardia due to atrioventricular nodal reentry by radiofrequency catheter ablation of slow pathway conduction. *N Engl J Med* 1992;327:313–318.

49. Wathen M, Natale A, Wolfe K, et al. An anatomically guided approach to A.V. mode: slow pathway ablation. *Am J Cardiol* 1992;70:886–889.

50. Wu D, Yeh ST, Wang CC, et al. A simple technique for selective radiofrequency ablation of the slow pathway in atrioventricular node reentrant tachycardia. *J Am Coll Cardiol* 1993;21:1612–1621.

Chapter 10

Update of the Treatment of Atrial Flutter

Nadir Saoudi, MD, Hervé Poty, MD,
Mohan Nair, MD, Ahmed Abdel-Azziz, MD,
Brice Letac, MD

Introduction

In the routine practice of cardiology "common flutter" refers to a regular right atrial tachycardia at a rate of 300 beats per minute with the striking particularity of being not only monomorphic, but also almost identical from one patient to another. The electrocardiographic hallmark of this arrhythmia is the saw tooth pattern of the flutter waves. In the inferior leads, this is manifested by a frank negative portion that is followed, after a slightly positive notch, by a descending plateau, which then joins a new negative deflection. In fact, recent work from our laboratory and others has shown that this ECG pattern may vary slightly, reflecting different types of atrial tachycardias, rendering the frontiers with atrial fibrillation (AF) at times when it is difficult to clearly individualize. This chapter deals only with the common form of atrial flutter. Both these arrhythmias are common and frequently drug resistant, particularly with respect to the prevention of recurrences in the intermittent forms. We shall first speak of the treatment of acute attacks of atrial flutter, and later of their prevention with particular emphasis on catheter ablation techniques.

Treatment of an Acute Episode of Atrial Flutter

Overdrive Atrial Pacing

In our opinion, it is the elective treatment of atrial flutter attacks. The pacing site may be the left atrium via the transesophageal route, or the right

From *Practical Management of Cardiac Arrhythmias* edited by Nabil El-Sherif, and Jean Lekieffre. Futura Publishing Co., Armonk, NY, © 1997.

atrial endocardium by the transvenous approach. In a series of 102 transesophageal pacing attempts in 83 patients (79 common flutters), Gallay et al observed a 61% sinus rhythm restoration rate, with intervening transient AF in 47% of the cases.[1] Stable AF was encountered in 8% of the cases and failure due to intolerance or lack of atrial capture occurred in 31% of the cases. The idiopathic or postoperative forms seem particularly suitable for stimulation. It has been suggested that antiarrhythmic drug loading prior to pacing would enhance the rate of pacing termination, but this point has never been clearly evaluated in a controlled study. The advantages of the transesophageal approach are its simplicity and innocuity, but besides the fact that pacing is initiated far from the (right atrial) reentrant circuit, its main disadvantage is that it can be painful and is often disagreeable to the patient.

The insertion under local anesthesia of a multipolar catheter electrode that can be easily positioned in the right atrium (RA) is our preferred approach. The steerability of the recent generation catheters, further facilitates precise positioning inside the reentrant circuit. This can be the area located between the coronary sinus ostium (CSO) and the tricuspid annulus (TA) or any area in the lower portion of the RA, provided that the endocardial contact is good enough to allow consistent atrial capture and that the catheter is close to the TA.

Depending on the pacing rate, the so-called transient entrainment phenomenon preceding tachycardia termination, will be observed.[2] In the late 1970s, the modalities of flutter termination with straightforward pacing at a rate faster than that of tachycardia were carefully studied. It was clearly established that a critical pacing rate is required in order to terminate atrial flutter. If the pacing rate, although faster than that of the tachycardia, is too low, atrial flutter will be transiently entrained but never terminated. On the contrary, too fast a pacing rate will rapidly precipitate AF. In clinical practice, we start pacing at a rate of 20 beats per minute above that of the flutter and deliver the run for a minimum of 15 seconds, at least 5 times. In case of failure, the pacing rate is slowly incremented by steps of 10 beats per minute and a new series of runs is attempted. Usually, in the initial attempts, tachycardia is not interrupted but on the contrary seems to accelerate with pacing, while resuming at its previous rate upon pacing cessation. This "transient entrainment" phenomenon may be recognized on the surface electrocardiogram, if the pacing site is outside the reentrant circuit (in the right atrial appendage for example). In this case, the morphology of the paced atrial electrogram is that of a fusion beat, i.e., intermediate between that of the "native" flutter wave and that of the pure paced beat that would have occurred, had the stimulation been initiated at this rate and at this site during sinus rhythm. In this condition, atrial flutter termination may also be recognized by the sudden disappearance of the atrial fusion complexes that is followed by the emergence of pure paced atrial beats. It should be noted that careful application of this protocol does not always prevent the unwanted emergence of AF. However, this rhythm is frequently less stable than that of atrial flutter, and frequently sinus rhythm is spontaneously restored in the subsequent hours. We think that this technique is superior to that of the transesophageal one, because in our experience, the sinus rhythm restoration rate is higher (probably because of the better pacing site), and also because it is painless. Also, patients having experienced both, prefer the transvenous approach.

The extreme sensitivity of atrial flutter to pacing has led to attempts at control by the implantation of an antitachycardia pacemaker. Barold et al have used this approach in five symptomatic and drug refractory patients.[3] In three cases after manual activation, the pacemaker delivered fixed pacing runs, and in two others it was fully automatic. After 4 years of follow-up, the vast majority of attacks had been controlled (although with concomitant antiarrhythmic drug intake), and patients claimed to be satisfied. Although attractive because of its specificity, and the avoidance of potentially dangerous secondary drug-related effects, this technique is expensive, purely palliative, and it appears appropriate to turn to direct atrial ablation techniques in case of frequent recurrence.

Direct Current Countershock

Although seldom used in France, DC countershock is often used as first-line therapy in the United States. The energy requirement is usually low (50 Joules) and it can be delivered on an outpatient basis.[4] One of its advantages over pacing, is the possibility of delivering immediately another shock, if the first shock fails or results in AF. The overall efficacy of this intervention is excellent and approaches 100%, the main drawback being that it requires general anesthesia.

Pharmacological Conversion of Atrial Flutter

Although we are now dealing with one of the oldest forms of therapy, this is also the less well-known. There is indeed almost no study where atrial flutter and AF have not been mixed, so that the effects of antiarrhythmic drugs on atrial flutter alone are not really known. In the cardiology textbooks, it is common to read that the injection of a short-acting digitalis preparation occasionally results in sinus rhythm restoration.[5] Because of the lack of controlled study, the prevalence of this phenomenon is unknown but it is unlikely that cardiotonic glycosides can be reproducibly efficacious in this situation. A recent nonrandomized study estimates at 33% the sinus rhythm restoration rate in recent onset of atrial flutter after intravenous injection of 2 mg/kg of propafenone.[6] Another recent study comparing flecainide and propafenone in atrial arrhythmias (flutter and fibrillation) has yielded comparable results (40% success rate) in the latest analysis of the flutter population.[7] Both beta-blockers and calcium antagonists have also been proposed, but they do not seem to affect the atrial rate in atrial flutter. Classically recommended high doses of quinidine derivatives have been responsible for frank aggravation of the hemodynamic status.[8] The combination of the slowing of intra-atrial propagation of impulse (class I effect) prolonging atrial flutter cycle length, along with the enhancement of atrioventricular (AV) nodal conduction (associated vagolytic effect), has resulted in the acceleration of the ventricular rate by the transformation of a fast flutter with 2:1 AV transmission into a flutter with a slower atrial cycle length with 1:1 AV transmission. This phenomenon has also been observed with class IC antiarrhythmic drugs.

In a noncontrolled study evaluating the effect of intravenous class I and class III drugs on the excitable gap of atrial flutter, "spontaneous" flutter termination with the drug has not been observed.[9] In fact, chemical cardioversion of atrial flutter has been almost abandoned in favor of pacing techniques which are faster, safer, and more efficacious.

Prevention of Late Recurrences: Catheter Ablation of Atrial Flutter

Other than cases that have a curable etiology, pharmacological prevention is usually disappointing. Two factors are recognized to have strong predictive value, these are: arrhythmia duration; and the size of the atria. Of note, is that here again in the prognostic evaluation, flutter has not been distinguished from fibrillation in most of the studies.[10,11] In the controlled studies, the commonly available antiarrhythmic drugs have shown a relatively poor efficacy, although they are still superior to that of placebo. However, owing to the heterogeneity of the study protocols, it is in our opinion, and currently it is not possible to individualize a specific drug or dosage that would reasonably prevent relapses without significant side effects on a long-term basis. This relative resistance to pharmacological drug therapy has prompted the development of new curative techniques.

Until the end of the 1980s, the simplest and most radical treatment of refractory atrial arrhythmias was the delivery under general anesthesia, of a unipolar DC current shock between the tip of a catheter positioned against the AV node—His bundle (His bundle fulguration) region and a cutaneous back paddle. The technique later evolved into the use of radiofrequency energy, but both resulted in intentional complete AV block. This was particularly efficacious in the amelioration of symptoms, but had the obvious drawback of the requirement of a permanent pacemaker on which the patient was dependent, while the atrial arrhythmia continued to be present.

Fulguration of Atrial Flutter

In order to circumvent these shortcomings, a technique was developed in 1987 that consisted of delivering the fulguration shocks inside the atrial reentrant circuit itself.[12,13] This was rendered possible by a better understanding of the circuit of atrial flutter due to improvement in catheter mapping techniques. The first attempts at definite ablation were directed towards low voltage, prolonged and fragmented electrograms in the area surrounding the CSO. These potentials were interpreted, by analogy with what is usually seen in ventricular tachycardia, as being indicative of the slow conduction zone responsible for the reentrant circuit. Late results of fulguration shocks delivered in this area in 14 patients were relatively poor, as after 3 years, only 50% of the patients were free of recurrence.

Radiofrequency Ablation of Atrial Flutter

Because of the very small size of the lesion, and thanks to the lack of simultaneous tachycardia cardioversion, the introduction of the radiofrequency technique has further helped in the understanding of the flutter circuit. It was rapidly clear that the appropriate selection of a target should be accompanied by tachycardia termination during the pulse. Further improvement of circuit understanding was facilitated by the availability of steerable multipolar catheters, and by the appearance of systems with computerized analysis that allowed simultaneous, rather than sequential recording of a high number of endocardial points. For example, we currently use a duodecapolar (20 poles), a decapolar, and two quadripolar catheters for a routine flutter mapping and ablation procedure.

Following the early work of Puech,[14] Cosio has shown that during atrial flutter, the impulse traverses the anterolateral right atrial wall downward (at the level of the pectinate muscles) to reach the isthmus located between the inferior vena cava and the TA (IVC-TA).[15] It then propagates towards the CSO and to depolarize the interatrial septum ascendingly. He is also the first worker to have clearly demonstrated that ablation of the isthmus between the IVC and the TA, interrupts and definitely cures AF by preventing its recurrences. In 1992, almost simultaneously, several series were reported confirming this phenomenon.[16-20] The idea of a purely anatomically guided ablation became therefore clear, and the search for specific electrophysiological criteria was abandoned by most authors.[21] The experience of the authors' institution is detailed below.

Patient Population

Fifty-two patients with type I Atrial flutter have undergone radiofrequency catheter ablation at our center. There were 44 males and 8 females in this population and their ages ranged from 26 to 76 years (mean 58.1 + 12.6 years). An underlying heart disease was present in 22 (40%) patients.

Atrial Flutter Mapping

Figure 1 shows the usual catheter positions for this procedure as seen in the right anterior oblique projection (left panel), along with the corresponding electrograms (right panel). A multipolar catheter is inserted via the left subcla-

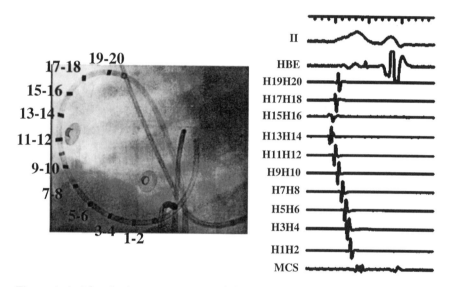

Figure 1. Atrial activation sequence recorded during sinus rhythm. Catheter position is shown in the left part of this and subsequent figures. A 20 poles "Halo" (H) catheter records the anterolateral right atrial wall down to the IVC-TR isthmus. The other catheters that are routinely inserted in our laboratory are a quadripolar electrodes at the His bundle recording site, and a quadri polar specially designed for the ablation procedure (4, 6 or 8 mm distal tip). During sinus rhythm (right part), the impulse emerges from the sinus node area (poles H13H14) and propagates downward towards the distal poles of the halo while simultaneously it also reaches a more septal portion of the high right atrium (poles H19H20) and travels down to reach the His bundle area. Other labels in this and subsequent figures are coronary sinus, His bundle (HBE) and an ablation (here with an 8 mm tip) catheter positioned at the ablation site in a relatively septal location (Abl). Abbreviations are for this and subsequent figures. II = standard ECG lead II; PCS = proximal coronary sinus; DCS = distal coronary sinus; MCS = middle coronary sinus; H = Halo. Numbers indicated the sequential dipoles of the Halo catheter.

vian vein. This traverses the RA in an oblique manner and catheterizes the coronary sinus. It is used for recording the left atrial activation and for pacing the proximal coronary sinus. Three electrodes are introduced via the right femoral vein. One (quadripolar) is used for recording the His bundle activation. Another catheter (duodecapolar, halo) has a special design that allows it to form a loop within the RA. This facilitates mapping of activation covering a large area, starting in the high RA, close to the superior vena cava (poles H19H20), down to the mid-part of the IVC-TA isthmus (poles H1H2). The fourth catheter is a special quadripolar ablation catheter with an extra large (8 mm) tip that in this figure is shown and positioned in the septal end of the IVC-TA isthmus. During sinus rhythm (right part), the impulse emerges from the sinus node area (poles H13H14) and propagates downward towards the distal poles of the halo (which corresponds to the descending depolarization of the pectineate muscles). In the mean time, the impulse also reaches a more septal portion of the high RA (poles H19H20) and travels down to reach the His bundle area. The coronary sinus is activated later, after completion of the right atrial depolarization.

Figure 2 shows the recording of atrial activation during atrial flutter. As depicted by the circled arrow, during flutter, the impulse is ascending in the

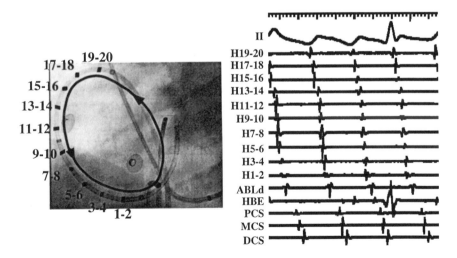

Figure 2. Atrial activation sequence recorded during common flutter. As depicted by the circled arrow, during flutter the impulse is ascending in the septum (from the ablation site to the His bundle area to the poles H19H20) and descending in the lateral wall (from the proximal to the distal poles of the halo catheter). Note that the atrial electrogram at the ablation site follows that of the distal (H1H2) of the halo and precedes that of the proximal coronary sinus and His bundle.

septum (from the ablation site to the His bundle area to the poles H19H20), and descending in the lateral wall (from the proximal to the distal poles of the halo catheter). Note that the atrial electrogram at the ablation site follows that of the distal (H1H2) pole of the halo and precedes that of the proximal coronary sinus and His bundle.

Delivery of Radiofrequency Pulses

The radiofrequency pulse is delivered using either an extra large tip (8 mm EPT blazer) or a thermistor tip catheter. The power output while using the 8-mm tip catheter is kept at 50 watts, and the temperature cut-off during the use of the thermistor control is set at 70° C. The ablating catheter is first introduced into the right ventricle and then withdrawn under fluoroscopic guidance to the tricuspid edge of the IVC-TA isthmus. At this point, there is a small atrial and a large ventricular electrogram recording at the distal dipole of the catheter. Radiofrequency energy delivery is commenced at this point and continued along a line, joining the TA to the IVC. Each pulse is given for a duration of 90 seconds, except when it has to be prematurely

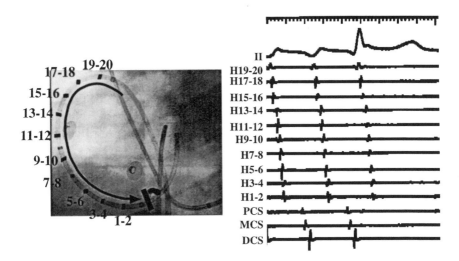

Figure 3. Counterclockwise AFL termination during the radiofrequency pulse. During AFL, a descending wavefront is observed at the lateral RA (H17–18 to H5–6) and then activation crosses the IVC-TA isthmus to reach the low septum (H3–4 to PCS). Suddenly, AFL interruption occurs at the ablation site (IVC-TA isthmus) between H1–2 and the PCS (i.e., immediately after the distal pole of the halo has been activated). This prevents further activation of the circuit and flutter can no longer occur.

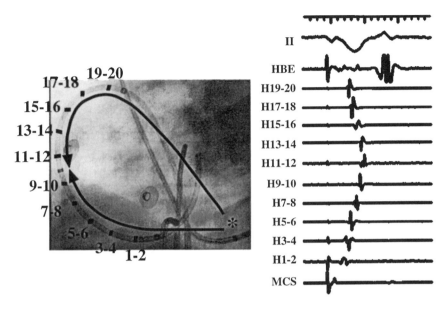

Figure 4. Mapping of atrial activation sequence during proximal coronary sinus pacing initiated during sinus rhythm after flutter termination, but without conduction block at the isthmus. Two wavefronts can be seen along the lateral right atrial wall, on that, after septal ascension, travels downward from the high right atrium, and another one that travels upward from the low right atrium. A collision of the two wavefronts can be observed at the mid-lateral right atrium (here at the level of poles 11–12). This pattern can also be observed when pacing is initiated during sinus rhythm before ablation.

interrupted due to impedance rise. In case the desired end-point of flutter termination and complete isthmus block is not achieved, further pulses are delivered around the same region.

Figure 3 depicts flutter termination during the radiofrequency pulse. The flutter circuit suddenly terminates exactly at the ablation site (i.e., immediately after the distal pole of the halo has been activated). This prevents further activation of the circuit, and flutter can no longer occur.

The more recent developments in mapping and assessment of conduction at the IVC-TA isthmus are depicted in the subsequent figures.[22] Figure 4 depicts the typical activation sequence that is seen during proximal coronary sinus pacing, when there is no impairment of conduction at the isthmus (for example, before the delivery of radiofrequency energy, or after delivery of a pulse that results in flutter termination but not IVC-TA conduction block). Two wavefronts can be seen, one that ascends in the interatrial septum, activating sequentially the His Bundle area and the proximal poles of the halo to propagate towards the sinus node area. Simultaneously, another wavefront crosses the IVC-TA isthmus and activates the distal poles of the halo catheter before ascending. Thus, there is a collision of these two wavefronts at the level of poles (H11H12). In contrast, when complete IVC-TA annulus isthmus block has been obtained, the pattern of right atrial depolarization is completely changed, as can be seen in Figure 5. There is now no wavefront that traverses the isthmus, and ascends along the lateral right atrial wall. This, therefore, leaves a single wavefront that is entirely descending along the lateral right atrial wall up to the ablation site. Thus the distal poles (H19H20) of the halo catheter which were the earliest to be activated while pacing from the proximal coronary sinus, are now activated last.

The block in the other direction is depicted in Figure 6. Pacing from the other side of block on the lateral part of the isthmus (i.e., now from the

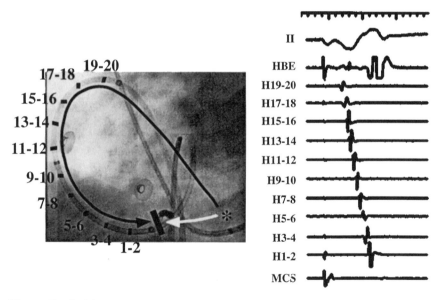

Figure 5. Atrial activation sequence during proximal coronary sinus pacing after having achieved conduction block at the isthmus. When complete inferior vena cava tricuspid annulus isthmus block has been obtained, the pattern of right atrial depolarization is completely changed. There is now no more wavefront traversing the isthmus and ascending along the lateral right atrial wall. Therefore a single wavefront is entirely descending along the lateral right atrial wall travels now down to the other side of the ablation site. Thus the distal poles (H1H2) of the halo catheter, (which were the earliest to be activated while pacing from the proximal coronary sinus before block) are now activated the last.

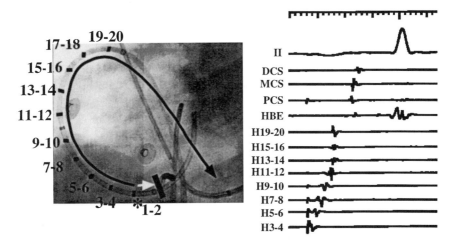

Figure 6. Block in the counterclockwise direction during low lateral right atrial pacing. Pacing from the other side of block on the lateral part of the isthmus (i.e., now from the distal dipole of the halo catheter, H1H2) shows a late and descending septal depolarization, whereas, in the absence of block it should be ascending due to the proximity of the pacing site. As a consequence, the activation of the coronary sinus occurs now latest, after activation of the His bundle area. Note that the morphology of the paced P wave is biphasic in lead II with a slight negativity that is synchronous with the right atrial ascension, followed by a positivity corresponding to the descending septal wavefront and to the left atrial depolarization.

distal dipole of the halo catheter, H1H2) shows a late and descending septal depolarization, whereas, in the absence of block it should be ascending due to the proximity of the pacing site. Note that the activation of the coronary sinus is even later.

Late Follow-Up

Forty-three patients have now been followed-up for a mean of 13 months (range 3–18). Three (9%) patients have had recurrence of atrial flutter, one of whom had a second successful ablation. A systematic controlled electrophysiological study has been performed at a mean of 4 months (range 1–29) after ablation in 17 out of 43 patients. The block of conduction at the IVC-TA isthmus was seen to persist in all the patients. Incremental atrial pacing (up to a cycle length of 180 msecs.), from the PCS-induced atypical atrial flutter in two patients and atrial fibrillation in six patients, but common atrial flutter could not be induced in any.

Conclusion

In 1996, the treatment of acute flutter has dramatically evolved, because for the first time in the history of this tachycardia, a reliable and reproducible curative treatment has been individualized. This in fact is not specific to atrial flutter, because due to the emergence of DC catheter ablation techniques in the 1980s, and radiofrequency ablation in the 1990s, a whole new therapeutic field has emerged. However, the individualization of the target as well as the various steps of the ablation protocol have been more difficult for atrial flutter than it has been for AV nodal reentry tachycardia, or accessory pathways ablation. These encouraging results are indeed paving the way toward a better understanding of flutter tachycardias. We recently reported that the above-described ablation technique also applies to the reversed form of AF, which is also slightly different on surface electrocardiogram than the common (counterclockwise) form, indeed share the same right atrial reentrant circuit.[23] Finally, a good understanding of atrial flutter mechanisms and ablation therapy, is in our opinion, the first but mandatory step that will really open the door to AF ablation.

References

1. Gallay P, Bertinchant JP, Lehujeur C, et al. La stimulation trans oesophagienne dans le traitement du flutter et de la tachysystolie auriculaire. *Arch Mal Coeur* 1985; 78:311–316.
2. Waldo AL, Mac Lean WAH, Karp RB, et al. Entrainment and interruption of atrial flutter with atrial pacing; Studies in man following open heart surgery. *Circulation* 1977;56:737–745.
3. Barold SS, Whyndham CRC, Kappenberger LL, et al. Implanted atrial pacemakers for paroxysmal atrial flutter. Long term efficacy. *Ann Intern Med* 1987;107: 144–149.
4. Lesser MF. Safety and efficacy of in office cardioversion for treatment of supraventricular arrhythmias. *Am J Cardiol* 1990;66:1267–1268.
5. Zipes DP. Specific arrhythmias: Diagnosis and treatment. In: Braunwald E (ed): *Heart Disease: A Textbook of Cardiovascular Medicine*. Philadelphia, PA: WB Saunders Company, 1988, pp 658–716.
6. Bianconi L, Boccadamo R, Pappalardo A, Gentili C, Pistolese M. Effectiveness of intravenous propafenone for conversion of atrial fibrillation and flutter of recent onset. *Am J Cardiol* 1989;64:335–337.
7. Suttorp MJ, Herre Kingma J, Jessurun ER, Lie-A-Huen L, Van Hemel NM. The value of class 1C antiarrhythmic drugs for acute conversion of paroxysmal atrial fibrillation or flutter to sinus rhythm. *J Am Coll Cardiol* 1990;16:1772–1777.
8. Coplen SE, Antmann EM, Berlin JA, Hewitt P, Chalmers TC. Efficacy and safety of quinidine therapy for maintaining sinus rhythm after cardioversion. *Circulation* 1990;82:1106–1116.
9. Della Bella P, Marenzi GC, Tondo C, Doni F, Lauri GF, Guazzi MD. Effect of different antiarrhythmic drugs on atrial flutter excitable gap: implications for arrhythmia termination. *Eur Heart J* 1989;10:377 (Abstract).

10. Hentl orn RW, Waldo AL, Anderson JL, et al. Flecainide acetate prevents recurrence of symptomatic supraventricular tachycardia. *Circulation* 1991;83:119–125.
11. Müller SJ, Edvardsson N, Rehnqvist-Alberg N. Sotalol versus quinidine for the maintenance of sinus rhythm after direct current cardioversion of atrial fibrillation. *Circulation* 1990;82:1932–1939.
12. Saoudi N, Mouton Schleiffer D, Cribier A, Letac B. Direct catheter fulguration of atrial flutter. *Lancet* 1987;2:568–569.
13. Saoudi N, Atallah G, Kirkorian G, Touboul P. Catheter fulguration of the atrial myocardium in human type I atrial flutter. *Circulation* 1990;81:762.
14. Puech P, Latour H, Grolleau R. Le flutter et ses limites. *Arch Mal Coeur* 1970; 61:116.
15. Cosio FG, Lopez Gil M, Arribas F, et al. Mechanisms of entrainment of human common flutter studied with multiple endocardial recordings. *Circulation* 1994; 89:2117–2125.
16. Cosio FG, Lopez Gil M, Goicolea A, et al. Radiofrequency ablation of the inferior vena cava-tricuspid valve isthmus in common atrial flutter. *Am J Cardiol* 1993; 71:705–709.
17. Feld GK, Fleck P, Peng-Shen C, et al. Radiofrequency catheter ablation for the treatment of atrial flutter. Identification of a critical zone in the reentrant circuit by endocardial mapping techniques. *Circulation* 1992;86:1233–1240.
18. Lesh Md, Van Hare GF, Epstein LM, et al. Radiofrequency catheter ablation of atrial arrhythmias: Results and mechanisms. *Circulation* 1994;89:1074–1089.
19. Calkins H, Leon AR, Deam G, et al. Catheter ablation of atrial flutter using radiofrequency energy. *Am J Cardiol* 1994;73:353–356.
20. Interian A, Cox M, Jimenez RA, et al. A shared pathway in atrioventricular nodal reentrant tachycardia and atrial flutter: Implications for pathophysiology and therapy. *Am J Cardiol* 1993;71:297–303.
21. Saoudi N, Derumeaux G, Cribier A, et al. The role of catheter ablation techniques in the treatment of classic (type I) atrial flutter. *PACE* 1991;14;2022–2027.
22. Poty H, Saoudi N, Abdel Azziz A, Nair M, Letac B. Radiofrequency catheter ablation of type I flutter. Prediction of late success by electrophysiological criteria. *Circulation* 1995;92:89–92.
23. Saoudi N, Poty H, Anselme F, Letac B. Electrocardiographic and electrophysiologic characteristics of antidromic type I atrial flutter. *PACE* 1995;18:257.

Chapter 11

Radiofrequency Current Therapy in AV Nodal Reentrant Tachycardias

Michel Haïssaguerre, MD, Dipen C. Shah, MD,
Pierre Jaïs, MD, Laurent Gencel, MD,
Mélèze Hocini, MD, Bruno Fischer, MD,
Jacques Clémenty, MD

Introduction

Atrioventricular nodal reentrant tachycardia (AVNRT) is acknowledged to be the most common form of paroxysmal supraventricular tachycardia.[1] For a long period, the only therapeutic measures included vagal maneuvers and pharmacological therapy. Nonpharmacological measures such as antitachycardia pacemakers are limited by inconsistent efficacy and the necessity of a long-duration intravascular implant. For desperate drug resistant tachycardias, surgical atrioventricular (AV) node ablation has been performed in the past, however, with the obvious disadvantages of requiring open heart surgery as well as a permanent pacemaker.

As a sequel of one such surgical attempt, Pritchett et al in 1979, noted preserved antegrade AV conduction, a prolonged PR interval and relief from the tachycardia.[2] This first inadvertent surgical ablation of the "fast pathway" showed the way for the pioneering surgical efforts of Ross et al (in skeletonizing the AV node),[3] and Cox et al (perinodal cryosurgery).[4] They established that it was possible to treat/cure AVNRT by modifying the AV node without producing AV block.

Techniques of catheter ablation developed along similar lines; DC shocks used initially to ablate the AV node were applied to the retrograde fast pathway exit site, with resultant abolition or impairment of retrograde nodal conduction and relief from tachycardia.[5] The ability of radiofrequency (RF) cur-

From *Practical Management of Cardiac Arrhythmias* edited by Nabil El-Sherif, and Jean Lekieffre. Futura Publishing Co., Armonk, NY, © 1997.

rent to produce smaller, more homogeneous and titrable lesions, allowed electrophysiologists to selectively target different segments of the reentrant circuit.[6]

Early efforts such as those of Goy et al, met with limited success,[7] while contemporary workers benefitting from previous experiences have successfully modified the AV node in > 90 % of cases.

Reentrant Circuit

There is considerable debate about anatomical delimitations, but it is generally accepted that this tachycardia is the result of a reentrant circuit in the AV junctional region.[8] Functional heterogeneity of these tissues—primarily with respect to conduction velocity, "pathway" length, and refractory periods—permits the sustenance of an excitable gap reentry circuit. Though Mendez and Moe proposed the involvement of perinodal tissue as early as 1966,[9] the strongest support for this to date has been the success of therapeutic approaches (both surgical and catheter ablation techniques), selectively directed at the atrionodal approaches.[10–15]

A contemporary view envisages at least 3 types of AVNRTs characterized by different circuits[10]: (1) slow antegrade/fast retrograde; (2) fast antegrade/slow retrograde; and (3) slow antegrade/slow retrograde. In addition to differences in conduction velocity and refractory periods, the fast and slow pathways manifest relatively disparate anterior and posterior retrograde exit sites. Recent evidence suggests the presence of multiple posteriorly situated pathways[11] or probably a network; however, there are no detectable anatomical differences in patients with AVNRT. Nonhomogeneous anisotropic conduction has therefore been hypothesized to account for such behavior.[12]

Classically, a premature impulse blocking antegradely in the fast pathway, is conducted over the slow pathway and reenters the fast pathway retrogradely. An anterior exit of this pathway from the compact AV node is thought to allow the impulse to circulate posteriorly (probably through the perinodal atrium) and enter the posterior atrionodal approach/approaches; the lower turnaround point in common typical AVNRT is considered within the compact AV node. This relatively straightforward model has been amended to involve at least one more pathway—another "slow" pathway with a posterior exit,— thus accounting for multiple reentry circuits. The term "pathway" is used in a broad sense, insomuch as no distinct pathway has ever been demonstrated. In the fast/slow form of atypical AVNRT, the impulse is thought to proceed anterogradely down the fast pathway and retrogradely up the slow pathway; the third variant (slow/slow) uses one part of the slow "network" for antegrade and another part for retrograde conduction.

Indications

Early investigators proposed catheter modification of the AV node for patients with multiple drug-resistant/refractory AVNRT; however, with present day success rates and operator experience, this may be more liberally advocated. Symptomatic patients wishing to be free of drugs or intolerant of standard drug therapy may be offered this intervention.[13] Because of the small but finite risk of AV block, the procedure should probably not be performed for initial or infrequent episodes of AVNRT.

Techniques

As alluded to above, the recognition of earliest retrograde activation at the anterosuperior tricuspid annulus (TA) during typical AVNRT allowed localization of the fast pathway exit site, and similarly retrograde activation near the posteromedial TA during fast-slow AVNRT, localized the slow pathway exit.

Techniques of AV nodal modification have therefore targeted these sites in an effort to produce selective fast or slow pathway ablation.[13]

Fast Pathway Ablation

The first report of RF energy modification of the AV node described fast pathway ablation in eight patients with modest success.[7] Since the retrograde fast pathway exit is usually located near the anterosuperior TA, this region can be localized by slow withdrawal of the catheter a few millimeters from the His bundle position[5] while concurrently applying clockwise torque to maintain good septal contact. A monitoring catheter kept in the His bundle recording position may be a convenient reference. There are no accepted electrogram markers of fast pathway activation; thus indirect parameters such as an AV electrogram amplitude ratio > 1, His deflection < 0.05 mV are used to assure relative separation from the His bundle. We have however noted localized potentials, bridging the AH interval at the site of the most proximal His deflection in some cases, and we believe that they may represent fast pathway activation (Figure 1). An alternative technique may be to utilize the site of earliest retrograde atrial activation during tachycardia—provided that a significant His bundle deflection is not recorded. Radiofrequency current applied here for a short period, usually results in PR prolongation and elimination, or marked attenuation of retrograde ventriculoatrial (VA) conduction. Frequently a junctional tachycardia is noted: requiring atrial pacing to allow monitoring of AV conduction. PR interval prolongation by > 50 % or AV block are indicators for prompt discontinuation of RF application.

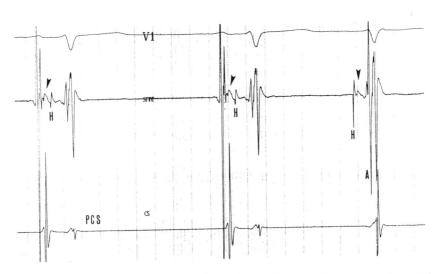

Figure 1. Possible potential of fast pathway (**arrows**) intervening between the atrial and His bundle electrograms. The third beat is junctional with the fast pathway potential now intervening between H and A potentials.

Because of the higher incidence of procedural AV blocks, a titrated delivery of RF power output has been advocated. Beginning with 10 W, the output is increased by 2 to 4 W every 10 to 15 seconds to a maximum of 30 W in the absence of PR prolongation or junctional ectopy. If the PR prolongs or junctional ectopy occurs, the power is held constant for 15 to 30 seconds or until the PR increases markedly (> 50 % or AV block). This approach has allowed selective fast pathway ablation in a group of 38 consecutive patients without complete AV block.[16]

Electrophysiological evaluation following fast pathway ablation, characteristically reveals abolition or marked attenuation of VA conduction accompanied by an increase in the AH interval and elimination of dual AV nodal physiology.[5] Data from the literature indicate that ventricular atrial (VA) conduction is eliminated in more than a third of patients while the VA block cycle length is increased in the remainder. Similarly the (atrio-Hisian) AH prolongs significantly (< 50 % in the majority) but there is no significant change in the HV interval, AV nodal effective refractory period (ERP), or anterograde Wenckebach cycle length. The shorter refractory period of the slow pathway explains the latter findings. A small group of patients undergoing fast pathway ablation lose VA conduction without elimination of dual AV node physiology or a change in AH intervals. This may represent truly selective retrograde fast pathway ablation.[17]

In about 5% of patients, fast pathway ablation can unmask a fast-slow or slow-slow variant AVNRT[18]; since this is usually inducible only with ventricular pacing with isoproterenol, it may be left alone without additional ablation or drug therapy. This phenomenon is further evidence for multiple potential pathways in the AV junction and has been used as an argument to favor slow pathway ablation.

Results

Published series[18,19] all report successful ablation in > 90% of patients. However complete AV block is the most important complication that was reported in up to 21% of patients in one series.[18] Stepwise increments in RF power application with vigilant monitoring of PR intervals and the use of atrial pacing during junctional tachycardia may avoid or reduce the incidence of this problem.[20] An important issue is the timing of AV block: while most instances are apparent during the procedure, there are reports of delayed/late complete AV block[18] (at 24 hours or later after the procedure). As a result, in-patient telemetric monitoring may be advisable for 1 to 2 days after fast pathway ablation. Lesion extension (at the edges) due to microvascular injury or cellular inflammation has been held responsible. Sporadic evidence also suggests that at late electrophysiological study, some further (minor) deterioration of parameters of antegrade AV nodal conduction may be noted. Whether this has any specific clinical connotation is presently unknown. Other complications such as deep-vein thrombosis, pulmonary embolism, or cardiac tamponade (common to any invasive intravascular procedure) are not unexpected, but infrequent.

Recurrence

From the available evidence, it is not clear whether recurrence of the tachycardia represents insufficient ablation or regeneration of the fast pathway. Clinically, the recurrence rate after fast pathway ablation is usually < 15% and most recurrences are noted within 3 months.[5] No consistent markers for recurrence have however been noted, and repeat ablation procedures are usually effective.

Slow Pathway Ablation

In analogous fashion to the fast pathway, recognition of the posterior exit of the slow pathway led to it being targeted for selective ablation. In the first published report, Roman et al described a 100% success rate in a small group of patients without any instance of complete AV block.[21] Since then, slow pathway ablation has become the therapeutic procedure of choice.[13]

Two approaches have been utilized: the anatomical and the electrophysiological approach.[22]

Anatomical fluoroscopic landmarks are used in the first approach to guide positioning of the ablation catheter. While different groups have described slightly differing target areas most of these are either near the junction of the mid- and posterior thirds of the medial interatrial septum, at the level of the TA or in the vicinity of coronary sinus ostium (CSO). An A:V ratio of 0.5 or < 1 is desirable and RF energy is delivered (beginning at more posterior areas) for 60 to 90 seconds. This is followed by electrophysiological assessment of the slow pathway and attempted induction of AVNRT. If unsuccessful, subsequent pulses are applied closer to the AV node (i.e., more anteriorly). Although some authors have described a direct mid-septal approach[23] with good results, we believe that the most posterior successful ablation site is the safest.

The other approach utilizes the mapping of earliest atrial activation during retrograde slow pathway conduction (during fast/slow AVNRT or ventricular pacing), and is limited by difficulty in inducing consistent retrograde slow pathway conduction adequate for precise mapping. The bulk of the published experience suggests that this is possible only in a minority of patients.[19] Thus, this approach, in spite of its sound pathophysiological basis is infrequently used. More commonly, however, characteristic electrograms considered representative of slow pathway conduction have been used to guide RF energy application. Two distinct morphologies of slow pathway potentials have been described.

Jackman et al described a sharp spike-like "Asp" potential preceded by a lower frequency, lower amplitude A potential during sinus rhythm.[24] Asp usually follows A after 10 to 40 msec and these double potentials are recorded in the vicinity of the CSO close to the TA. The electrophysiological behavior of these potentials is characteristic of signals with a different origin. During retrograde conduction over the slow pathway (fast-slow AVNRT, reverse ventricular echo beats, or ventricular pacing with retrograde block in the fast pathway) the sequence of these double potentials is reversed (i.e., Asp now precedes A). Moreover, we have also shown that atrial stimulation at different sites in sinus rhythm alters the relationship of the two components[25] (Figure 2). Radiofrequency current applied at the site recording the sharpest, longest, and latest Asp potential close to the TA (small A, large V) successfully eliminated AVNRT in 99% of patients (with only one instance of AV block). Significant attenuation of the Asp potential was noted after successful RF application in some cases. The same group observed such potentials in 98% of a cohort without AVNRT as well.

Experimental work in pigs and dogs correlating intracellular and extracellular recordings has established that similar double potentials are produced by asynchronous activation of muscle bundles flanking the mouth of the coronary sinus. These cells appear histologically to be atrial and intracellular recordings

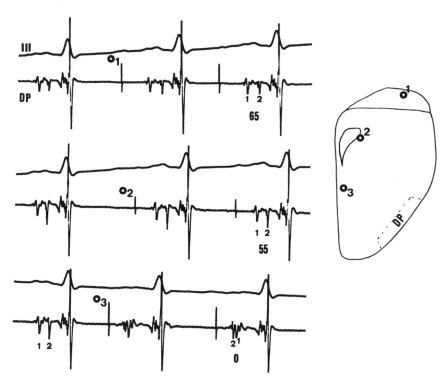

Figure 2. The effect of pacing from different sites in the right atrium (RA) on double potentials recorded near the coronary sinus ostium. Top trace depicts an interspike interval of 65 msec during pacing from the high RA (❸ 1) which is longer than in sinus rhythm. Middle trace: the interspike interval remains the same (55 msec, as in sinus rhythm) during pacing from the region of the sinus node (❸ 2). With pacing from the low RA, spike potential 2 precedes potential 1 and both nearly fuse. The lower the site of pacing, the greater the anticipation of the second spike (not shown) leading to reversal of the double potential sequence. This behavior is characteristic of different functional tracts originating from the sinus region and activating potentials 1 and 2. DP = double potentials.

indicate a rapid upstroke potential (phase 0) without decremental behavior during stimulation. Such potentials therefore appear to be markers for the region between the coronary sinus orifice and the TA.[26]

In contrast to the dominant high frequency content of the foregoing potentials, we described low amplitude low frequency signals.[27] These potentials are characteristically concealed within or follow the atrial electrogram and can occupy some or all of the AV interval in sinus rhythm. Requiring high amplification (0.1 to 0.2 mV/cm), they are readily recorded by withdrawing the catheter posteriorly from the His bundle position. They may be uni-phasic, biphasic or like a double hump, but in the posterior septum they are usually hump shaped, while more anteriorly they are rapid, less broad, often biphasic and with a superimposed His bundle deflection. It is uncommon to record such slow potentials posterior to the ostium of the coronary sinus and they are most typical at the junction of the anterior two-third and the posterior one-third of the area between the His bundle and the coronary sinus ostium. They are also recordable in the majority of patients without AVNRT (16/20 of a control group). While the potentials described by Jackman et al,[24] are not altered morphologically by atrial pacing, these slow potentials typically separate from within already complex and fractionated atrial electrograms with pacing (Figure 3), prolong in duration and decline in amplitude. They

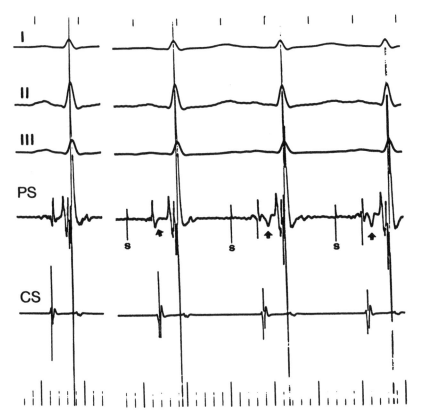

Figure 3. A slow potential **(arrows)** totally concealed within the atrial electrogram is revealed by rapid atrial pacing. PS = posterior septum; CS = coronary sinus; S = stimulus artifact.

Table 1

Differences in the Potentials Utilized in Slow Pathway Mapping

	Slow Potentials	Spike Potentials
Anatomical location	Generally mid- and posteroseptal	Generally posteroseptal
Prevalence in humans	100%	85%
Morphology	High then slow frequency double potential	Low then high frequency double potential
Electrophysiological behavior is characteristic:		
site of atrial pacing	No alteration (sometimes inversion of polarity)	Increase, or fuse, or reverse the double potential sequence
rate of atrial pacing	Separation from atrial electrogram Attenuation then disappearance of slow potentials	No change (in rare cases, the spike potential can be dissociated)
micro-electrode recording	Presence of a plateau Decremental property	Sharp action potential No decremental property
Origin	Superficial transitional cells Lack of connexin 43	Atrial cells

fractionate and disappear at rapid pacing rates so that they are not discernable during tachycardia. The differences between these two potentials are summarized in Table 1.

Guided by slow potentials, we successfully eliminated AVNRT in all 64 patients without AV block. Correlative animal studies using simultaneous intra and extracellular recordings, indicate that such low frequency signals coincide with the activation of cells around the TA, possessing AV node-like properties—including adenosine responsiveness and lack of connexin 43. During reverse ventricular echoes these cells are activated before earliest atrial activation during retrograde slow pathway, but fail to be activated during antegrade conduction over the fast pathway.[28] Because they may be recorded over a relatively wide area, such low frequency signals might in some instances represent activation of dead-end pathways.[29]

Evaluation after successful ablation indicated an increase in the antegrade AV block cycle length and in the AV nodal refractory period without a change in the AH interval or retrograde conduction. The maximum AH interval during incremental atrial pacing is also characteristically curtailed.[27] However there is evidence of residual slow pathway function in approximately 50% of patients with persistent antegrade AV nodal duality and/or single AV nodal echoes. AVNRT nevertheless remains noninducible, even with an infusion of isoproterenol.

Results

Comparisons of the anatomical and the electrogram mapping approach have not been systematically performed but success rates and complications (i.e., AV block) are reported to be similar, although more applications of RF energy appear to be necessary with the anatomical approach.[22] The only prospective randomized study comparing the two approaches, demonstrated that the successful site with both approaches possessed more "complex" electrograms, and suggested that in some patients the effective target site may be outside the area of the anatomical approach, requiring electrogram mapping for successful ablation.[30] Our experience of slow pathway ablation guided by slow potentials (until August 1995) in 364 patients is detailed in Table 2.

Complete AV block during slow pathway ablation is definitely uncommon, but since inadvertent fast pathway ablation has been posterior, it is important to monitor the PR interval during RF application.[30]

Table 2
Slow Pathway Ablation for AVNRT: Experience in 364 Patients
(Until August 1995)

No. of RF applications: one in 55%, one or two in 75%

Outcome: 1 AV block
          2 failures
          361 successes

          Recurrences
          ╱   ╲
2% with slow   6% with slow
pathway ablation   pathway modification

Our experience of slow pathway ablation using radiofrequency current in 364 patients. Using the slow potential guided approach, 75% of patients required only one or two applications of RF energy for successful ablation.

Avoiding AV Block During Slow Pathway Ablation

In our experience, a careful search for the most posterior site (between the His bundle and the CSO) with typical slow potentials is an important prerequisite. Needless to say, a His deflection must not be recordable at the site; moreover, we believe that hump-like or biphasic potentials occurring towards the end of the AV interval and persisting during rapid atrial pacing represent nodal potentials and therefore sites with such electrograms should also be avoided (Figure 4).

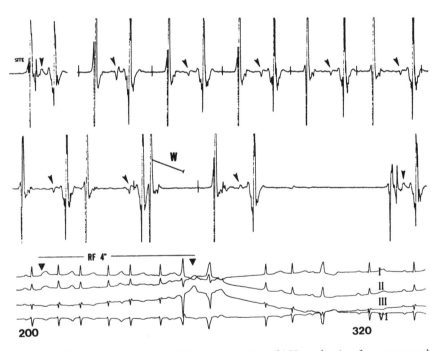

Figure 4. This patient was referred for interruption of AV conduction for paroxysmal atrial fibrillation. Nodal potentials **(arrowheads)** and the effect of applying RF energy at such a site are shown. The biphasic potential occuring progressively later in the A-V interval and persisting at rapid rates (except with one blocked atrial impulse [W]) is representative of potentials arising from the AV node. In the panel below, RF energy (10 watts) is applied at this site for 4 seconds producing a prolongation of the PR interval (from 200 to 320 msec).

Successful ablation of the slow pathway is associated with junctional ectopy at 70% to 90 % of effective sites and atrial mapping indicates that the ectopy originates in the AV node, not from the site of slow pathway ablation.[31] It is important to monitor VA conduction during such rhythms with right atrial electrograms—especially if the junctional rhythm is rapid. Junctional tachycardia with a faster rate and VA block has been recognized as a useful marker of impending AV block.[32] If in doubt, it may be wise to stop RF energy delivery to check the PR interval during sinus rhythm and if necessary to continue during overdrive atrial pacing. AV block may occur with only a few seconds of RF energy application and therefore in such situations, gradual titration of power/temperature is recommended; if AV block does occur, early recovery of AV conduction (< 2 to 3 minutes) bodes a good prognosis. In any event, even transient abnormalities of AV conduction probably mandate rhythm monitoring for several days.

Two to six percent of patients in our experience develop a recurrence after successful slow pathway ablation (see Figure 3) and this occurs more frequently in case of persistent slow pathway function after ablation. This does not justify pursuit of complete slow pathway ablation provided that no tachycardia is inducible; even with isoproterenol. In our opinion, it is probably physiologically better to succeed with preservation of at least a part of the slow network.

Fast or Slow Pathway Ablation?

Our experience and that of others, indicates a lower incidence of complete AV block with slow pathway ablation. This makes slow pathway ablation the preferred approach for curing AVNRT, primarily because of the larger margin of safety. Slow pathway ablation also does not result in the prolongation of the PR interval, and allows the monitoring of VA conduction during junctional ectopic activity to warn of impending AV block. Fast pathway ablation has however been advocated when the slow pathway approach is ineffective or when the efficacy of slow pathway ablation is difficult to assess because induction of AVNRT is not reproducible.[33] Successful fast pathway ablation can be rapidly assessed by checking VA conduction during ventricular pacing.

Atypical AVNRT ("Fast-slow" and "Slow-slow"AVNRT)[10,11]

Fast-slow and slow-slow AVNRT are both characterized by earliest retrograde atrial activation during tachycardia near the CSO. The AH:HA ratio is < 1 in fast-slow tachycardias but may be > 1 for some slow-slow tachycardias. The PR/RP relationships vary accordingly. However, these tachycardias are clinically uncommon (< 10 %) and the limited available clinical data suggests that slow pathway ablation is the treatment of choice. It is important to note that uncommon or fast-slow AVNRT is more readily induced by ventricular extrastimulation. The long RP relationship makes it necessary to rule out both a concealed accessory pathway, participating in an orthodromic tachycardia as well as atrial tachycardia. Also, a slow-slow tachycardia may sometimes mimic a typical slow-fast AVNRT in case of a delay in conduction (possibly along the lower common pathway). This has been termed a pseudo slow-fast AVNRT.

In a study of 15 cases of atypical AVNRT, we have found evidence which may indicate an accessory atrionodal pathway.[34] In half of these patients, we found a very localized spike potential (much smaller than the Jackman spike) during mapping of the retrograde atrial activation site (Figure 5); this could

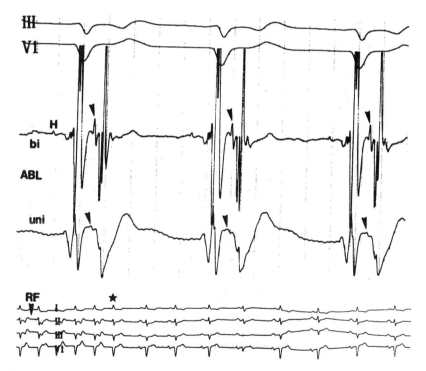

Figure 5. During atypical AVNRT (a variant of slow-slow AVNRT with an AH > HA) the bipolar electrogram at the site of ablation reveals a spike potential preceding atrial activation. This is associated with initial positivity on the simultaneous unipolar electrogram recorded from the distal electrode (see text). In the lower panel, RF energy applied at the site terminates the tachycardia by producing a retrograde block (*). Note the absence of junctional rhythm.

be traced for a few millimeters posteriorly from the AV node and in two cases, dissociated from the local atrial electrogram. On the unipolar electrogram, the spike potential was associated with initial positivity, suggesting a discrete. Moreover, successful RF delivery at the site was not associated with junctional ectopy, and parameters of antegrade slow pathway conduction remained unchanged after successful ablation. These features in our opinion warrant consideration of atrionodal fibers.

Conclusion

Radiofrequency current catheter ablation has evolved into a well-accepted, established, and low-risk modality for treatment of AVNRT. Because of the lesser risk of AV block, slow pathway ablation is the preferred approach. Both the anatomical and potentially guided approaches appear to be equally efficacious, but the electrophysiological approach is more anatomical in terms of RF applications.

References

1. Josephson ME, Wellens HJJ. Differential diagnosis of supraventricular tachycardia. *Cardiol Clin* 1990;8(3):411–442.
2. Pritchett LC, Anderson RR, Benditt DG, et al. Reentry within the atrioventricular node: surgical cure with preservation of atrioventricular conduction. *Circulation* 1979;60:440–446.
3. Ross DL, Johnson DC, Denniss AR, et al. Curative surgery for atrioventricular junctional ("AV nodal") reentrant tachycardia. *J Am Coll Cardiol* 1985;6: 1383–1392.
4. Cox JL, Holman WL, Cain ME. Cryosurgical treatment of atrioventricular node reentrant tachycardia. *Circulation* 1987;73:1329–1336.
5. Haïssaguerre M, Warin JF, Le Métayer P, et al. Closed-chest ablation of retrograde conduction in patients with atrioventricular nodal reentrant tachycardias. *N Engl J Med* 1989;320:426–433.
6. Wittkampf FHM, Hauer RNW, Robles de Medina EO. Control of radiofrequency lesion size by power regulation. *Circulation* 1989;80:962–968.
7. Goy JJ, Fromer M, Schlaepfer J, et al. Clinical efficacy of radiofrequency current in the treatment of patients with atrioventricular node reentrant tachycardia. *J Am Coll Cardiol* 1990;16:418–423.
8. McGuire MA, Janse MJ. New insights on anatomical location of components of the reentrant circuit and ablation therapy for atrioventricular junctional reentrant tachycardia. *Curr Opin Cardiol* 1995;10:3–8.
9. Mendez C, Moe GK. Demonstration of a dual A-V nodal conduction system in the isolated rabbit heart. *Circ Res* 1966;19:378–393.
10. Jackman WM, Nakagawa H, Heidbuchel H, et al. Three forms of atrioventricular nodal (junctional) reentrant tachycardia: differential diagnosis, electrophysiological characteristics and implications for anatomy of the reentrant circuit. In: Zipes D, Jalife JJ, (eds): *Cardiac Electrophysiology: From Cell to the Bedside*, 2nd edition. 1995, pp 620–637.

11. Wu D, Yeh S, Wang C, et al. Double loop figure-of-8 reentry as the mechanism of multiple atrioventricular node reentry tachycardias. *Am Heart J* 1994;127:83–95.
12. Spach MS, Josephson ME. Initiating reentry: the role of non uniform anisotropy in small circuits. *J Cardiovasc Electrophysiol* 1994;5:182–209.
13. Akhtar M, Jazayeri MR, Sra J, et al: Atrioventricular nodal reentry : Clinical, electrophysiological and therapeutic considerations. *Circulation* 1993;88:282–295.
14. Janse MJ, Anderson RH, McGuire MA, et al. "AV nodal" reentry: Part I : "AV nodal" reentry revisited. *J Cardiovasc Electrophysiol* 1993;4:561–572.
15. McGuire MA, Janse MJ, Ross DL. "AV nodal" reentry: Part II : AV nodal, AV junctional or atrionodal reentry? *J Cardiovasc Electrophysiol* 1993;4:573–586.
16. Langberg JJ, Harvey M, Calkins H, et al. Titration of power output during radiofrequency catheter ablation of atrioventricular nodal reentrant tachycardia. *PACE* 1993;16:465–470.
17. Wu D, Yeh S, Chieh, et al. Nature of dual atrioventricular node pathways and the tachycardia circuit as defined by radiofrequency ablation technique. *J Am Coll Cardiol* 1992;20:884–895.
18. Jazayeri MR, Hempe SL, Sra JS, et al. Selective transcatheter ablation of the fast and slow pathways using radiofrequency energy in patients with atrioventricular nodal reentrant tachycardia. *Circulation* 1992;85:1318–1328.
19. Calkins H, Sousa J, El-Atassi R, et al. Diagnosis and cure of the Wolff-Parkinson-White syndrome or paroxysmal supraventricular tachycardias during a single electrophysiologic test. *N Engl J Med* 1991;324:1612–1618.
20. Kottkamp H, Hindricks G, Willerns S, et al. An anatomically and electrogram guided stepwise approach for effective and safe catheter ablation of the fast pathway for elimination of atrioventricular node reentrant tachycardia. *J Am Coll Cardiol* 1995;25:974–981.
21. Roman CA, Wang X, Friday KJ, et al. Catheter technique for selective ablation of slow pathway in AV nodal reentrant tachycardia. *PACE* 1990;13:498 (Abstract).
22. Haïssaguerre M, Fischer B, Marcus FI, et al. Role of catheter ablation for treatment of supraventricular tachyarrhythmias. In: Mandel WJ (ed): *Cardiac Arrhythmias*, 3rd edition. Philadelphia: JB Lippincott Company, 1995;939–962.
23. Epstein LM, Lesh MD, Griffin JC, et al. A direct midseptal approach to slow atrioventricular nodal pathway ablation. *PACE* 1995;18(I):57–64.
24. Jackman WM, Beckman KJ, McClelland JH, et al. Treatment of supraventricular tachycardia due to atrioventricular nodal reentry by radiofrequency catheter ablation of slow pathway conduction. *N Engl J Med* 1992;327:313–318.
25. Haïssaguerre M, Fischer B, Le Métayer P, et al. Double potentials recorded during sinus rhythm in the triangle of Koch. Evidence for functional dissociation from pacing of various right atrial sites. *PACE* 1993;16(II)10–1101 (Abstract).
26. McGuire MA, de Bakker JMT, Vermeulen JT, Opthof T, et al. Origin and significance of double potentials near the atrioventricular node. Correlation of intracellular potentials and histology. *Circulation* 1994;89:2351–2360.
27. Haïssaguerre M, Gaita F, Fischer B, et al. Elimination of atrioventricular nodal reentrant tachycardia using discrete slow potentials to guide application of radiofrequency energy. *Circulation* 1992;85:2162–2175.
28. McGuire MA, Loh P, de Bakker JMT, et al. Atrioventricular junctional tissue—discrepancy between histological and electrophysiological characteristics. *Circulation* 1996;94:571–577.
29. De Bakker JMT, Coronel R, McGuire MA, et al. Slow potentials in the atrioven-

tricular junctional area of patients operated on for atrioventricular node tachycardias and in isolated porcine hearts. *J Am Coll Cardiol* 1994;23:709–715.

30. Kalbfleisch SJ, Strickberger SA, Williamson B, et al. Randomized comparison of anatomic and electrogram mapping approaches to ablation of the slow pathway of atrioventricular node reentrant tachycardia. *J Am Coll Cardiol* 1994;23:716–723.

31. Boyle NG, Zardini M, Monahan KM, et al. Origin of junctional rhythm during radiofrequency ablation for atrioventricular nodal reentrant tachycardia. *Circulation* 1994;90:1157 (Abstract).

32. Thakur RK, Klein GJ, Yee R, et al. Junctional tachycardia: a useful marker during radiofrequency ablation for atrioventricular node reentrant tachycardia. *J Am Coll Cardiol* 1993;22:1706–1710.

33. Morady F. Fast pathway ablation for atrioventricular node reentrant tachycardia. *J Am Coll Cardiol* 1995:25:982–983 (Editorial Comment).

34. Haïssaguerre M, Coromilas J, Poquet F, et al. Observations suggesting the involvement of an atrionodal tract-like structure in atypical AV junctional reentrant tachycardia (AVJRT). *PACE* 1995;18:819 (Abstract).

Chapter 12

Radiofrequency Ablation of Atrioventricular Accessory Pathways: Respective Value of Unipolar and Bipolar Recording Modes

Nicolas Sadoul, MD, Christian de Chillou, MD, Etienne Aliot, MD

Introduction

For many years, the sole therapeutic options for patients suffering from arrhythmias due to atrioventricular (AV) accessory pathways were antiarrhythmic drugs or surgery. Surgery, despite its high success rate, its low morbidity and mortality, has been increasingly abandoned due to the advent of ablation techniques, especially with the advent of radiofrequency (RF) energy. Since the early 1990s, RF catheter ablation has become the nonpharmacological therapy of choice for patients with symptomatic accessory pathway-mediated tachycardias.[1-3]

In experienced hands, the success rate appears to be considerably above 90%, independently of the location of the accessory pathway. Serious complications such as tamponade due to myocardial perforation, or coronary artery spasm are rare. The incidence of death related to the procedure appears to be under 0.5%.[4-6]

Several reviews on the subject of RF ablation of AV accessory pathways have been recently published.[4,5,7] In this chapter, after a short technical account, we will mainly focus on the respective value of unipolar and bipolar recording modes to determine the optimal ablation site, based on our experience of 250 accessory pathway ablations.

From *Practical Management of Cardiac Arrhythmias* edited by Nabil El-Sherif, and Jean Lekieffre. Futura Publishing Co., Armonk, NY, © 1997.

Technical Account

Conventional electrophysiological (EP) studies and ablation of accessory pathways are usually performed as a single procedure.

The first part of the EP study is always dedicated to: (1) the identification of the mechanism of the clinical tachycardia; and (2) the confirmation that the APs are part of the reentrant circuit. The second part of the procedure is dedicated to the accurate mapping of the accessory pathway, which is the key to success. A steerable catheter with a large-tip electrode is used for mapping.[4,5]

The conventional EP catheters that were first used for ablation had a low success rate. The development of new catheters is largely responsible for the improvement and the widespread use of ablation techniques. These 5- to 7-French ablation catheters have a steerable distal platinum electrode, 4 mm in length. This steerability improves their maneuverability around the tricuspid and the mitral annuli. Several types of catheters, with varying radius of curvature and varying temperature profiles are now available.[8] For example, catheters capable of rotation and deflection are used to ablate left-sided accessory pathways. In contrast, catheters with a bigger dumb-bell shaped distal electrode which allows the delivery of higher energy, and which facilitates the positioning and the stability on the tricuspid annulus are used for ablating right free-wall accessory pathways.

This greater size of tip allows higher energy to be applied (25 to 50 W) without an increase in impedance and consequent lack of coagulum formation.

The primary cause of tissue injury induced by RF is heat generated at the electrode tissue interfact. The size of the lesion is related to: (1) the power and total energy delivered; (2) the area of contact between the distal electrode and the tissue; (3) the electrode-tissue impedance; and (4) the type of electrode used.

The choice of the initial energy remains rather empirical. However, it is accepted that a minimum temperature of 45°C and a mean temperature of 62°C are mandatory to produce tissue injury and destroy the accessory pathway. On the other hand, temperatures > 95° to 100°C produce boiling and a rise in impedance which causes the generator to automatically terminate RF delivery. For this reason, most of the currently available catheters and RF generators are temperature controlled to modulate energy delivery. This temperature control is obtained via a thermistor or a thermocouple located at the distal tip of the ablation catheter. The highest temperature which does not lead to impedance rise is generally used. When the ablation electrode is positioned in a region where the blood flow is limited, such as the coronary sinus or below the mitral valve, the heat loss by convection is reduced. These catheter positions are therefore the most prone to impedance rise, even when limited energy deliveries ($<$ 30 W) are applied. In contrast, when the ablation catheter is positioned on the tricuspid annulus or on the atrial aspect of the mitral valve, the risk of impedance rise is limited, even when high energies are used (50 W).

In most cases, RF delivery is discontinued when preexcitation (or retrograde conduction in the case of concealed accessory pathways) fails to be eliminated soon ($<$ 10 seconds) after the onset of energy. However, it is prolonged to 30 or 60 seconds when preexcitation (or retrograde conduction) disappears early ($<$ 10 seconds). Monitoring of impedance, current, and voltage during RF delivery are mandatory. Radiofrequency generators are preprogrammed to automatically discontinue RF delivery in the event of impedance rise or decrease in current. Current commercially available RF generators have a feedback loop that maintains the distal ablation electrode at a fixed pre-selected temperature (below the boiling point) in order to avoid coagulum formation. However, temperature measurement at the tip of the ablation catheter may not accurately reflect the temperature at the electrode-tissue interface when the contact between the electrode and the tissue is poor.[5]

Predictive Value of the Different Electrogram Parameters in Determining the Optimal Ablation Site

While the serious complications due to RF ablation remain rare, the long-term effects of RF delivery on the myocardium are unclear. It is therefore important to limit the number of RF deliveries during ablation procedures. This requires accurate mapping of the AV groove in order to determine the "optimal" ablation site. Several electrogram characteristics have been described.[5,7]

In the case of an overt accessory pathway, careful mapping is performed in order to determine the ventricular insertion site of the accessory pathway. This ventricular insertion site is characterized by: (1) a short AV interval; (2) a local ventricular electrogram preceding the delta wave on the surface electrocardiogram (ECG); and (3) the presence of an accessory pathway potential located between the atrial and the ventricular electrograms. In addition, ablation on the ventricular insertion site of an accessory pathway requires the presence of an atrial electrogram with a small amplitude associated with a large ventricular electrogram (Figure 1).

The shortest possible AV conduction time on preexcited beats is one of the most commonly used parameters to identify the optimal ablation site. While "long" AV intervals ($>$ 50 msec from peak to peak) are nearly always predictive of failure, "short" AV intervals are not always predictive of success.[5,7] Indeed, in our experience, this parameter used in isolation has a low

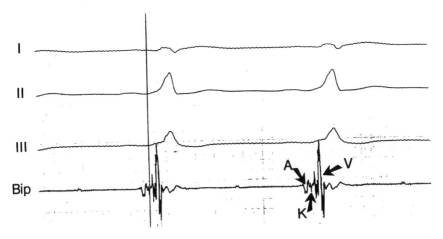

Figure 1. Ablation of a left free-wall accessory pathway. Bipolar electrogram recorded at the mitral annulus. A: atrial potential; V: ventricular potential; and K: possible accessory pathway potential. Note the small amplitude of A (ablation catheter positioned on the ventricular site) and the continuous electrical activity. The vertical line is inscribed at the beginning of the delta wave on the 12-lead ECG.

positive predictive value, even though some authors consider this parameter as the one with the highest predictive value.[9]

Localizing the ventricular site of the insertion of the accessory pathway is also obtained by measuring the interval between the ventricular electrogram, and the beginning of the delta wave on the surface ECG (V-delta). The degree of prematurity of the ventricular electrograms depends on the location of the accessory pathway. The shortest V delta intervals are observed with right free wall and right anteroseptal (negative V-delta), as compared to left free-wall accessory pathways (V-delta close to zero).

The recording of an accessory pathway potential is a precise marker of a successful ablation site. However, the validation of such an accessory pathway potentials is long and difficult (Figure 1). For this reason, an accessory pathway potential is often defined in the literature as: (1) "probable" if the accessory pathway deflection precedes the onset of the QRS complex and is distinct from the atrial and ventricular components of the local electrogram; and (2) as "possible" if the accessory pathway deflection precedes the onset of the QRS complex and merges with the atrial or ventricular components of the local electrogram.[10] This potential is considered by many authors as a parameter with a particularly high predictive value of success.[10-15] However, the lack of concordance in its recognition by blinded observers probably explains why its specificity is low.[12]

Localizing the atrial insertion site of the accessory pathway requires orthodromic reciprocating tachycardia (ORT) or ventricular pacing. This site is defined by the shortest ventriculoatrial (VA) time (and hence the earliest atrial activation). An accessory pathway potential can sometimes be found within the VA interval. However, in most cases, continuous electrical activity is recorded.[5,10,12] When ventricular pacing is performed, the possibility of fusion between retrograde conduction via the AV node and retrograde conduction via the accessory pathway must be taken into account. In the case of a concealed accessory pathway, only the atrial site of the accessory pathway can be identified since there is no delta wave (and no anterograde conduction) on the surface ECG. Finally, in the case of an overt accessory pathway, Fisher and Swartz[16] have recently proposed, using unipolar recordings, the reversal of the atrial electrogram polarity as the catheter passed the atrial insertion site as a parameter to localize the site for ablation.

Finally, the stability of the ablation catheter is another important predictor of success. It is determined by the stability of 3 to 5 consecutive local electrograms as well as by the movement of the catheter seen on fluoroscopy.

In conclusion, the reduction in the number of energy deliveries and of total energy delivered, requires accurate mapping in order to determine the "optimal" ablation site. Several authors have reported, based on bipolar recordings, the electrogram parameters predictive of RF ablation outcome.[9–11,14,17,18] However, the exclusive use of such bipolar recordings is hampered by several limitations: (1) the morphology of the electrogram wave depends on interelectrode distance; (2) the accurate determination of local activation times based on peak electrogram deflection can be ambiguous and inaccurate due to the frequent occurrence of polyphasic electrograms (Figures 2 and 3); and (3) low frequency responses are entirely lost with the use of a high pass filter. For all these reasons, we consider that bipolar recordings have a poor reproducibility in determining the optimal ablation site.

In a recent study from our department, three blinded observers have analyzed 233 bipolar electrograms.[19] The reproducibility of the measurements was poor, because only 50% of the intervals (AoVo, AaVa, V-delta) were measured within a 10-msec margin. From this study, it appears that the most reproducible interval is AoVo (from the onset of the A wave to the onset of the V wave), whereas the least reproducible interval is V-delta. In our opinion, this poor reproducibility is a major limiting factor in the use of bipolar recordings to determine the optimal ablation site.

According to Calkins et al,[10] the best predictors of outcome are: (1) the electrogram stability; (2) the presence of an accessory pathway potential; (3) the interval between activation of the local ventricular electrogram and the onset of the QRS complex (V-delta) in the case of an overt accessory pathway;

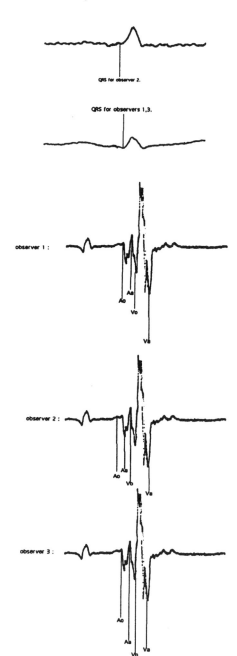

Figure 2. Simultaneous recordings of the endocardial bipolar electrogram and leads I and II immediately prior to RF delivery. This is an example of poor interobserver reproducibility in defining the onset of the atrial electrogram (Ao), or the local atrial activity (Aa), or the onset of the ventricular electrogram (Vo) or the local ventricular activity (Va) or the beginning of the delta wave on the surface ECG among the three blinded observers.

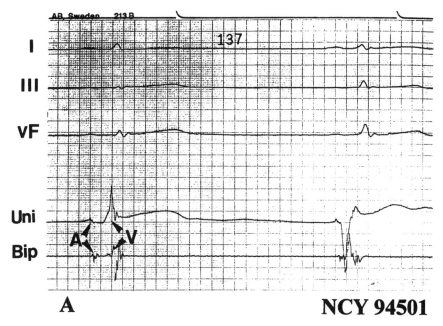

Figure 3. Example of the difficulty in separating atrial (A) activity from ventricular (V) activity due to continuous electrical activity between A and V. Electrograms recorded during the ablation of an intermittent left free-wall accessory pathways with minor preexcitation. The intermittent block in the accessory pathway allows to precisely determine the beginning of the ventricular activation on the unipolar and bipolar recordings. **A:** paper speed = 100 mm/s on the left, the ventricular complex is not preexcited while it is preexcited on the right. Note the different aspect in the unipolar and the bipolar recording modes.

and (4) the presence of continuous electrical activity in the case of a concealed accessory pathway. In a multivariate analysis, Bashir et al[17] reported that the V-delta interval and the presence of a possible accessory pathway potential were the only independent factors predictive of success. The requirement for both of these 2 factors decreased the sensitivity but did not increase the positive predictive value to above 25%. According to Silka et al,[9] the best bipolar predictive parameter of success is a local AV interval < 40 msec. For several other authors, the best predictive parameter of success is the presence of an accessory pathway potential with a positive predictive value ranging from 35% to 82%.[10–12,14,15] These differences may be explained by the use of different ablation catheters with an interelectrode distance, ranging from 2 to 5 mm in these studies as well as by the difficulty in validating the accessory potential.

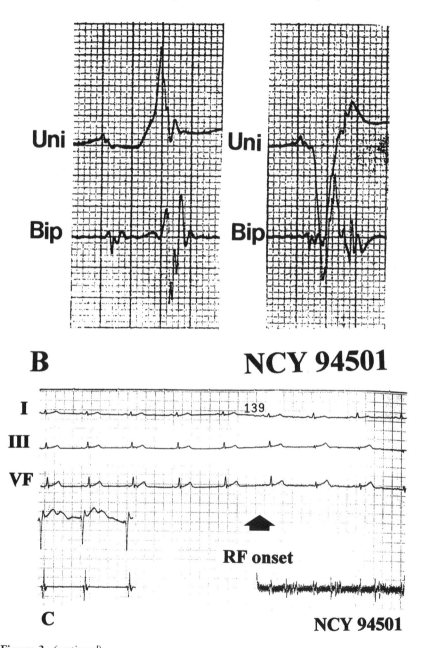

Figure 3. *(continued)*
B: enlargement of the endocardial electrograms from Figure 3A. **C:** radiofrequency delivery is associated with an immediate block in the accessory pathway.

Unipolar Recordings

The lack of reproducibility in the interpretation of bipolar electrograms, and the difficulty in accurately determining the onset of the delta wave has lead some authors to use unfiltered unipolar electrograms[13,14] (Figures 3 and 4).

Unlike bipolar recordings, unipolar electrograms provide a recording directly from the distal electrode of the ablation catheter which is used to deliver energy. The use of the intrinsic deflection of the unipolar electrogram gives more precise local activation timing (especially for the ventricle) than bipolar recordings. Unipolar recordings also allow in combination with bipolar recordings, a separation of the atrial and the ventricular components when continuous electrical activity is recorded. Following Spach's experimental studies,[20] Gallagher[21] has clearly shown that it is possible to define the accessory pathway location by the morphology of the unipolar ventricular electrogram. A purely negative QS pattern indicates proximity of the ventricular activation origin, whereas, an rS pattern (with a clear positive initial deflection) in the unipolar ventricular waveform indicates the presence of myocardial tissue between the recording electrode and the origin of ventricular excitation. However, an rS pattern at a successful ablation site has been described in some left free-wall accessory pathways suggesting an oblique course of the pathway.

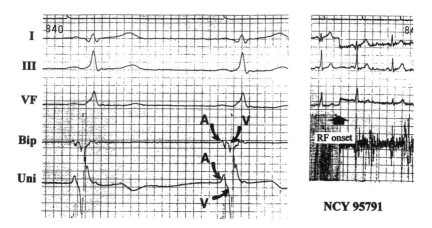

Figure 4. Unipolar and bipolar electrogram recorded immediately prior to a successful ablation of a left free-wall accessory pathway. Utility of the unipolar recording associated with the bipolar recording. In the bipolar mode, there is no continuous electrical activity with an AV interval measuring 50 msec. In unipolar mode, the AV interval is shorter.

Using unipolar recordings, Simmers et al have defined two multivariate models.[13] The first model (Model I) employing the 3 following parameters: accessory pathway potential; AV interval (; 30 ms; and catheter stability was associated with a prediction of successful ablation of 76%. The second model (Model II) employing the 3 following parameters: initial ventricular positivity (1) 0.1 mV; AV interval; (2) 0.1 mV; AV interval, and (3) 30 msec and catheter stability was associated with a prediction of successful ablation of 63%. Furthermore, as the catheter tip moves toward the insertion site, the progressive decrease of the positive initial deflection of the QRS complex as well as the progressive shortening of the AV interval, provides dynamic criteria to determine the optimal ablation site. Finally, Haïssaguerre et al recommend avoiding RF delivery when the initial R wave of the unipolar recording is > 0.1 mV. For this author, although the accessory pathway potential is best seen with bipolar recordings, unipolar recordings allow the validation of accessory pathway potentials in most cases.[5,7,14]

In another retrospective study from our department, three blinded observers studied 147 unipolar and bipolar electrograms recorded simultaneously, and immediately before RF delivery. This study showed that the sensitivity of unipolar recordings was not statistically different from that of bipolar recordings. However, the specificity of unipolar recordings was higher than that of bipolar recordings. Our results suggest that the use of unipolar recordings allows a more accurate determination of inappropriate sites, thus decreasing the number of unsuccessful RF deliveries.[22] However, it should be emphasized that the decision to deliver energy should not be made exclusively on the basis of the morphology of the electrograms. Other parameters, such as the ablation catheter position, its stability during fluoroscopy, and the changes in the electrogram during small movements of the ablation catheter (especially changes in ventricular depolarization) must also be taken into account.

Improved mapping techniques are required in order to increase the predictive value of electrograms. One of the major limitations of studies devoted to electrogram criteria predictive of ablation success, is that accessory pathways are considered as a uniform entity with a statistical analysis applied only to the electrogram recordings. Other variables, such as the anatomy of the AV groove, the geometry and the location of the accessory pathway, as well as the orientation of the ablation catheter in relation to the accessory pathway should also be considered.

Specific Considerations According to Accessory Pathway Location

Accessory pathways have an atrial insertion and a ventricular insertion. Although right-sided accessory pathways are found to be more vulnerable at their atrial insertion site, generally, while left-sided accessory pathways are more vulnerable at their ventricular insertion[23]; in practice, ablation may be successfully performed at either site.

Left "Free-Wall" Accessory Pathways

These pathways represent a fairly uniform entity, allowing a systematic approach. Their locations may be anterior, lateral, or posterior. They have a particularly localized ventricular insertion site and are mainly subendocardial. A multielectrode EP catheter located in the coronary sinus facilitates the localization of these accessory pathways and is often used as a fluoroscopic reference. However, some experienced authors recommend ablation with a single catheter technique[24] which can only be used for an overt accessory pathway. The placement of the ablation catheter within the left ventricle, high against the mitral annulus, is verified by the recording of an atrial potential of at least 25% of the amplitude of the ventricular potential. Correct positioning is confirmed by the recording of an accessory pathway potential. However, this technique has several limitations: (1) the validation of the accessory pathway potential is impossible; (2) the presence of retrograde conduction cannot be tested at the end of the procedure; and (3) the mechanism of any inducible tachycardia following successful ablation cannot be determined. However, in experienced hands, this technique appears to be highly effective, and decreases fluoroscopy time and hence radiation exposure. Most centers use the conventional arterial retrograde approach, but some centers prefer to employ the transseptal approach. Each technique has its advantages and drawbacks. The potential advantages of the retrograde approach are: catheter positioning within the left ventricle, it is also familiar to most electrophysiologists. The stability of the ablation catheter below the mitral valve is usually excellent, thus enhancing the probability of success, and ablation can also be performed above the mitral valve (atrial insertion site). Moreover, complications of transseptal punctures are avoided. However, catheter manipulation around the mitral valve is sometimes difficult, especially if the left ventricular cavity is small. In addition, both the aortic valve and the coronary arteries may be damaged by the ablation catheter. Finally, this technique requires femoral artery puncture with the enhanced likelihood of vascular complications. With the transseptal technique, arterial cannulation is not required. Radiofrequency energy is generally applied to the atrial site, thus possibly reducing any long-term, ventricular arrhythmogenic potential of ablation. Finally, the positioning of the catheter at the mitral annulus is generally easy, thus allowing accessory pathway localization by unipolar atrial electrogram polarity reversal.[16] In fact, these two techniques appear to be complementary. Their respective success rates, complication rates and radiation exposure durations are almost identical.[25]

Both transseptal and retrograde approaches may be unsuccessful with epicardially located accessory pathways. In some patients, AV intervals recorded within the coronary sinus may be shorter and ventricular activation earlier as compared to AV intervals recorded via the ablation catheter. This suggests an epicardial location of the accessory pathway.

When a V-delta interval < -10 msec is recorded, a ventricular epicardial insertion should also be suspected and ablation performed at the atrial insertion site. Finally, a transient block despite "optimal" placement may indicate the presence of a large ventricular insertion, and successful ablation may require prolonged energy delivery.

Right-Sided Accessory Pathways

These pathways may be ablated using a superior (through the superior vena cava) or inferior (through the inferior vena cava) approach. The ablation site can be approached on the atrial site, directly on the AV groove or on the ventricular insertion site via a loop in the right ventricle. For right posterolateral or posterior accessory pathways, the inferior approach is most commonly used. For right anteroseptal and right anterolateral accessory pathways, a superior approach allows better catheter positioning. These pathways are often difficult to ablate, owing to catheter instability and poor tissue contact. Furthermore, the ablation catheter is most often positioned above or on the tricuspid valve where heat convective loss is greater. Higher energy outputs are therefore usually required to achieve the same temperature as used for left-sided accessory pathways.[7] Enhanced stability may be obtained by using long sheaths or ablation catheters with a "dumb-bell" distal electrode or with a long distal curve.[5] Finally, some workers recommend the use of a reference or mapping catheter introduced into the right coronary artery. However, this clearly does not solve the problem of ablation catheter instability.

Paraseptal Accessory Pathways

The ablation of paraseptal accessory pathways requires low energy deliveries in order to preserve the normal AV conduction system. Anteroseptal fibers are located above and anteriorly to the normal conduction system, whereas "mid-septal" fibers are located in the zone between the His bundle and the coronary sinus.[27] For anteroseptal pathways in particular, although the ablation catheter can be positioned below the tricuspid valve using the femoral vein approach, a superior is more commonly used. These two types of accessory pathways must be differentiated from the normal AV conduction tissue[26,27] and to avoid damage to the normal conduction system, several guidelines are applicable[5,7]: (1) minimize the number of RF deliveries by using the optimal predictive criteria; (2) check the absence of a significant (> 0.1 mV amplitude) His bundle potential by inducing, whenever possible, a narrow QRS complex tachycardia; (3) terminate RF delivery at 10 seconds if preexcitation is still present; and (4) terminate RF delivery immediately in the event of a sustained junctional rhythm.

It must be emphasized that transient block in the accessory pathway is often obtained merely mechanically by movement of the ablation catheter, owing to the superficial sub-endocardial location of these accessory pathways.

Mid-Septal Accessory Pathways

The mid-septal accessory pathways can be ablated just above the coronary sinus, using the same approach employed for posteroseptal accessory pathways (see below). However, some true mid-septal pathways, adjacent to the His bundle (para-Hisian) or immediately posterior to the His bundle, close to the AV node (paranodal) present difficulties. Ablating such pathways requires particularly low energy delivery to preserve the normal conduction system.[5]

Posteroseptal Accessory Pathways

The anatomy of the posterior space is complex. Fibers joining the posteromedian region of the atrium to the interventricular septum after crossing the posteroseptal pyramidal region are defined as posteroseptal accessory pathways. Such pathways can be ablated in various sites using a variety of approaches depending on the fibers' orientation. Using the femoral venous (inferior) approach, effective ablation sites can be on the tricuspid annulus, at the margin of the coronary sinus ostium, within the proximal coronary sinus, or one of the coronary sinus venous branches.[1-4,28] A retrograde arterial or a transseptal approach must be used for left-sided posteroseptal accessory pathways. In some patients, RF pulses must be applied from both sides of the septum to completely eliminate anterograde and retrograde conduction. On the surface ECG, a predominantly negative, and maximally preexcited QRS complex in lead V1 suggest a right-sided posteroseptal accessory pathway with the likelihood of successful ablation at the endocardium, or within the proximal coronary sinus using a right (venous) approach. A predominantly positive and maximally preexcited complex in lead V1 is in favor of a left-sided accessory pathway, but such pathways can be ablated at the right endocardium, the proximal coronary sinus, or the left endocardium. Other ECG parameters have been described in order to further differentiate right-sided from left-sided posteroseptal accessory pathways.[5,29]

Permanent Junctional Reciprocating Tachycardia

Some concealed accessory pathway connections have decremental conduction properties analogous to the AV node. They are responsible for permanent junctional tachycardias[30] with a negative P wave inscribed in leads II, III, aVF and V3 to V6 with a "long RP" interval. Such tachycardias can be ablated, leading to the cure of tachycardia-induced cardiomyopathy that is frequently encountered in these patients. The earliest site of retrograde activation of the atrium represents the optimal ablation site. It must be emphasized that the VA interval at the optimal ablation site is long, due to the decremental conduction properties. An accessory pathway potential is sometimes recorded at the successful ablation site. Such pathways are most often located in the posteroseptal region, but other locations around the tricuspid or the mitral annulus have also been described.[5,31] Analysis of the P wave on the 12-lead ECG may be a useful adjunct to localize the accessory pathway. A negative P wave in lead I, associated with a positive P wave in V1 is in favor of a left-sided location. A biphasic P wave in lead I associated with a negative P wave in V1 is in favor of a posteroseptal location.

Mahaim Fibers

The advent of catheter ablation of Mahaim fibers has led to a better understanding of the anatomy and the electrophysiological properties of such fibers. Originally, Mahaim fibers were thought to connect the AV node and either the intraventricular conduction system (nodofascicular fibers) or the ventricle (nodoventricular fibers). In fact, most of the ventricular insertion sites of Mahaim fibers appear to be around the right bundle branch, and their origin is from the free portion of the tricuspid annulus. They must therefore be considered as atrioventricular fibers.[32-35] They have anterograde decremental conduction properties and can be ablated at their atrial or ventricular insertion sites. Since they do not conduct in a retrograde fashion, they can only mediate antidromic tachycardias. The conventional approach for ablation is performed at the atrial insertion site, guided by the shortest atrial stimulus to delta wave interval. This technique, associated with direct recording of a Mahaim potential and the occurrence of a mechanical block in the accessory pathway is effective in most cases. If unsuccessful, the same approach can be used with the ablation catheter positioned below the tricuspid valve. Finally, ablation can also be performed at the ventricular insertion site, guided by the earliest ventricular potential, relative to preexcitation onset and by an accessory pathway potential recording.

Conclusions

Radiofrequency catheter ablation is widely used to treat patients with a tachycardia, due to AV accessory pathways with a high degree of success. Future improvements will include a decrease in procedure time and a decrease in the number of RF deliveries, which will minimize the morbidity and any potential long-term adverse effect of RF delivery. The use of both new energy sources and new ablation catheters in conjunction with improvements in the determination of the optimal ablation site, with a greater positive predictive value, should allow us to reach these objectives.

References

1. Jackmann WM, Wang X, Friday KJ, et al. Catheter ablation of accessory atrioventricular pathways (Wolff-Parkinson-White syndrome) by radiofrequency current. *N Engl J Med* 1991;324:1605–1611.
2. Kuck KH, Schlüter M, Geiger M, et al. Radiofrequency current catheter ablation of accessory atrioventricular pathways. *Lancet* 1991;337:1557–1561.
3. Calkins H, Sousa J, Rosenbeck S, et al. Diagnosis and cure of the Wolff-Parkinson-White syndrome or paroxysmal supraventricular tachycardias during a single electrophysiologic test. *N Engl J Med* 1991;324:1612–1618.
4. Plumb VJ. Catheter ablation of the accessory pathways of the Wolff-Parkinson-White Syndrome and its variants. *Progr Cardiovasc Dis* 1995;5:295–306.
5. Haïssaguerre M, Gaïta F, Marcus FI, et al. Radiofrequency catheter ablation of accessory pathways: a contemporary review. *J Cardiovasc Electrophysiol* 1994;5: 532–552.
6. Hindricks G, on behalf of the multicenter European Radiofrequency Survey Investigators of the Working Group on Arrhythmias of the European Society of Cardiology. The multicenter European Radiofrequency Survey (MERFS): complications of radiofrequency catheter ablation of arrhythmias. *Eur Heart J* 1993; 4:1644–1653.
7. Haïssaguerre M, Gencel L, Fisher B, et al. Ablation des voies accessoires par courants de radiofréquence. *Arch Mal Coeur* 1994;87:1563–1570.
8. Langberg JJ, Calkins H, El-Atassi R, et al. Temperature monitoring during radiofrequency catheter ablation of accessory pathways. *Circulation* 1992;86: 1469–1474.
9. Silka MJ, Kron J, Halperin BD, et al. Analysis of local electrocardiogram characteristics correlated with successful radiofrequency catheter ablation of accessory atrioventricular pathways. *PACE* 1992;15:1000–1006.
10. Calkins H, Kim YN, Schmatz S, et al. Electrocardiogram criteria for identification of appropriate target sites for radiofrequency catheter ablation of accessory atrioventricular connections. *Circulation* 1992;85:565–573.
11. Chen X, Borggrefe M, Hindricks G, et al. Radiofrequency ablation of accessory pathways: characteristics of transiently and permanently effective pulses. *PACE* 1992;15:1000–1007.
12. Villacastin J, Almendral J, Arenal A, et al. Interobserver variability in the appreciation of Kent potentials at successful sites for RF ablation of accessory AV pathways. *PACE* 1995;18(II): 914.

13. Simmers TA, Hauer NW, Wever FE, et al. Unipolar electrocardiogram models for prediction of outcome in radiofrequency ablation of accessory pathways. *PACE* 1994;17:86–97.
14. Haïssaguerre M, Fisher N, Warin JF, et al. Electrocardiogram patterns predictive of successful radiofrequency catheter ablation of accessory pathways. *PACE* 1992; 15(II):2138–2145.
15. Calkins H, Langberg J, Sousa J, et al. Radiofrequency catheter ablation of accessory atrioventricular connections in 250 patients: abbreviated therapeutic approach to Wolff-Parkinson-White syndrome. *Circulation* 1992;85:1337–1346.
16. Fisher WG, Swartz JF. Three dimensional electrogram mapping improves ablation of left-sided AP. *PACE* 1992;15:2344–2356.
17. Bashir Y, Heald SC, Katritsis D, et al. Radiofrequency ablation of accessory atrioventricular pathways. Predictive value of local electrocardiogram characteristics for the identification of successful target sites. *Br Heart J* 1993;69:315–321.
18. Haïssaguerre M, Dartigues JF, Warin JF, et al. Electrocardiogram pattern predictive of successful ablation for radiofrequency catheter ablation of accessory atrioventricular connections. *Circulation* 1992;85:565–573.
19. de Chillou C, Magnin-Poull I, Sadoul N, et al. Reproducibility of bipolar endocavitary electrocardiogram measurements at sites of radiofrequency application in patients with the Wolff-Parkinson-White syndrome. *PACE* 1995;18(Part II):915.
20. Spach MS, Miller WT, Miller-Jones E, et al. Extracellular potentials related to intraventricular action potentials during impulse conduction in anisotropic canine cardiac muscle. *Circ Res* 1979;45:188–204.
21. Gallagher JJ, Kassel J, Cox JL, et al. Techniques of intraoperative electrophysiologic mapping. *Am J Cardiol* 1982;49:221–240.
22. Magnin-Poull I, de Chillou C, Sadoul N, et al. Valeur de l'enregistrement unipolaire et bipolaire dans l'ablation par radiofréquence des faisceaux accessoires auriculo-ventriculaires. *Arch Mal Coeur* (sous presse).
23. Kuck KH, Friday KJ, Kunze KP, et al. Sites of conduction block in accessory atrioventricular pathways. Basis for concealed accessory pathways. *Circulation* 1990;82:407–417.
24. Kuck KH, Schluter M. Single-catheter approach to radiofrequency ablation of left-sided accessory pathways in patients with Wolff-Parkinson-White syndrome. *Circulation* 1991;84:2366–2375.
25. Lesh MD, Van Hare GF, Scheinman MM, et al. Comparison of the retrograde and transseptal methods for ablation of left free wall accessory pathways. *J Am Coll Cardiol* 1993;22:542–549.
26. Schlüter M, Kuck KH. Catheter ablation from right atrium of anteroseptal accessory pathways using radiofrequency current. *J Am Coll Cardiol* 1992;19:663–670.
27. Kuck KH, Schlüter M, Gürsoy S. Preservation of atrioventricular nodal conduction during radiofrequency current catheter ablation of midseptal accessory pathways. *Circulation* 1992;86:1743–1752.
28. Wang X, Jackman W, McClelland J, et al. Sites of successful radiofrequency ablation of posteroseptal accessory pathways. *PACE* 1992;15:535 (Abstract).
29. Arruda M, Wang X, McClelland J, et al. ECG algorithm for predicting radiofrequency ablation site in posteroseptal accessory pathways. *PACE* 1992;15;535 (Abstract).
30. Coumel P, Cabrol C, Fabiato A, et al. Tachycardie permanente par rythme réciproque. *Arch Mal Coeur* 1967;60:1830–1864.
31. Ticho BS, Saul JP, Hulse JE, et al. Variable location of accessory pathways associ-

ated with the permanent form of junctional reciprocating tachycardia and confirmation with radiofrequency ablation. *Am J Cardiol* 1992;70:1559–1564.
32. Haïssaguerre M, Warin JF, Le Metayer Ph, et al. Catheter ablation of Mahaim fibers with preservation of atrioventricular nodal conduction. *Circulation* 1990;82: 418–427.
33. Klein GJ, Guiraudon GM, Kerr CR, et al. "Nodoventricular" accessory pathway: evidence for distinct accessory atrioventricular pathway with atrioventricular node-like properties. *J Am Coll Cardiol* 1988;11:1035–1040.
34. Tchou P, Lehmann MH, Jazayeri M, et al. Atriofascicular connection or a nodoventricular Mahaim fiber? Electrophysiological elucidation of the pathway and associated reentrant circuit. *Circulation* 1988;77:837–848.
35. Klein LS, Kackett FK, Zipes DP, et al. Radiofrequency catheter ablation of Mahaim fibers at the triscuspid annulus. *Circulation* 1993;87:738–747.

Chapter 13_____

Radiofrequency in the Treatment of Ventricular Tachycardia

Guy Fontaine, MD, Robert Frank, MD,
Joelci Tonet, MD, Yves Gallais, MD,
F. Rosas Andrade, MD, Gilles Lascault, MD,
P. Aouate, MD, F. Poulain, MD

Introduction

Radiofrequency (RF) ablation is based on the delivery of a RF current at the tip of an endocardial catheter placed on the arrhythmogenic substrate. This approach[1,2] has been used for the treatment of ventricular tachycardia (VT) resistant to antiarrhythmic drug therapy.[3-11] In a preliminary report, we have shown that this technique could be effective irrespective of the etiology of chronic VT.[3] In particular, this technique has been used successfully to treat VT in patients with structural as well as those who do not have structural heart diseases.[4] Therefore, ablation of VT by RF energy is preferred to direct current (DC) energy for this purpose. However, a form of DC ablation using reduced energy, is still used in patients that are resistant to RF ablation.[4,11]

The purpose of this chapter is to assess the effectiveness of RF energy in conjunction with reduced energy DC ablation in patients with or without structural heart disease. It is an extension of our previous work in which we reported 58 cases using this approach.[4]

Clinical Series

The study group is selected from a series of 96 consecutive cases referred to Jean Rostand Hospital, Ivry, France, for the treatment of chronic forms of VT. These patients were referred by other cardiological centers where they were considered to be resistant to antiarrhythmic drug therapy. All of

From *Practical Management of Cardiac Arrhythmias* edited by Nabil El-Sherif, and Jean Lekieffre. Futura Publishing Co., Armonk, NY, © 1997.

the patients were reassessed based on pharmacological protocols, developed by our group, using amiodarone alone or in combination, mostly with beta-blocking agents. Of the 96 patients, there were 68 who could not be treated adequately by antiarrhythmic drugs as assessed by Holter monitoring and/or programmed pacing, and who were considered eligible for the ablative techniques. There was no exclusion due to age, clinical condition, or other factors. The mean follow-up is 19.6 months.

Structural Heart Diseases

The etiology of VT (Figure 1) includes 31 patients (45.6%) with chronic coronary artery disease. The VT occurred as late as 10 years after the previous myocardial infarction. Thirteen patients (19.1%) had arrhythmogenic right ventricular dysplasia (ARVD), 5 (7.3%) had idiopathic dilated cardiomyopathy, and four (5.8%) had congenital anomalies (including tetralogy of Fallot

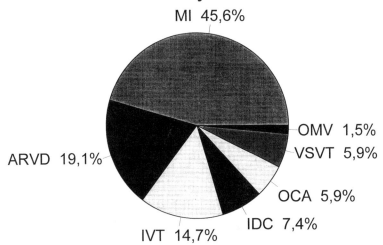

Figure 1. Etiologies of ventricular tachycardia (VT) showing the predominance of VT after myocardial infarction, arrhythmogenic right ventricular dysplasia, idiopathic dilated cardiomyopathies, followed by idiopathic VT and the nonstructural heart disease. MI = Myocardial infarction; VSVT = Verapamil sensitive ventricular tachycardia; IDC = Idiopathic dilated cardiomyopathy; ARVD = Arrhythmogenic right ventricular dysplasia; IVT = Idiopathic ventricular tachycardia; OCA = Operated congenital anomaly; OMV = Operated mitral valve.

and its variants; all of them had previous surgery with incision of the free wall of the right ventricle). One patient developed VT after a surgical intervention on the mitral valve, and one patient previously classified as hypertrophic cardiomyopathy was reclassified as having a dilated idiopathic cardiomyopathy.

Nonstructural Heart Disease

This series includes ten patients (14.7%) who had idiopathic VT, mostly localized in the right ventricular infundibular area, and four (5.8%) had fascic-

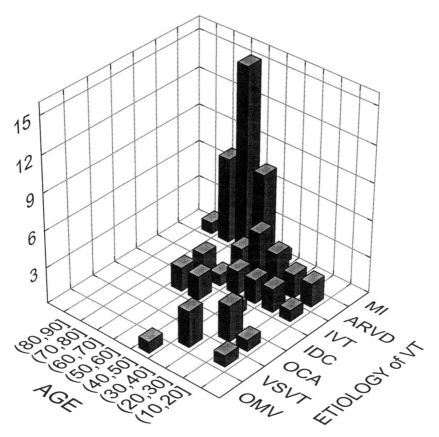

Figure 2. Tridimensional histogram showing the distribution of ages according to the ventricular tachycardia (VT) etiologies. The oldest ages are observed in patients with VT after myocardial infarction. The youngest correspond to patients with nonstructural heart diseases, arrhythmogenic right ventricular dysplasia, congenital heart diseases. Labeling of this figure is similar to Figure 1.

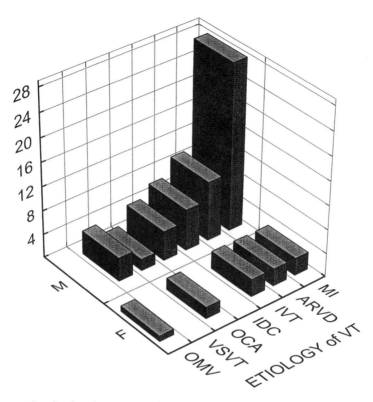

Figure 3. Gender distribution according to etiologies showing a strong predominance of males in cases of ventricular tachycardia (VT) after myocardial infarction and arrhythmogenic right ventricular dysplasia (ARVD).

ular VTs sensitive to verapamil with a right bundle branch block, and left axis deviation, also called Fauchier-Belhassen tachycardia. The clinical data of the patients is summarized in Figures 2 and 3.

Equipment

Our approach to mapping was originally developed for the surgical treatment of Wolf-Parkinson-White syndrome and VT. The techniques have evolved over the years, in particular, using steerable catheters with distal electrodes 4 mm in length, that are suitable for RF ablation.[12] More recently, we have used temperature-controlled catheters using equipment manufactured by Medtronic Cardiorhythm® (San Jose, CA, USA) and Cordis Webster™ (Baldwin Park, CA, USA).

The generator used for RF is produced by Osypka™ (Grenzach-Whylen, Germany) model HAT 200S, and the Medtronic Cardiorhythm generators. Each of the generators has microcomputers with the appropriate software for impedance and temperature monitoring which prevents temperatures in excess of 70°.

The return RF electrode is located beside the indifferent electrode used for fulguration or defibrillation.

The fulgurator is a Fulgucor™ (Odam, Wissembourg, France). The energy was delivered, except in three cases, according to a protocol modified from previous works.[3] It is now adjusted at 160 Joules in the cathodal mode. This decreases barotraumatism and increases the effect due to the flow of current as compared to the mechanical effects.[13]

During the procedures, the fluoroscopic events were recorded on a videotape, with a voice channel, and a second recorder obtained electrocardiographic tracings from four surface leads as well as the endocardial signals from an "Electronics for Medicine" VR12 recorder.

Radial blood pressure is monitored continuously during the procedure, and a Swan-Ganz catheter is placed in the pulmonary artery to monitor SVO2 pressures and to measure cardiac output and right ventricular ejection fraction (RVEF) by thermodilution techniques. Special attention is given in the electrophysiological laboratory to obtain satisfactory hemodynamical control over the procedure, before sending the patient to the recovery room. This approach decreases the subsequent monitoring.

Recently, we have found that monitoring of coronary sinus oxygen saturation seems to be a reliable marker for procedure tolerance.[14] In addition, monitoring of coagulation is performed during the procedure as soon as the catheter is introduced inside the left ventricle, by APTT Hemochrom™, (Bard, USA) (1.5 baseline).

Before ablation, class I antiarrhythmic drugs are interrupted for at least five half-lives. Amiodarone is continued. Only monomorphic sustained VTs are considered for attempted ablation. Ablation is performed under anesthesia to obtain good relaxation of the patient, to control myocardial function, and to monitor thrombogenicity by transesophageal echocardiography. The level of anesthesia is increased during delivery of DC shocks. Ventricular tachycardia is generally induced by programmed pacing, and in some cases after isoprenaline injection.

The classic approach to mapping is to record the site of origin of VT based on the recording of earliest potentials before the QRS complex is visible on the surface tracing during VT. This coupling interval is usually short in the range of ≥ 30 msec in patients with nonstructural heart disease. Pace mapping is also used and should exactly reproduce in the twelve leads morphology of QRS complexes during spontaneous VT. Pace mapping can be achieved by overdrive pacing during VT at a slightly higher rate using the same catheter that will deliver the electrical energy for ablation. In addition, VT should be still present after the interruption of pacing. In patients with a structural heart disease and a reentrant intraventricular phenomenon, special attention has to be given to treat the area of slow conduction which is frequently represented by fragmented potentials located between two ventricular QRS complexes. Additional features facilitate the identification of the zone of slow conduction which is a necessary link for the perpetuation of the arrhythmia.[15-21]

Radiofrequency is first used at all ablation attempts. If it is ineffective, or if there is an impedance rise or lack of increase of temperature, one or several DC energy shocks are delivered through the same catheter. The DC ablation signal of voltage and current is displayed on the screen of a two-channel digital Tektronix 5116 oscilloscope (Beaverton, OR). This validates the assumption that the energy of each shock was correctly delivered, and that there was no damage of the catheter which could be used for the next shock if necessary.[22]

The statistical methods used in this work are based on the Student t-test and the Chi-square test. A p value ≤ 0.05 is considered to be significant.

The In-Hospital Follow-Up Period

The in-hospital follow-up period, because of better control of postoperative hemodynamic parameters has been simplified and consists of the monitoring of arterial radial blood pressure for a period of 24 hours. A left subclavian electrode catheter is placed at the apex of the right ventricle and is left in place for up to 10 days. During this time, a repeated electrophysiology study is generally performed at the bedside to determine if the tachycardia is still inducible. During a period of 10 days, the surface ECG is monitored continuously by computerized telemetry using Hewlett-Packard equipment.

Control of the cardiac arrhythmia is generally assessed before discharge of the patient by 24-hour Holter recording, stress testing, and in patients with inducible VT, by programmed pacing, using up to three extrastimuli at basic cycle drive lengths going up to 400 msec.

Definition of Results

If a VT identical or similar to the previous attacks in rate as well as in morphology occurs spontaneously, or is inducible by the same previously defined protocols, the case is considered as a "failure" and further pharmacological attempts are made to prevent the arrhythmia. The same dosages and drugs as before the ablative session are attempted. When this drug treatment is effective, it is classified as a "partial success," because the ablation may prevent ventricular arrhythmias by modifying the arrhythmogenic substrate. Therefore, patients in whom antiarrhythmic treatment that is different from that which is used before the ablation, that led to the control of VT, are considered as "uninterpretable."

The case is classified as a "success" when drugs are no longer needed and when patients are noninducible after ablation. Antiarrhythmic drugs may be continued for safety reasons (rapid VT or ventricular fibrillation, or to treat ventricular or supraventricular extrasystoles). The final clinical assessment of the arrhythmias: "clinical efficacy" is represented by the sum of "success" and "partial success."

Follow-Up

After hospital discharge, the follow-up is systematically assessed by a computer-based system. Follow-up consists of discussion with the referring physician or the referring hospital, as well as by direct phone calls to the patient or family members. Follow-up is based on the time interval between the first ablation procedure and the latest information obtained for each patient with a minimal follow-up of 1 month. The follow-up (mean ± sd) was 18 ± 11.5 months.

Calculation of Results

A microcomputer software system is used to calculate and graph the results to perform statistical analysis.

Results

VTs in Patients with Structural Heart Disease

This series consists of 54 cases including 45 males, with a mean age of 54.2 years (ranging from 14 to 85 years) (Figure 2). The mean left ventricular ejection fraction (LVEF) obtained in 46 cases was 38% ± 19% ranging from 15% to 80% (Figure 4). Twenty-five patients had more than 20 independent episodes of VT. In 53 cases, the VT was monomorphic in 22 cases; 13 patients had 2 morphologies; 10 had 3 morphologies; 8 had more than 3 morphologies, of which 1 case had up to 12 morphologies (Figure 5).

Two sessions were necessary in 13 cases (24%); and three sessions in one case (1.8%). The site of ablation of VT was on the left ventricle in 29 cases (53.7%); the right ventricle in 22 (40.7%); and in both ventricles in 3 cases (5.5%) (Figure 6).

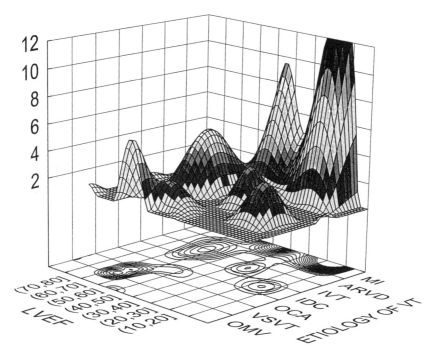

Figure 4. Distribution of ejection fractions in different ventricular tachycardia (VT) etiologies. The lowest values are observed in patients of VT after myocardial infarction, idiopathic dilated cardiomyopathy, and the largest number of cases is below 30%. The best ejection fractions are observed in nonstructural heart diseases and arrhythmogenic right ventricular dysplasia (ARVD).

In 38 cases where this data was available, the tachycardia was incessant in 9 (17%); and the shortest interval between two attacks was daily in 7 cases (18.4%); weekly in 5 (13.2%); monthly in 13 (34.2%); and yearly in 4 (10.5%). Among the longest intervals, an interval between two attacks of 1 month was observed in 11 cases and of 1 year in 18 cases.

The First Ablation Session

The first RF session was classified as successful in 17 patients and unsuccessful in 36 patients. One case was uninterpretable. This resulted in a clinical efficacy of 31.5% (Figure 7). The use of DC ablation after an ineffective RF ablation during the first session was attempted in 30 cases and led to 15 successes, 10 failures, and 3 partial successes. Two cases were uninterpretable. This resulted in a clinical efficacy of 60% for these patients (Figure 8).

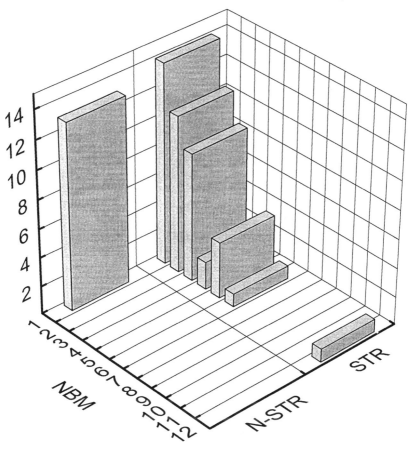

Figure 5. The number of morphologies in structural and nonstructural heart diseases, showing a high predominance of the largest number of morphologies in structural heart diseases (STR). STR = Structural heart disease; N-STR = Nonstructural heart disease.

Complications

There was one case of pericardial tamponade due to the perforation of the right ventricular wall. This occurred due to mechanical manipulation of the mapping catheter inside the right ventricle, before the delivery of any energy. Another case had this complication after fulguration, prior to modification of the amount of DC energy, and before employing the present proto-

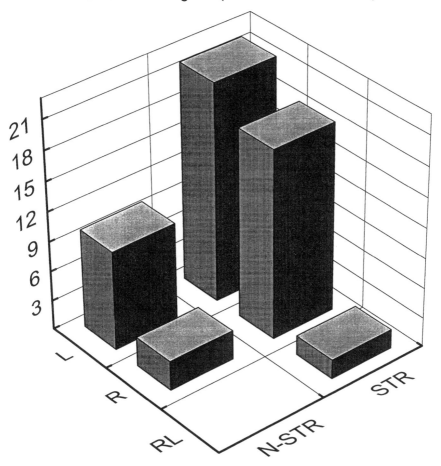

Figure 6. Site of ablation versus VT etiology (R = right ; L = left). This histogram is built in percentage of the number of cases observed in each category, structural and non structural heart diseases. The homogeneity of the results is obvious.

col. These two problems of pericardial tamponade were successfully treated by percutaneous drainage of the pericardium.

There was one case of cerebral thromboembolism which partially regressed.

Second Ablative Session

A second ablative session was attempted in nine cases. One of them was a partial success after the first session, however a new ablation was attempted.

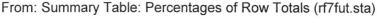

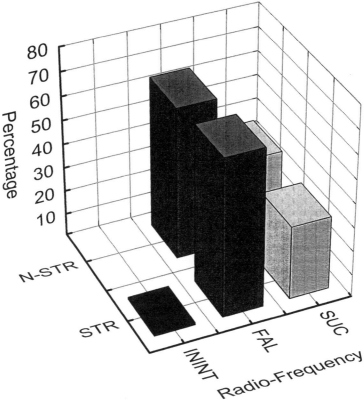

Figure 7. Results of a single session of RF ablation compared with the classification of myocardial diseases expressed in the percentage of number of cases in each category, structural or nonstructural heart diseases. This representation is also used for Figures 8 and 9, and shows at the first sight the idea of the homogeneity of the results in the two categories. FAL = failure; ININT = uninterpretable result; SUC = success.

Radiofrequency did not improve the previous result in all these cases. A new fulguration procedure using the new protocols was then delivered in all cases leading to five failures and four successes, with a clinical efficacy of 44% in this subgroup. There were no complications.

Third Ablative Session

A third session of ablation was used in one case who had 12 morphologies of VT after ineffective RF application. This case was finally controlled with complete success after use of the fulguration procedure.

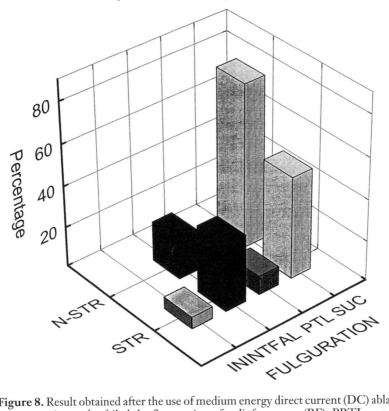

From: Summary Table: Percentages of Row Totals (rf7fut.sta)

Figure 8. Result obtained after the use of medium energy direct current (DC) ablation, in some patients who failed the first session of radiofrequency (RF). PRTL = partial success.

The global results of this series of 54 cases of structural heart disease are 37 successes (68.5%), 14 failures (26%), and one partial success (1.8%). Two cases were uninterpretable (3.7%) (Figure 9).

Early Mortality

There was only one case of early mortality due to low output failure on the 3rd day after ablation, following an intravenous injection of disopyramide for recurrent VT.

Long-Term Follow-Up

The long term follow-up of 44 survivors was a mean of 15 ± 12 months. There were two patients who had VT after myocardial infarction that were lost to follow-up.

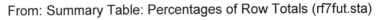

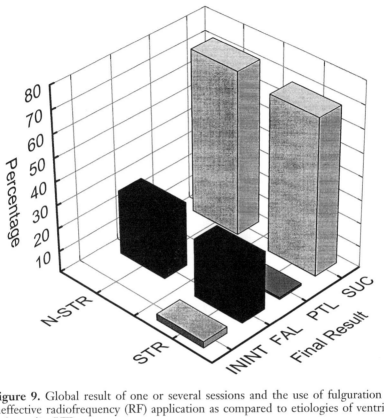

Figure 9. Global result of one or several sessions and the use of fulguration after ineffective radiofrequency (RF) application as compared to etiologies of ventricular tachycardia (VT).

Late Mortality

During long-term follow-up, we have observed seven deaths including 2 sudden deaths after 1 month and 21 months (one classified as a success, the other as a failure;) and four deaths due to congestive heart failure between 2 and 7 months; and one due to low output failure after recurrence of acute myocardial infarction after 6 months (Figure 10).

Results at the End of Follow-Up

However, six cases considered as failures at the end of previous protocols have had disppearance of their VT, and are now considered as success or partial success (one case). This led at the end of follow-up to a clinical efficacy

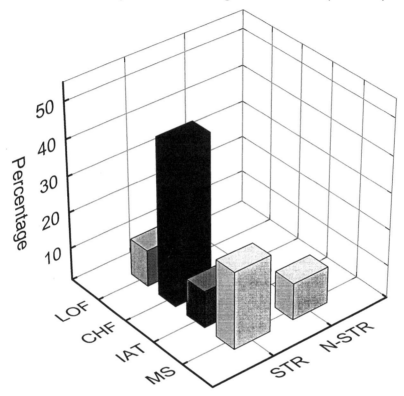

From: Summary Table: Percentages of Total N=9 (rf7fut.sta)

Figure 10. Distribution of causes of death according to the classification of myocardial diseases, whatever the result of ablative techniques. This histogram is built in the percentage of all groups, as opposed to the cases observed in each category of myocardial disease. This could have led to a bar of 100% of sudden death in the nonstructural heart diseases, although there is only a single case in this category. Congestive heart failure appears to be the predominant cause. LOF = Low output; IAT = iatrogenic antiarrhythmic therapy; CHF = congestive heart failure; SD = sudden death.

of 77.7%, keeping in mind that three patients are uninterpretable, and two patients are lost of follow-up (because of the long follow-up, the two patients who died suddenly were not considered as failures but development of "new" arrhythmia).

Ventricular Tachycardia Independent of a Structural Heart Disease

This series consists of 14 cases, including 11 males. Their clinical data are reported in Table 1. Their mean age was 39 years, ranging from 14 to

Table 1
The First Session of Radiofrequency

	MI	ARVD	VSVT	IVT
MI	1	0.64	0.64	1
ARVD	0.64	1	0.8	0.7
VSVT	0.64	0.8	1	0.92
IVT	1	0.7	0.92	1

ARVD = Arrhythmogenic right ventricular dysplasia
MI = Myocardial infarction
IVT = Idiopathic ventricular tachycardia
VSVT = Verapamil sensitive ventricular tachycardia

69 years (Figures 2 and 3). The LVEF available in 13 cases was a mean of 61% ± 13% ranging from 36% to 70% (Figure 4). Three patients had incessant VT. Nine patients had more than 20 independent episodes of VT. In all the cases VT was monomorphic (Figure 5).

Two sessions were used in one case. The site of VT was located in the right ventricle in three cases and in the left ventricle in 11 (Figure 6).

The result of the first delivery of RF has led to five successes and nine failures, with a clinical efficacy of 36% (Figure 7). The use of fulguration after ineffective RF during the first session was used in five cases leading to four successes and one failure (Figure 8). Failure persisted after a second RF attempt, as well as after a second fulguration procedure.

At this point in time, a clinical efficacy was obtained in ten cases (71.4%), and failure in four cases (29%) (Figure 9).

Complications

One patient had a coronary spasm. The same patient had a cerebrovascular accident after a second RF session, followed by fulguration.

Early Mortality

There was no early mortality.

Long-Term Follow-Up

The mean follow-up is 23 ± 13 months. These results remain stable over the follow-up period.

Late Mortality

There was only a single case of late mortality in a patient who had an idiopathic VT not controlled by a single session of RF ablation. The patient refused a second session and died 7 months later of sudden death after multiple episodes of VT (Figure 10).

Study of Subgroups

Ventricular Tachycardia After Myocardial Infarction

This series of 31 patients who had VT after chronic myocardial ischemia consisted of 28 males and 3 females, mean age 66 years, ranging from 50 to 85 years. The mean LVEF available in 26 cases, was 30%, ranging from 15% to 56%. The distribution of the LVEF is presented together with the other etiologies in Figure 3. Six patients had incessant VT. For the 19 other cases in whom this parameter was available, the longest interval between two attacks was 1 day in one case; 1 week in two; 1 month in eight; 1 year in eight. Thirteen patients survived more than 20 independent episodes of VT.

In 12 patients, VT was monomorphic, seven had respectively two and three morphologies; and five more than three morphologies. Two patients had up to six morphologies (Figure 4).

Six patients had two sessions, one close to 2 months after discharge, the others during the same hospital stay, which did not exceed more than 10 days between the two sessions.

In five cases, the ablation was performed only in the right ventricle, in two patients in both ventricles. The 24 remaining cases had ablation in the left ventricle.

After the 1st session of RF, 19 failures and 11 successes (35.5%) were observed. One result was uninterpretable (3.2%). The clinical efficacy of RF was 35%. After use of the fulguration procedure, performed in 15 cases, 10 successes (66%) and 4 failures (26.6%) were obtained. One result was uninterpretable (6.6%).

Second Session

After the use of RF attempted at the beginning of the second session on three cases, success on two patients was obtained after the modified fulguration procedure. The sequential use of these two methods on 31 cases has led to 22 successes (70.9%), seven failures (22.2%), and two uninterpretable results (6.4%).

The Long-Term Evolution

At the end of the follow-up period, with a mean value of 13 months, going up to 34, no spontaneous improvement was observed. However, two patients who were classified as failures, have been lost to follow-up.

Early Mortality

One patient died the 3rd day after intravenous injection of disopyramide, 3 days after a failed attempt to ablate incessant VT.

Complications

Pericardial tamponade was observed in one case, during the first session. This was observed in a 61-year-old patient and was controlled by percutaneous drainage.

Late Mortality

Four patients died during the follow-up period in less than 1 year, in one case by low output failure, in one case after a new myocardial infarction 6.5 months after the procedure, and the two other cases due to congestive heart failure. The survival curve using the Kaplan-Meier method is presented in Figure 11.

Arrhythmogenic Right Ventricular Dysplasia

The 13 patients affected by ARVD include 10 males and three females. Their mean age was 36 years, ranging from 19 to 57 (Figure 2). Their mean

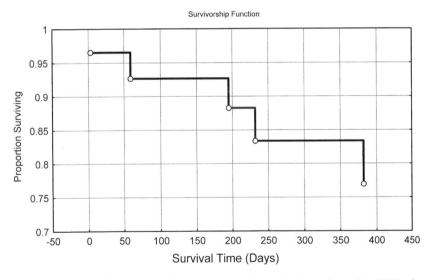

Figure 11. Survival curves of the treatment of ventricular tachycardia (VT) after myocardial infarction. Despite the limited sampling, and the short period of follow-up, the result is globally identical to those previously reported with the use of high energy direct current (DC) ablation.

LVEF available in eight cases was 61% ± 13% and was always above 40% (Figure 3).

The longest interval between two independent episodes of VT was 1 year in seven cases. Eight patients had more than 20 independent episodes of VT and three patients had incessant VT. One patient had an implantable defibrillator but had too many frequent shocks and was therefore considered for the treatment of tachycardia episodes which were increasingly poorly tolerated.

Ventricular tachycardia was monomorphic in five patients, and seven patients had from two to five morphologies. One had 12 morphologies. Three patients had two sessions, the ablations were delivered in all the cases in the right ventricle, except one who had tachycardias of septal origin and for whom ablation was attempted at the level of the left ventricle. In the seven patients in whom this information was available, ablation was performed in the pulmonary infundibulum in six and once at the apex.

First Ablation Session

After the first RF application, four successes and nine failures were observed. Therefore, the clinical efficacy was 31% after the first session.

On the eight failures, a fulguration was performed during the same session, leading to two partial successes, three failures and one uninterpretable result. The clinical effectiveness of RF followed by fulguration is 55% of successes and 44% of failures.

Second Ablation Session

A second ablation session was attempted in three cases and an effectiveness of fulguration after failure of RF was observed in two cases, therefore the clinical efficacy at discharge of the hospital was nine successes (76.8%), one partial success, and three failures.

However, a favorable evolution was observed during the follow-up period with a mean value of 20 ± 13 months, going up to 39 months leading to a clinical efficacy of 92%, and finally a single failure in a patient referred from a foreign country and who was not managed by a second session.

Long-Term Follow-Up

There was neither early mortality nor complications in this series. The follow-up period of the 13 cases has a mean value of 20 months going up to 39 months. No late deaths were observed.

Identification of a Subgroup with a High Success Rate

The study of the subgroup of patients with incessant VT demonstrates that in this subgroup, the use of a single session of RF led to 9 successes out of 12 cases, eight of them pertaining to the group of patients with structural heart disease (5 postinfarction VT and 3 cases of ARVD).

Discussion

The use of RF ablation is important for the treatment of cardiac arrhythmias, leading to dramatic results in the treatment of supraventricular tachycardia.[23-25] Its application to the treatment of VT of different etiologies was the result of several improvements.

Evolution of Equipment

One of the probable benefits provided by RF has been the achievement of steerable catheters with a terminal tip of 4 mm.[12] This explains why one of our ARVD patients who failed a previous session of fulguration was treated effectively by RF, because the steerable catheter could be guided to an area that could not be reached with the regular electrophysiological catheters used for the fulguration procedure. The temperature control used 33 times in this series may have contributed to efficacy (p = 0.2) (Figure 12).[26]

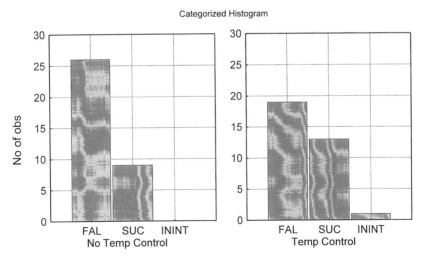

Figure 12. The distribution of results obtained during the first radiofrequency (RF) ablation session, with or without temperature control.

Evolution of the Methods

The protocols used at the beginning of high energy DC ablation have led to complications almost always explainable and corrected. This new study demonstrates on a series of 32 cases where the moderate energy DC was used, that this approach was no longer associated with the operative mortality and major complications that were previously reported. The amount of energy delivered by this new protocol is less than that previously used in high energy DC ablation. In addition, the electrical behavior of RF catheters is different as compared to those previously used for electrophysiology. This could explain the slight decrease of efficacy observed in this series as compared to high energy shocks,[3] although the difference between these two methods does not reach the level of statistical significance (p = 0.09).

Identification of the Zone for Ablation

In this series, there is no case in which a systematic attempt made by RF at the beginning of the second session proved successful. In all the cases, it was necessary to use fulguration to obtain success. This suggests that the methods used to localize the zone for ablation are properly identified.[15-21] However, the insufficient amount of energy needed for ablation justifies the use of fulguration after ineffective RF procedure.

Global Clinical Efficacy

This study confirms the relative lack of efficacy of RF energy for ablation of VT. In these two groups, there is a failure rate of 64%. There are several explanations: (1) the inclusion of the learning phase; (2) temperature-controlled catheters were not used at the beginning of the series; (3) the influence of favorable results obtained with the fulguration procedure leading to switch to DC to shorten the session; and (4) in the series of patients with non structural heart diseases, the fact that the nonlife-threatening feature of VT and its good control by antiarrhythmic drugs (the ablation attempt was made to avoid long-term drug treatment) has led to postponing or even abandoning a new session.

The relatively limited damage of myocardial tissue produced by RF in order to modify the critical tissue for the perpetuation of cardiac arrhythmia should also be considered. At the level of left ventricle, the thickness of the myocardial wall where it is known that reentry phenomenon could be generated between endocardium and epicardium, may not be modified by RF, if the reentrant circuit is located close to the epicardium. The same is true for the treatment of VT originating in the interventricular septum[3] as well as in the infundibular area in ARVD and some cases of idiopathic dilated cardiomyopathy, where it is difficult to maintain the catheter with a good contact against the wall during ablation. We found that in difficult cases, the Medtronic Cardiorhythm catheter appeared to result in a more stable position for ablation of VT.

Perioperative and Early Mortality

The use of RF for the treatment of VT seems to be safer as compared to fulguration. However, in this series the procedural mortality is zero, despite the decrease in LVEF identical to those observed in previous series of patients treated by our group with DC energy ablation. Postoperative early mortality was observed in only one case and was related to the negative inotropic effect of class I-a antiarrhythmic drugs.

Late Mortality

Three cases of sudden death were observed, one of them before a scheduled procedure. Acute or chronic congestive heart failure was the most frequent cause of late death related to the underlying heart disease.

Complications

Complications which were generally attributed to mapping are still possible in patients in whom it was planned to ablate with RF energy. In this series, there was one case of myocardial perforation of the right ventricle before the delivery of energy. In fact, this complication was detected first by fluoroscopy during the session, but more easily with transesophageal echocardiography, and finally by careful study of hemodynamic parameters. Treatment should be performed as soon as possible by percutaneous drainage of the hemopericardium.

Thromboembolism is the main concern in the ablation using RF energy. This was observed in two cases. In one, it is possible to discuss the possible role played by the fulguration which was delivered during the same session, after application of multiple ineffective RF ablation. The barotraumatic shock of fulguration could have displayed a mural thrombus that was observed on the myocardial wall after multiple RF applications. However, in the other case, RF was used alone.

Structural and Nonstructural Heart Diseases

Effectiveness of RF used alone was mostly studied in VT related to nonstructural heart disease.[27,28] However, other studies have reported the effec-

Table 2
Final Results After Fulguration

	MI	ARVD	VSVT	IVT
MI	1	0.95	0.39	0.9
ARVD	0.95	1	0.36	0.9
VSVT	0.39	0.36	1	0.39
UVT	0.9	0.9	0.39	1

ARVD = Arrhythmogenic right
MI = Myocardial infarction
IVT = Idiopathic ventricular tachycardia
VSVT = Verapamil sensitive ventricular tachycardia

tiveness of the ablative techniques which were encouraging even in patients with postinfarction VT.[29] Our results show that the number of complete or partial successes as compared to the failures is not significantly different between these two groups. In addition, the result seems valuable not only for structural and nonstructural heart diseases, generally considered in their role, but in the study of subgroups of patients like postmyocardial infarction VT or complicating ARVD (Tables 1 and 2).

Limits of the Study

In this study, the follow-up of a significant number of cases is not longer than the longest interval between attacks.

The experience gained after the use of ICDs demonstrated that in some patients the episodes of VT could decrease spontaneously over a period of time, and could lead to spontaneous regression.

The treatment of VT by ablative techniques should not be compared with the treatment of supraventricular rhythms where there are clear cut electrophysiological parameters to guide this therapy. In supraventricular tachycardia, the site of ablation is usually unique and the pathological structure is of a small size. In addition, the heart is basically normal and the ablation will lead to a complete "cure" of the disease. These cases are the closest to VT not related to a nonstructural heart disease. They are in a strong contrast with structural diseases where multiple and diffuse alterations of myocardium are present, producing zones of fibrosis and/or of adipocytes. These features may prevent the physical effect of the ablative energy with the exception of VT due to bundle branch to branch reentry.[30,31] In structural heart diseases, the number of VTs is more diffuse, and multiple morphologies could be observed during the procedure, which in any case will last longer than for the treatment of supraventricular tachycardias. This parameter has not been included in this study.

Finally, the ablative techniques by themselves that are in our center are only one aspect of the treatment of VT. In the success of results, it is also necessary to consider the expertise of our group in the use of antiarrhythmic drugs, especially in the preparation of the patients before the ablative techniques. This is why in a patient with poorly tolerated VT, or degenerating rapidly in ventricular fibrillation, the loading dose of amiodarone used as a first approach will lead in most of the cases to the induction of sustained monomorphic VT, well-tolerated, which is effectively treated by the ablative technique.

Conclusion

Radiofrequency may be used for the treatment of chronic VT resistant to drug therapy. However, its clinical efficacy used alone in 68 cases was limited to 32%.

This technique could be followed by the fulguration using an intermediate energy of cathodal 160 Joules shocks, leading to clinical effectiveness in 70% of cases at discharge of the hospital and 76% at the end of a mean follow-up period of 17 months up to 44 months.

Medium energy DC ablation used with new technical and anesthesiological protocols in 32 cases is not followed by any case of perioperative mortality.

The clinical efficacy of the first session of RF alone or followed by medium energy DC ablation shows no significant difference whatever the substrate, structural or nonstructural, particularly in a patient with VT after myocardial infarction or ARVD ($p \geq 0.6$).

A clinical efficacy is obtained in a single session of RF in 9 cases out of 12 incessant VTs in which 8 were observed in structural heart disease.

References

1. Huang SK, Jordan N, Graham AR, et al. Closed chest catheter dessication of atrioventricular junction using radiofrequency energy—a new method of catheter ablation. *Circulation* 1985;72(Suppl 3):389.
2. Gewillig M, Aubert AE, Witters E, Ector H, De Geest H. Transvenous electro-desiccation of the atrioventricular conduction system in the dog. *Stimucoeur* 1986; 14:219–225.
3. Fontaine G, Frank R, Gallais Y, et al. Fulguration et radiofréquence dans la tachycardie ventriculaire. *Arch Mal Coeur* 1994;87:1589–1607.
4. Fontaine G, Frank R, Gallais Y, et al. La radiofréquence dans le traitement de la tachycardie ventriculaire. *Arch Mal Coeur* 1996 (In press).
5. Kuck KH, Schluter M, Geiger M, Siebels J. Successful catheter ablation of human

ventricular tachycardia with radiofrequency current guided by an endocardial map of the area of slow conduction. *PACE* 1991;14:1060–1071.

6. Oeff M, Langberg J, Chin M, Finkbeiner WE, Scheinman MM. Ablation of ventricular tachycardia using multiple sequential transcatheter application of radiofrequency energy. *PACE* 1992;15:1167–1176.

7. Borggrefe M, Willems S, Chen X, et al. Catheter ablation of ventricular tachycardia using radiofrequency current. *Hertz* 1992;17:171–178.

8. Jordaens L, Vertongen P, Provenier F. Radiofrequency ablation of incessant ventricular tachycardia to prevent multiple defibrillator shocks. *Int J Cardiol* 1992; 37:117–120.

9. Gursoy S, Chiladakis I, Kuck KH. First lessons from radiofrequency catheter ablation in patients with ventricular tachycardia. *PACE* 1993;16:687–691.

10. Morady F, Harvey M, Kalbfleisch S, El-Atassi R, Calkins H, Langberg J. Radiofrequency catheter ablation of ventricular tachycardia in patients with coronary artery disease. *Circulation* 1993;87:363–372.

11. Gonska BD, Cao K, Schaumann A, Dorszewski A, Von Zur Muehlen F, Kreuzer H. Catheter ablation of ventricular tachycardia in 136 patients with coronary artery disease: results and long term follow-up. *J Am Coll Cardiol* 1994;24: 1506–1514.

12. Langberg J, Lee MA, Chin M, Rosenqvist M. Radiofrequency catheter ablation : the effect of electrode size on lesion volume in Vivo. *PACE* 1990;13:1242–1248.

13. Fontaine G, Umemura J, Iwa T, Aldakar M, Grosgogeat Y. Aspects physiques et biophysiques des decharges electriques intracardiaques a haute energie. IV-Effets des bulles de fulguration en milieu diphasique isotrope. *Ann Cardiol Angeiol* 1991; 40:515–525.

14. Gallais Y, Lascault G, Tonet J, et al. Continuous measurement of coronary sinus oxygen saturation during ventricular tachycardia. *Eur Heart J* 1993;14(Suppl):368 (Abstract).

15. Fitzgerald DM, Friday KJ, Wah JA, Lazzara R, Jackman WM. Electrogram patterns predicting successful catheter ablation of ventricular tachycardia. *Circulation* 1988;77:806–814.

16. Fontaine G, Frank R, Tonet J, Grosgogeat Y. Identification of a zone of slow conduction appropriate for VT ablation. Theoretical and practical considerations. *PACE* 1989;12(Pt II):262–267.

17. Stevenson WG, Weiss JN, Wiener I, et al. Resetting of ventricular tachycardia: implications for localizing the area of slow conduction. *J Am Coll Cardiol* 1988; 11:522–529.

18. Morady F, Kadish AH, Rosenheck S, et al. Concealed entrainment as a guide for catheter ablation of ventricular tachycardia in patients with prior myocardial infarction. *J Am Coll Cardiol* 1991;17:678–689.

19. Stevenson WG, Klein H, Sager P, et al. Identification of reentry circuit sites during catheter mapping and radiofrequency ablation of ventricular tachycardia late after myocardial infarction. *Circulation* 1993;88:1647–1670.

20. Aizawa Y, Naitoh N, Kitazawa H, et al. Frequency of presumed reentry with an excitable gap in sustained ventricular tachycardia unassociated with coronary artery disease. *Am J Cardiol* 1993;72:916–921.

21. Aizawa Y, Chinushi M, Naitoh N, Kitazawa H, et al. Catheter ablation of ventricular tachycardia with radiofrequency currents, with special reference to the termination and minor morphologic change of reinduced ventricular tachycardia. *Am J Cardiol* 1995;76:574–579.

22. Fontaine G, Cansell A, Lampe L, et al. Endocavitary Fulguration (electrode catheter ablation): equipment-related problems. In: Fontaine G, Scheinman MM (eds): *Ablation in Cardiac Arrhythmias*. Mount Kisco, NY: Futura Publishing Co., 1987, pp 85–100.
23. Borggrefe M, Budde Th, Podczeck A, Breithardt G. High frequency alternating current ablation of an accessory pathway in humans. *J Am Coll Cardiol* 1987;10: 576–582.
24. Jackman WM, Kuck KH, Naccarelli GV, Pitha J, Carmen L. Catheter ablation at the tricuspid annulus using radiofrequency current in canines. *J Am Coll Cardiol* 1987;9:99-A (Abstract).
25. Lavergne Th, Guize L, Le Heuzey JY, et al. Transvenous ablation of the atrioventricular junction in human with high-frequency energy. *J Am Coll Cardiol* 1987; 9:99-A (Abstract).
26. Langberg J, Calkins H, El-Atassi R, et al. Temperature monitoring during radiofrequency catheter ablation of accessory Pathways. *Circulation* 1992;86: 1469–1474.
27. Coggins DL, Lee RJ, Sweeney J, et al. Radiofrequency catheter ablation as a cure for idiopathic tachycardia of both left and right ventricular origin. *J Am Coll Cardiol* 1994;23:1333–1341.
28. Klein LS, Shih HT, Hackett K, Zipes DP, Miles WM. Radiofrequency catheter ablation of ventricular tachycardia in patients without structural heart disease. *Circulation* 1992;85:1666–1674.
29. Trappe HJ, Klein H, Auricchio A, Lichtlen PR. Catheter ablation of ventricular tachycardia: role of the underlying etiology and the site of energy deliveries. *PACE* 1992;15:411–424.
30. Touboul P, Kirkorian G, Atallah G, et al. Bundle branch reentrant tachycardia treated by electrical ablation of the right bundle Branch. *J Am Coll Cardiol* 1986; 7:1404–1409.
31. Tchou P, Jazayeri M, Denker S, Dongas J, Caceres J, Akhtar M. Transcatheter electrical ablation of right bundle branch. A method of treating macroreentrant ventricular tachycardia attributed to bundle branch reentry. *Circulation* 1988;78: 246–257.

PART III

Antiarrhythmic Surgical Treatment: Implantable Cardioverter Defibrillator

Chapter 14

Usefulness of Mapping in Ventricular Tachycardia Surgery

Dominique Lacroix, MD, Didier Klug, MD, Henri
Warembourg, MD, Régis Logier, PhD, Daniel
Grandmougin, MD,
Jean-Luc Hennequin, MD,
Philippe Delfaut, MD, Salem Kacet, MD,
Jean Lekieffre, MD, FACC

Introduction

Although the automatic implantable defibrillator has had an important impact on the management of drug-refractory sustained ventricular tachycardia (VT), the individual patient remains prone to clinical recurrences of arrhythmia, a fact that is at least intellectually dissatisfying.[1] The paradigm for ablative therapy of arrhythmias involves accurate definition and localization of the arrhythmia circuit or origin, followed by application of the ablative technique. Intraoperative mapping has played a fundamental role in the development of this paradigm, it has been demonstrated that mapping data permit to elucidate VT mechanisms and to design the surgical ablative procedure. In early studies, intraoperative left ventricular endocardial mapping localizes the regions that are critical for the initiation and maintenance of VT, and provides guidance for surgical ablation.[2-6] As experience is growing, it is recognized that endocardial ablation of larger volumes of tissue increases the surgical cure rate over procedures guided by the exclusive mapping of the left endocardium.[7] More recent studies demonstrate that some patients may have an infarct with anatomical and electrophysiological characteristics different from those of patients with a typical aneurysm to allow reentry that is not dependent on the endocardium but rather on the epicardium, the deep myocardium or both.[8,9] During mapping studies in which hand-held electrodes are used to record sequentially from individual sites during VT,[10] the

From *Practical Management of Cardiac Arrhythmias* edited by Nabil El-Sherif, and Jean Lekieffre. Futura Publishing Co., Armonk, NY, © 1997.

procedure is limited by the time. With the current state of development of computer technology, multipoint mapping systems enhance the ability to map VT and aim at a favorable influence on the trade-off between curative ablation of arrhythmogenic tissue and excessive loss of normal bordering myocardium, which is needed to sustain adequate ventricular function. In the present study, we retrospectively analyze data obtained during surgery in 17 patients with postinfarction VT to evaluate the interest of simultaneous mapping of the left ventricular endocardium and of the entire epicardial surface of both ventricles.

Methods

Patients Characteristics and Management

Seventeen consecutive patients recruited from April 1993 to September 1995, underwent intraoperative computerized activation mapping to guide therapy of refractory sustained (i.e., >30 seconds) monomorphic VT. Their characteristics are listed in Table 1. All patients had a history of previous myocardial infarction with documented sustained monomorphic VT in 16 patients and documented ventricular fibrillation in the remaining patient. In 16 patients receiving amiodarone, the drug had been stopped 4 to 25 days (mean 18) before surgery. Standard preoperative electrophysiological testing including a train of 8 paced beats at 3 basic cycle lengths, and introduction of up to 3 extrastimuli, delivered at 2 right ventricular sites was used to demonstrate the inducibility of sustained monomorphic VT in all 17 patients. The patients had VT refractory to pharmacological regimens or catheter ablation as judged by spontaneous recurrences or electrophysiological studies or both. No patient was excluded from surgery on the basis of infarct location, presence or absence of an aneurysm, number of VT configurations, or electrocardiographic characteristics of spontaneous VTs. A total of 57 episodes of VT corresponding to 1 to 6 (mean 3.33) episodes per patient, were mapped during surgery. All patients underwent subendocardial resection and regional cryoablation of the endocardial or epicardial sites of earliest activation during VT. When complete reentry was detected, the surgical ablation was extended to include the sites of delayed activity during VT that were adjacent to the primary breakthrough. Coronary artery bypass grafting, aneurysmectomy and mitral valve replacement were performed when necessary. Postoperative electrophysiological studies were conducted off antiarrhythmic drugs and β-blockers in all survivors with the same methodology. The institutional committee on human research approved the study protocol.

Intraoperative Mapping

Under normothermic cardiopulmonary bypass, activation epicardial, then combined epicardial and endocardial mapping were accomplished during

Table 1
Patients' Characteristics

Patient	Age:Sex (yrs)	MI	Age of MI (months)	Coronary Lesions	Scar	LVEF (%)	NYHA	VT-CL (msec)	Syncope	Drug Regimen	VT Episodes
1	45:M	ANT	3.4	1	Ak	39	II	461	No	1	3
2	61:M	ANT	52	2	An	9	II	333	No	1	1
3	64:M	INF	176	2	Ak	43	I	342	No	4	4
4	64:F	ANT	41.5	1	An	20	III	VF	VF	1	1
5	64:M	INF	237	1	Ak	42	II	384	No	8	6
6	61:M	INF	4.9	2	An	37	I	352	No	3	2
7	53:M	ANT	180	1	Ak	56	I	333	No	2	1
8	67:M	INF	N/A	1	Ak	47	I	306	No	4	7
9	64:M	ANT	28.3	2	An	31	II	300	Yes	3	20
10	67:F	ANT	65.1	2	An	10	II	300	No	2	1
11	71:M	INF	34.1	2	An	52	II	300	Yes	2	1
12	69:M	INF	213	1	An	29	I	300	Yes	1	6
13	57:M	ANT	172	2	An	32	II	307	No	2	4
14	57:M	INF	0.4	1	Ak	31	I	461	No	1	1
15	66:M	ANT	55.2	1	An	20	II	324	Yes	2	1
16	66:M	ANT	224	2	An	43	I	342	No	3	1
17	59:M	ANT	N/A	1	An	28	II	444	No	2	3
M±SD	62±6.2		99.2±86.2	1.3±0.7		33±13		349±56		2.5±1.7	3.8±4.7

Ak = akinetic; An = aneurysm; ANT = anterior; CL = cycle length; F = female; INF = inferior; LVEF = angiographically determined left ventricular ejection fraction; M = male; MI = myocardial infarction; N/A = not available; NYHA = functional status according to the NYHA classification; VF = ventricular fibrillation; VT = ventricular tachycardia.

sinus rhythm, then during sustained monomorphic VT, induced by programmed stimulation either from the right or the left epicardium, in 16 patients. In the remaining patient, only nonsustained episodes of monomorphic VT were obtained intraoperatively. Simultaneous multiple unipolar recordings were obtained by use of epicardial shock and endocardial balloon arrays. The shock electrode array consisted of 63 evenly-spaced (interelectrode distance 0.9–2.0 cm) unipolar contacts mounted on a nylon mesh. The balloon array comprised 63 unipolar electrodes (interelectrode distance 0.7–1.2 cm) mounted on an inflatable latex support. The deflated balloon array was passed through a left atriotomy across the mitral valve into the left ventricle. It was inflated with a 9% saline solution at a pressure below 25 mm Hg. Projections of left anterior and posterior descending coronary arteries on the shock array and position of the reference mark of the balloon array were noted as anatomical landmarks.

The unipolar signals with reference to Wilson's central terminal were amplified, filtered with a bandpass of 0.05–200 Hz, multiplexed, sampled at 500 Hz, and converted to a 10-bit digital format. We used the *Cardiomap II* software[11] (Institut de Génie Biomédical, Université de Montréal) based on a VAX-4000[TM] host computer (Digital Equipment Corp., Maynard, Mass. USA). Files containing either 1 second or 26 seconds of continuous data were selected and stored on hard disk during surgery. Data were analyzed in a 1-second time window selected from the stored material. The computer automatically detected the local activation time on each electrogram, at the point of most rapid potential decrease (i.e., the intrinsic deflection). The threshold for local activation was set at -0.5 V/sec.[12] Each activation map was generated for a single beat over a time interval corresponding to the duration of one VT cycle. The zero activation time was defined as the earliest activation time detected within the time window. In case of continuous activity from beat to beat, the zero activation marked the beginning of the activation of the noninfarcted myocardium (the exit point of the return pathway located over scar tissue). Slowly conducted activity corresponding to the so-called "presystolic" or "mid-diastolic" activity was arbitrarily expressed as delayed activity, and detected as low-amplitude notched deflections with slopes between -0.1 to -0.5 V/sec. Sites at which electrograms did not fulfill these criteria were considered to be unexcitable. The results were manually edited for correction of any artefacts, acceptance of activation times < -0.5 V/sec and selection of appropriate activation times in cases of multiple deflections. Isochronal maps depicting the cardiac activation sequence were plotted in a polar format with apex at the center and base along the circumference.

Definitions

Distinct VTs were defined by electrocardiographic configurations showing controlateral bundle branch block patterns, frontal axis differences of at least 60° or cycle length changes greater than 50 msec. Onset of the activation of the normal (noninfarcted) myocardium, either on the epicardial or the endocardial surface was called a breakthrough. The earliest breakthrough was called the leading breakthrough. The time-span from the earliest activation (leading breakthrough) to the latest local activation on either mapped surface was called the total activation time and expressed in percentage of the VT cycle length. Complete superficial reentry was thought to be adequately mapped when the total activation time was greater than 90% of VT cycle length and when latest and earliest activity were recorded on adjacent electrodes. Surgical success was defined as the absence of any inducible monomorphic VT at early and delayed postoperative studies, failure to induce polymorphic VT or fibrillation prior to the use of 3 extrastimuli in patients who had only monomorphic VT preoperatively and obviously as the absence of sudden death or VT recurrence postoperatively.

Mapping Limitations

We did not attempt any intervention at the site of delayed activity (i.e., pacing, cryothermia or digital pressure) to try to terminate, reset or entrain the arrhythmia. Second, we did not perform intramural recordings to analyze the spread of activation. Third, the spatial resolution of our mapping system may account for the lack of mapping of some complete reentry patterns.

Results

A total of 55 distinct morphologies of VT was obtained intraoperatively. Out of these episodes, 48 were adequately mapped with simultaneous recordings from the epicardial and endocardial surfaces in 16 patients. Twenty seven tachycardias were mapped in 9 patients with anterior myocardial infarction (Table 2), 21 tachycardias were mapped in the 7 patients with inferior myocardial infarction (Table 3). Thirteen morphologies corresponded to spontaneous episodes (clinical tachycardias), 10 had been induced preoperatively, 25 new morphologies were obtained intraoperatively. Nonsustained runs of VT were mapped in 5 morphologies, the remaining 43 episodes were sustained (i.e., >30 sec), the mean cycle length was 293 ± 55 msec. Based on the temporal epicardial to left endocardial relation, we distinguished 30 VT morphologies with onset of activation at the left endocardium (septal in 15 cases, free wall in 9 cases, apex in 3 cases and papillary muscle in the remaining 3 cases) from 15 VT morphologies arising from the left ventricular epicardium (paraseptal in 8 cases, free wall in 4 cases and apex in 3 cases). In the remaining 3 cases the first activation was detected on the right ventricular epicardium.

Table 2
Ventricular Tachycardias Mapped in Patients with Anterior Myocardial Infarction

Pt #	VT	Dur	Axis (°)	ECG Pattern	Status	CL (msec)	Leader	Site	Follower	Site	Delay	Map Pattern	TAT (msec)	%
1	A	S	120	R	Clin	260	LV-Epi	AS	LV-Endo	AS	96	Mono-R	172	66
	B	S	105	+Conc	EP-Lab	226	LV-Endo	F	LV-Epi	F	34	Bi-R	142	63
	C	S	-135	R	EP-Lab	259	LV-Endo	AS	LV-Epi	IS	56	Mono-R	194	75
2	A	S	-125	R	EP-Lab	322	LV-Epi	F	LV-Endo	S	72	Mono-R	216	67
	B	S	185	-Conc	EP-Lab	220	LV-Epi	AP	LV-Endo	S	46	Figure-8	198	90
	C	NS	130	R	New	244	LV-Epi	AP	LV-Endo	AP	24	Figure-8	126	52
	D	S	30	L	New	348	LV-Epi	AS	LV-Endo	AP	78	Figure-8	314	90
4	A	S	-90	R	EP-Lab	286	LV-Epi	AS	LV-Endo	S	18	Figure-8	192	67
	B	S	-110	R	EP-Lab	246	LV-Endo	S	LV-Epi	IS/F	20	Bi-R	220	89
	C	S	-75	+Conc	EP-Lab	290	LV-Endo	S	RV-Epi	F	56	Circle	202	70
	D	S	-60	L	EP-Lab	384	LV-Epi	AP	LV-Endo	S	26	Figure-8	354	92
	E	S	90	R	New	250	LV-Endo	F	LV-Epi	F	24	Circle	184	74
	F	S	-90	L	New	330	LV-Endo	S	LV-Epi	AS	52	Circle	318	96

7	A	S	−90	R	Clin	307	LV-Endo	AP	LV-Epi	IS	6	Mono-R	64	21
	B	NS	120	R	EP-Lab	272	LV-Endo	F	LV-Epi	F	34	Bi-R	82	30
	C	NS	90	R	New	296	LV-Endo	F	LV-Epi	AS	6	Mono-R	44	15
9	A	NS	−115	R	Clin	196	LV-Endo	IS	LV-Epi	IS	4	Mono-R	62	32
10	A	S	−45	−Conc	Clin	220	LV-Endo	IS	LV-Epi	AS	0	Figure-8	208	95
	B	S	−90	R	EP-Lab	308	LV-Endo	S	LV-Epi	IS	80	Figure-8	276	90
	C	S	120	L	New	278	LV-Epi	F	LV-Endo	AS	2	Circle	274	99
13	A	S	−90	R	Clin	338	LV-Endo	F	LV-Epi	IS	25	Bi-R	90	27
	B	S	115	+Conc	EP-Lab	370	LV-Endo	AS	LV-Epi	AS	70	Circle	220	59
15	A	S	−30	L	Clin	322	LV-Endo	S	RV-Epi	F	0	Figure-8	192	60
	B	S	−90	R	EP-Lab	276	LV-Endo	AS	LV-Epi	F	52	Mono-R	86	31
17	A	S	90	L	Clin	316	LV-Endo	AS	LV-Epi	AS	38	Mono-R	100	32
	B	S	−150	−Conc	EP-Lab	454	RV-Epi	F	LV-Endo	S	76	Bi-R	114	25
	C	S	30	L	EP-Lab	212	LV-Endo	AS	RV-Epi	F	2	Bi-R	206	97

Abbreviations: AP: apex, AS: anteroseptal, Bi-R: bi-regional activation pattern, CL: cycle length, Clin: clinical, Endo: endocardium, Epi: epicardium, EP-Lab: VT morphology induced during electrophysiological study, F: free wall, Figure-8: figure-of-eight reentrant pattern, IS: inferoseptal, L: left bundle branch block pattern, LV: left ventricle, Mono-R: mono regional activation pattern, NS: nonsustained, R: right bundle branch block pattern, RV: right ventricle, S: septal, S: sustained, TAT: total activation time, +Conc: positive concordance, −Conc: negative concordance, %: TAT expressed as a percentage of VT cycle.

Table 3

Ventricular Tachycardias Mapped in Patients with Inferior Myocardial Infarction

Pt #	VT	Dur	Axis (°)	ECG Pattern	Status	CL (msec)	Leader	Site	Follower	Site	Delay	Map Pattern	TAT (msec)	%
3	A	S	-75	R	Clin	302	LV-Endo	APM	LV-Epi	IS	48	Mono-R	96	32
	B	S	-150	R	EP-Lab	276	LV-Endo	PPM	LV-Epi	F	52	Mono-R	N/A	N/A
	C	S	-110	R	EP-Lab	326	LV-Endo	PPM	LV-Epi	F	18	Mono-R	N/A	N/A
	D	S	135	L	New	317	LV-Endo	IS	LV-Epi	F	36	Mono-R	190	60
5	A	S	-60	+Conc	Clin	286	LV-Epi	IS	LV-Endo	S	24	Mono-R	12	42
	B	S	150	R	EP-Lab	260	LV-Endo	AP	LV-Epi	IS	0	Mono-R	122	47
	C	S	15	L	EP-Lab	216	LV-Endo	S	RV-Epi	F	36	Mono-R	132	61
6	A	S	-50	+Conc	Clin	270	RV-Epi	IS	LV-Endo	IS	22	Mono-R	104	39
	B	S	-90	R	EP-Lab	230	LV-Endo	AP	LV-Epi	AP	22	Mono-R	70	30
	C	S	-130	R	EP-Lab	222	LV-Epi	F	LV-Endo	F	88	Mono-R	198	89
	D	S	-70	R	New	278	LV-Epi	IS	LV-Endo	S	20	Bi-R	108	39
8	A	NS	120	+Conc	Clin	336	LV-Endo	F	LV-Epi	F	18	Mono-R	104	31
11	A	S	30	L	EP-Lab	328	LV-Endo	IS	RV-Epi	F	18	Mono-R	86	26
	B	S	-45	+Conc	EP-Lab	320	LV-Epi	IS	LV-Endo	F	42	Mono-R	124	39
	C	S	-120	R	EP-Lab	460	LV-Endo	F	LV-Epi	F	34	Mono-R	64	14
12	A	S	-30	+Conc	Clin	274	LV-Epi	IS	LV-Endo	IS	52	Circle	244	89
	B	S	90	R	EP-Lab	314	LV-Endo	F	LV-Epi	F	16	Mono-R	144	46
14	A	S	-120	R	Clin	310	LV-Endo	S	LV-Epi	AS	16	Mono-R	210	68
	B	S	-90	-Conc	EP-Lab	300	LV-Epi	IS	LV-Endo	AP	44	Circle	218	73
	C	S	-60	L	New	310	RV-Epi	IS	LV-Endo	IS	76	Circle	244	79
	D	S	165	R	New	320	LV-Epi	F	LV-Endo	F	30	Circle	298	90

Abbreviations: same as in Table 2.

Subendocardial Substrates

In the majority of VT morphologies (30 out of 48), the earliest break-through of activation was recorded on the left ventricular endocardium and preceded the onset of epicardial activation. In 26 cases, there was no evidence of complete reentry on either surface, conversely in 4 cases the endocardial map displayed a complete reentrant pattern (patient 4 morphology F, patient 10 morphologies A and B, patient 17 morphology C). The electrograms recorded at the endocardial level displayed a continuous sequence of local activations along the common pathway of a figure-of-eight pattern (n = 2), or along a leading circle with a single (n = 1) or double (n = 1) breakthrough. Among the 26 patterns without evidence of complete reentry, 4 of them displayed an incomplete figure-of-eight or leading circle (Figure 1), in the

ENDO

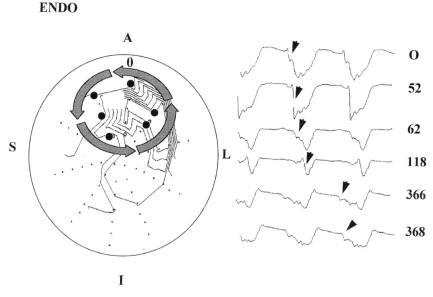

Figure 1. Upper panel: endocardial mapping (ENDO) during ventricular tachycardia in a patient with anterior myocardial infarction (patient #13, VT morphology B). The format of the map in polar with basal regions at the circumference and the apex at the center. Selected electrograms from recording sites indicated by dots are represented in the right part of the figure. Numbers and small arrows indicate activation times. Isochronal lines are traced at 50-msec intervals. Endocardial activation preceded epi-cardial activation by 70 msec. A counterclockwise circulating wavefront is indicated by arrows, however the reentrant mechanism is incompletely mapped with a missing gap >40% of the VT cycle length. "Presystolic activity" with activation times at 366 and 368 msec is visible in the last 2 electrograms.

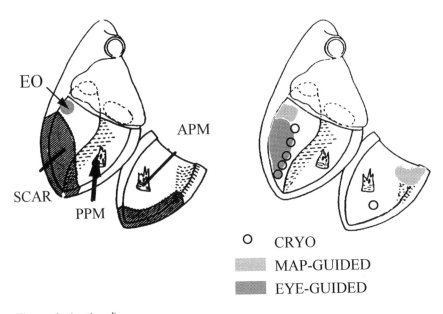

CRYO
MAP-GUIDED
EYE-GUIDED

Figure 1. *(continued)*
Ablative procedure in the same patient. The VT mechanism described above is indicated in the left part of the figure (EO) and located at the junction between the septum and the anterior wall of the left ventricle. Scarred tissue is indicated by dark shading. The left ventricular cavity is open through an imaginary cut along the anterior paraseptal wall. In the right part of the figure, circles show sites of map-guided cryoablation, dark shaded area indicates the visually guided subendocardial resection performed in the septum. The light shaded area is an additional map-guided subendocardial resection performed after the identification of the above-mentioned VT mechanism. A = anterior; APM = anterior papillary muscle; ENDO = endocardium; EO = endocardial origin; I = inferior; L = lateral; PPM = posterior papillary muscle; S = septal.

remaining cases a monoregional (n = 18) or biregional (n = 4) spread of activation was observed.[13]

Substrates Involving Papillary Muscles

In 3 VT morphologies obtained in the same patient (patient 3 in Table 3) with an inferior myocardial scar related to the occlusion of the circumflex artery, involvement of papillary muscles was observed. In the first morphology which corresponded to a clinical arrhythmia, the anterior papillary muscle was implicated whereas in the 2 other morphologies the mechanism of the tachycardia was located to the posterior papillary muscle (Figure 2). In each morphology a radial spread of activation centered on the papillary muscle

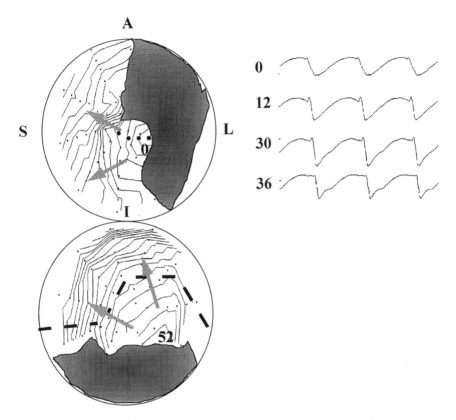

Figure 2. Example of VT originating in the posterior papillary muscle in a patient with a circumflex-related inferior infarction (patient #3, VT morphology B). Same polar format as in Figure 1. The upper map represents the left ventricular endocardial activation, the lower map represents the simultaneous epicardial activation of both ventricles. The epicardial breakthrough occurs 52 msec after the beginning of the endocardial activation. The pattern of epi/endocardial activation is a radial spread with concentric isochronal lines centered on the posterior papillary muscle and traced at 10-msec intervals. Selected electrograms recorded at sites indicated by black dots show sharp rS deflections in favor of a focal mechanism. Numbers on these signals refer to the activation times. Dark areas indicate scar tissue. Dashed line on the epicardial map represents the anatomical location of the left anterior and posterior descending coronary arteries. (Abbreviations: same as in Figure 1.)

was mapped endocardially. These mechanisms had been suspected preoperatively on the basis of magnetic resonance imaging showing incomplete necrosis of both papillary muscle.

Subepicardial Substrates

In some tachycardias (15 out of 48) the earliest endocardial activation followed the earliest epicardial activation (Figure 3). Strikingly, a high proportion of complete reentrant patterns was observed (i.e., 5 out of these 15 morphologies). In these episodes the electrograms recorded at the epicardial level displayed a continuous sequence of local activations along the common pathway of figure-of-eight pattern (n = 3), or along a leading circle with a single breakthrough (n = 2). Among the 10 patterns without evidence of complete reentry, 4 of them displayed an incomplete figure-of-eight or leading circle, in the remaining cases a monoregional (n = 5) or biregional (n = 1) spread of activation was observed. The vast majority of patients in whom a complete reentrant pattern was recorded either epicardially or endocardially, had an anterior myocardial scar (8 anterior versus 1 inferior infarct location).

Multiuse Reentry Substrates

This term has been proposed by Downar et al.[14] to describe a return path of reentry with multiple entry and exit points allowing for different paths at different times all in a same patient. Two of our patients (#10 and 14 in Tables 2 and 3) demonstrate such different VT morphologies sharing a same return path. In patient #10 who had an anterior infarction and 3 morphologies mapped peroperatively, 2 of these 3 morphologies demonstrated a complete subendocardial figure-of-eight reentrant pattern. These 2 patterns shared the same slowly conducting zone, whereas the VT cycle lengths varied (220 versus 308 msec) and the exit points were different (on the anterior and inferior part of the septum respectively). In patient #14, two morphologies (C and D in Table 3) were characterized by a superficial epicardial reentry (Figures 3 and 4). The first pattern propagated clockwise with a right ventricular breakthrough and the other pattern propagated counterclockwise with an exit area in the left ventricular free wall. The exit point of the first VT became the entry point of the second VT and *vice versa*.

Deep Septal Layers Involvement

In 2 tachycardias (patients #6 and 17 in Tables 3 and 2) a right epicardial breakthrough preceded the left endocardial breakthrough by 22 and 76 msec. This breakthrough occurred in the posterior paraseptal region in the first

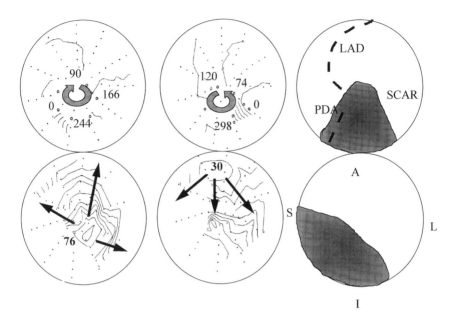

Figure 3. Diagrams and maps of two different VTs with subepicardial reentry in a same patient with inferior myocardial infarction (patient #14, tachycardias C and D). **Left and middle panels:** Upper diagrams are polar representations of left ventricular and right ventricular epicardial activations with the base of the heart at the circumference and its apex at the center. Lower diagrams are polar representations of the left ventricular endocardium. **Right panel:** Diagrams of the scar tissue (dark shaded areas) and of the left anterior and posterior descending coronary arteries (LAD and PDA). **Left panel** indicates that the earliest epicardial activation (zero time) was detected on the right margin of the epicardial scar between the apical and basal portion of the infarction in the first VT (episode C). From this area, activation spread out in a clockwise circulating front, circumvented an area of inexcitability centered on the apical portion of the scar and reentered at the lateral margin of the scar in the left ventricular free wall. The endocardial map (left panel, bottom) showed a mono regional activation pattern beginning 76 msec after the onset of epicardial activation. The second tachycardia (episode D) is represented in the middle panel. The earliest epicardial activation was detected on the left margin of the infarction, preceding the endocardial breakthrough by 30 msec. From this area a counterclockwise circulating wavefront was observed which circumvented the same area of inexcitability and reentered at the right margin of the scar. Activation patterns are detailed in Figure 4. (Abbreviations: same as in Figures 1 and 2.)

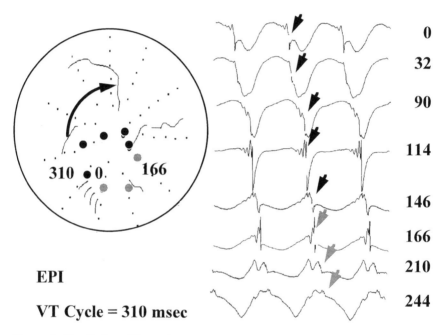

Figure 4. Details from Figure 3.
Epicardial activation observed in episode C. Isochronal lines drawn at 50-msec intervals depict a clockwise circular activation pattern. Selected electrograms are represented in the right part of the figure. The recording sites of the first five electrograms are indicated by black dots located in healthy myocardium. The activation times at these sites are indicated by numbers from 0 to 146 msec and black arrows. Shaded dots are the recording sites of the last three electrograms located along the return path, however, a missing gap is present from 244 msec to 310 msec (shaded arrows and numbers indicate activation times). The criteria for superficial complete reentry are therefore not fulfilled.

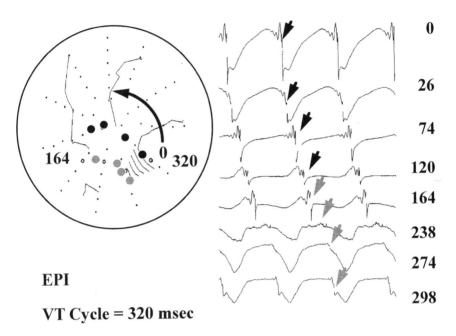

EPI

VT Cycle = 320 msec

Figure 4. *(continued)*
Epicardial activation observed in episode D. Isochronal lines drawn at 50-msec intervals depict a counterclockwise circular activation pattern. Similarly, selected electrograms are represented in the right part of the figure. The recording sites of the first four electrograms are indicated by black dots located in healthy myocardium. The activation times at these sites are indicated by numbers from 0 to 120 msec and the black arrows. Shaded dots are recording sites of the last four electrograms located along the return path (shaded arrows and numbers indicate activation times). The criteria for superficial complete reentry are fulfilled. The activation pattern mapped on the epicardium encompassed 93% of the VT cycle length (320 msec), and the earliest and latest activations were recorded from immediately adjacent electrodes. The earliest activity corresponded to the reentrant site of the preceding tachycardia, conversely the reentrant site of this episode was the exit point of the preceding morphology. Note that both episodes had similar cycle lengths and that the conduction across the scar covered approximately the same time intervals. Abbreviations: EPI: epicardium.

case and in the right ventricular free wall in the other case. The following left ventricular activation was found in the septum. These observations are throught to be related to a deep right-sided origin of the tachycardia.[8] A third case, already discussed above, of right ventricular epicardial breakthrough was observed in patient 14, tachycardia C, but the mechanism was different (i.e., superficial reentry).

Clinical Results

The surgical technique to ablate the substrates consisted in subendocardial resection combined with regional cryoablation. Subendocardial resection was limited to the septal fibrotic tissue in 5 patients, was extended to, or restricted to the the left ventricular free wall in 5 patients, involved the entire visible scar in 6 patients. In the remaining patient (patient #3 in Table 3) only the papillary muscles were resected. Cryosurgery was applied to endocardial site of earliest activation in 3 patients and to additional left epicardial sites in 11 patients. The remaining 5 patients received combined left endocardial, left epicardial and right epicardial cryolesions. One operative death was observed (patient #11). In 14 patients, VTs were no longer inducible; in patient #1 a single VT morphology (C in Table 2) was still induced without clinical recurrence during follow-up. In patient #10, two VTs (A and B in Table 2) were still inducible, one of them spontaneously recurred leading to implant an automatic cardioverter defibrillator. Overall, operative mortality rate and success rate were 5.9% and 87.5% respectively.

Discussion

Is Any Mapping Necessary?

Several groups[15-17] have proposed that intraoperative mapping can be totally eliminated if a visually guided resection of all visible endocardial scar is performed. In the series of Zee-Cheng,[15] 25 of the 43 operative survivors were treated with antiarrhythmic drugs. Late cardiac and sudden cardiac death rates were also high. In two other more recent series[16,17] (Landymore et al. and Sosa et al.) the results seem to be more favorable. However the patients were highly selected (notably inferior infarcts were excluded) and the number of patients was quite small. Our experience with visually guided procedures[18] is summarized in Table 4 and compared with the present series. This table shows that despite a longer pump time and a longer ischemic time in map-guided surgery, the operative mortality rate is not increased. Conversely, the postoperative rate of VT inducibility is dramatically lower in patients who underwent map-guided surgery.

Table 4
Comparison Between Visually Guided and Map-Guided Surgery

	Visually Guided	Map-Guided	p
n	23	17	
Age (years)	65 ± 6.2	62 ± 6.2	ns
LVEF (%)	33 ± 8.6	33 ± 13	ns
Aneurysm	18/23	11/17	ns
Ischemic time (min)	71 (48–100)	108 (78–143)	†
Bypass time (min)	100 (59–142)	208 (151–308)	†
VTs no longer inducible	8/22	14/16	*
Operative deaths	1/23	1/17	ns

LVEF = angiographically determined left ventricular ejection fraction; ns = nonsignificant; VT = ventricular tachycardia; *: $p < 0.01$; †: $p < 0.001$.

During two decades of experience with mapping of VT, an enormous amount has been learned about the mechanisms of this disorder. One of the last advances in that field is the recognition of "nonconventional" substrates. In this paper, we confirm the possible participation of subepicardial or deep intraseptal layers to the reentrant mechanism of a substantial number of post-infarction VTs. The prevalence of these atypical substrates is 37%, a proportion in agreement with studies previously published.[8,9,13] The identification of these substrates is highly dependent on the use simultaneous epicardial left endocardial mapping.

Is Computerized Mapping Helpful?

The potential advantages of computerized data acquisition and analysis systems seem to be obvious. Even a nonsustained episodes of VT can be completely mapped.[19] Since signals from all leads are simultaneously acquired, manipulation of the heart is no longer necessary. The use of a transmitral balloon array obviates the need for a ventriculotomy which may render a VT noninducible.[2–4,7] Finally, the total activation time can be determined within a short period of time, even though hundreds of points are included in the analysis. Disadvantages however exist. Noisy, double or fragmented electrograms may be difficult to analyze and may not be included in the final map. Mapping may help reduce bypass time if it is not made too complex and the electrophysiologist makes the correct interpretation. It may help reduce the amount of myocardium to be resected when the surgical-electrophysiological team has experience and mutual trust.

Atypical Reentrant Substrates

Reentry has long been recognized as a mechanism for arrhythmias, particularly those associated with infarcted myocardium. The key interplay among refractoriness, conduction velocity and the length of the circuit (i.e., the wavelength concept) has been emphasized. Many studies have concluded that the infarcted myocardium provides a substrate for slow conduction that is largely responsible for the genesis of reentry. Although human ventricular tachycardias are often generated subendocardially, some studies provide evidence that the reentrant circuits are not always confined to the subendocardium. De Bakker et al.[20–22] have demonstrated that segments of a reentrant circuit or even the entire reentrant circuit can be intramural or epicardial. The consequence is obvious: limiting mapping to the left endocardium may be insufficient to achieve successful identification of these circuits. The observations of the Duke University group[23] using three-dimensional intraoperative mapping of up to 156 intramural sites have confirmed that VT is often due to intramural reentry. The initiation usually occurs in the subendocardium or epicardium with prominent conduction delay as well as functional or anatomical block in the subendocardium and midmyocardium. These results explain, in part, the infrequent delineation of complete superficial (endocardial or epicardial) pathways even with combined epicardial and endocardial mapping.

For septal tachycardias, many reports have documented the existence of right septal tachycardias.[4,12,24] Despite the fact that the earliest activity was recorded on the right ventricular free wall, it is likely that the circuit was localized within the right half of the interventricular septum; the impulse might have been blocked in the infarcted left half of the septum and would then have exited toward the right normal myocardium. This interpretation is compatible with data obtained with right endocardial mapping showing that right septal endocardial activity preceded both right epicardial and left endocardial breakthroughs (Pagé et al. personal communication).

Conclusions

The three-dimensional view of the substrate of a given tachycardia can be derived from simultaneous epicardial and endocardial mapping data. This view provides the foundation for determining whether less extensive ablative procedures will be effective. On the other hand, in some cases, extension of the ablation into the septal midmyocardium or even epicardium may be required to eliminate VT. With multiple mechanisms possible in the same individual, the ablation of one mechanism could be followed by VT recurrence at a different site. Therefore, in guiding the ablative procedure intraoperative mapping help to treat the individual patient better surgically.

Acknowledgments

The authors wish to thank Pierre Pagé, MD, René Cardinal, PhD, Pierre Savard, BEng, PhD and Reginal Nadeau, MD, from the Sacré Cœur Hospital Research Center, Montreal Québec, for their constant support to the antiarrhythmic surgery program.

References

1. Fricchione GL, Vlay LC, Vlay SC. Cardiac psychiatry and the management of malignant ventricular arrhythmias with the internal cardioverter-defibrillator. *Am Heart J* 1994;128:1050–1059.
2. Ostermeyer J, Borggrefe M, Breithardt G, et al. Direct operations for the management of life-threatening ischemic ventricular tachycardia. *J Thorac Cardiovasc Surg* 1987;94:848–865.
3. Swerdlow CD, Mason JW, Stinson EB, et al. Results for operations for ventricular tachycardia in 105 patients. *J Thorac Cardiovasc Surg* 1986;92:105–113.
4. Krafchek J, Lawrie GM, Roberts R, et al. Surgical ablation of ventricular tachycardia: improved results with a map-directed regional approach. *Circulation* 1986;73: 1239–1247.
5. Miller JM, Kienzle MG, Harken AH. Subendocardial resection for ventricular tachycardia: predictors of surgical success. *Circulation* 1984;70:624–631.
6. Mason JW, Stinson EB, Winkle RA, et al. Surgery for ventricular tachycardia: efficacy of left ventricular aneurysm resection compared with operation guided by electrical activation mapping. *Circulation* 1982;65:1148–1155.
7. Cox JL. Patient selection criteria and results of surgery for refractory ischemic ventricular tachycardia. *Circulation* 1989;79(Suppl I):I-163–177.
8. Kaltenbrunner W, Cardinal R, Dubuc M, et al. Epicardial and endocardial mapping of ventricular tachycardia in patients with myocardial infarction. Is the origin of the tachycardia always subendocardially localized? *Circulation* 1991;84: 1058–1071.
9. Svenson RH, Littmann L, Gallagher JJ, et al. Termination of ventricular tachycardia with epicardial laser photocoagulation: a clinical comparison with patients undergoing successful endocardial ablation alone. *J Am Coll Cardiol* 1990;15: 163–170.
10. Josephson ME, Harken AH, Horowitz LN. Long-term results of endocardial resection for sustained ventricular tachycardia in coronary artery disease patients. *Am Heart J* 1982;104:51–57.
11. Bonneau G, Tremblay G, Savard P, et al. An integrated system for intraoperative cardiac activation mapping. *IEEE Trans Biomed Eng* 1987;34:415–423.
12. Durrer D, Van Lier AAW, Buler J. Epicardial and intramural excitation in chronic myocardial infarction. *Am Heart J* 1964;68:765–776.
13. Harris L, Downar D, Mickleborough L, et al. Activation sequences of ventricular tachycardia: endocardial and epicardial mapping studies in the human ventricle. *J Am Coll Cardiol* 1987;10:1040–1047.
14. Downar E, Kimber S, Harris L, et al. Endocardial mapping of ventricular tachycardia in the intact human heart. II. Evidence for multiuse reentry in a functional sheet of surviving myocardium. *J Am Coll Cardiol* 1992;20:869–888.

15. Zee-Cheng C, Kouchoukos NT, Connors JP, et al. Treatment of life-threatening ventricular arrhythmias with nonguided surgery supported by electrophysiologic testing and drug therapy. *J Am Coll Cardiol* 1989;13:153–162.

16. Landymore RW, Gardner MA, McIntyre AJ, et al. Surgical intervention for drug-resistant ventricular tachycardia. *J. Am Coll Cardiol* 1990;16:37–41.

17. Sosa E, Jatene A, Kaeriyama JV, et al. Recurrent ventricular tachycardia associated with postinfarction aneurysm. Results of left ventricular reconstruction. *J Thorac Cardiovasc Surg* 1992;103:855–860.

18. Aisenfarb JC, Kacet S, Lacroix D, et al. Thermoexclusion laser circonférentielle de tachycardies ventriculaires post-infarctus: à propos de 11 cas. *Arch Mal Coeur* 1991;84:1289–1295.

19. Branyas NA, Cain ME, Cox JL, et al. Transmural ventricular activation during consecutive cycles of sustained ventricular tachycardia associated with coronary artery disease. *Am J Cardiol* 1990;65:861–867.

20. De Bakker JMT, Van Cappelle FJL, Janse MJ, et al. Reentry as a cause of ventricular tachycardia in patients with chronic ischemic heart disease: Electrophysiologic and anatomic correlation. *Circulation* 1988;77:589–606.

21. De Bakker JMT, Coronel R, Tasseron S, et al. Ventricular tachycardia in the infarcted, Langendorff-perfused human heart: role of the arrangement of surviving cardiac fibers. *J Am Coll Cardiol* 1990;15:1594–1607.

22. De Bakker JMT, Van Capelle FJL, Janse MJ, et al. Macroreentry in the infarcted human heart: the mechanism of ventricular tachycardia with a "focal" activation pattern. *J Am Coll Cardiol* 1991;18:1005–1014.

23. Pogwizd SM, Hoyt RH, Saffitz JE, et al. Reentrant and focal mechanisms underlying ventricular tachycardia in the human heart. *Circulation* 1992;86:1872–1887.

24. Kaltenbrunner W, Veit F, Winter S, et al. Epicardial and left ventricular endocardial activation mapping of septal tachycardia in patients after myocardial infarction: Is estimation of the depth of origin feasible? In: Shenasa M, Borggrefe M, Breithardt G, (eds): *Cardiac Mapping*. Mount Kisco, NY: Futura Publishing Co, 1993, pp 467–494.

Chapter 15_____

Surgical Treatment of Ventricular Tachycardia:
Indications and Results

Pierre L. Pagé, MD

Introduction

The surgical approach to the treatment of arrhythmias at the ventricular level has been developed during a period when sustained monomorphic ventricular tachycardias (VTs) associated with postinfarction left ventricular scars were of major clinical concern and constituted an important paradigm in clinical cardiac electrophysiology.[1,2] Successful VT surgery was based on the concept that the arrhythmia could be induced and mapped intraoperatively and, therefore, it could be surgically corrected. However, the management of VT has evolved in the past several years into three distinct directions.[3] Two of these involve the ablation of the arrhythmogenic substrate through direct, open heart surgery, or a percutaneous catheter approach. The third is the implantation of devices capable of detecting and terminating ventricular arrhythmias with either pacing or high energy shock. The assumption that the latter two approaches bear a lower short-term mortality rate is only one reason explaining their increased use and the apparent decline in the number of VT surgery cases in several centers.

Clinical Use of Direct VT Surgery

It appears that the number of VT surgeries has declined by approximately 50% between 1990 and 1993.[4] Moreover, several centers have performed fewer than two such operations in the past year.[4] The number of patients referred for investigation of VT has declined, and in many cases, other treatment modalities were chosen on the same reference basis. At the present time, most clinical electrophysiologists taking care of VT patients believe that the

From *Practical Management of Cardiac Arrhythmias* edited by Nabil El-Sherif, and Jean Lekieffre. Futura Publishing Co., Armonk, NY, © 1997.

widespread use of thrombolysis in the management of acute myocardial infarction (MI) has resulted in fewer patients having large aneurysm, and hence, a reduced likelihood of ventricular arrhythmias.[5-7] Another reason for the change in arrhythmia management is the growing enthusiasm for other treatment options, including medical therapy. In many European and Canadian centers, ventricular arrhythmias are managed on the basis of an appropriate use of antiarrhythmic agents, notably amiodarone, either alone or in combination with beta-blockers.[8] In these centers, cardioverter defibrillator (ICD) implantation is rare and surgery is used in highly selected patients only. In the vast majority of the other centers, the preferred approach is the implantation of an ICD, despite the availability of highly competent electrophysiological surgery teams in their own center. Antitachycardia devices are now implanted transvenously, often in the prepectoral region, have better detection algorithms leading to a decreased incidence of inappropriate shocks, can terminate VT with pacing, thus avoiding painful high energy shocks, and are more efficacious due to better shock waveform configuration. In spite of these refinements, this form of treatment is still considered as palliative and most patients need to modify their lifestyle quite significantly (e.g., they are often not allowed to drive a car). Furthermore, the long-term benefits of this therapy in terms of total cardiac mortality are still under investigation.[3]

Clinical Decision-Making

Treatment outcomes in the management of ventricular arrhythmias include the return of the arrhythmia, either spontaneously or induced during programmed stimulation studies, the occurrence of sudden cardiac death, the life expectancy of the patients, and their functional status. In specific clinical situations, the prediction of a high operative mortality rate should not exclude the possibility of a greater therapeutic benefit with the operation than without.[9] In this chapter, the results of our own experience in VT surgery, initiated in 1983, will be reviewed in an attempt to delineate our current decision process in managing patients with malignant ventricular arrhythmias.

Our Experience

Patient Population

Between September 1983 and September 1995, we performed direct map-guided surgery in 100 patients. Their clinical characteristics are listed

Table 1
Patient Characteristics

	N = 100
Mean age (±SD, in years)	56.9 ± 9.8
Sex M/F	87/13
Mean EF	0.29 ± 0.09
NYHA I/II	71
NYHA III/IV	29
Cardiac Arrest	59
Episodes of VT preoperatively	
<3	51
4–10	43
>10	4
Infarct location	
Anterior	63
Inferior	37
Aneurysm	66
No Aneurysm	34
3 VD	35
1 VD	35
2 VD	28

EF = ejection fraction; VD = ventricular dysplasia.

in Table 1. All patients had an MI of 0.5 to 120 months prior to arrhythmia surgery. Seven patients had previous cardiac surgery. One to three morphologies of sustained monomorphic VT could be induced during the preoperative electrophysiological study.

Surgical Technique

Intraoperative electrophysiological mapping was performed using sequential recordings with a hand-held probe in the first 16 patients and with a multichannel computerized mapping system in the other 84 patients. Epicardial data were obtained with a shock electrode array containing 63 unipolar contacts and endocardial recordings were obtained with a 64-electrode balloon array introduced in the intact left ventricle through an incision in the left atrium at the right superior pulmonary vein. With this approach, VT could be induced and mapped intraoperatively in 100% of our patients. Epicardial and endocardial data were recorded simultaneously. This method allowed us to determine not only the site of earliest activation, but also the epicardial/endocardial timing relationship.[10] The localization of the arrhythmogenic substratum was deduced from three-dimensional interpretation of the global activation sequence of the two ventricles. This substratum was ablated under cold blood cardioplegia using endocardial resection alone in five patients, cryoablation alone in 63 patients, and cryoablation combined to endocardial resection in 22 patients. Coronary artery bypass grafting was done in 71 patients, aneurysmectomy in 66 and mitral valve replacement in 3.

Results

The postoperative results are presented in Table 2. Overall survival rates were 89% at 1 year, 72% at 5 years, and 59% at 10 years and included six (6%) in-hospital deaths (Figure 1). The freedom from sudden death was 98% at 5 years and remained constant until the 10th year of follow-up, since the only two sudden deaths occurred within the first 6 months after the operation. Univariate analysis indicated that two preoperative factors predicted operative mortality: previous cardiac surgery (two of six patients, 33%, 70% confidence intervals: 12% to 62%, $p < 0.01$) and 3 vessel disease (5 of 35 patients, 14%, 70% confidence intervals: 8% to 23%, $p < 0.01$). Age, ejection fraction, last MI to surgery interval, NYHA functional class, and pump time did not influence operative mortality rate. The presence of an aneurysm, as defined by intraoperative identification of a thinning of the left ventricular scar, significantly influenced the electrophysiological results, but not the operative mortality (Table 3). Interestingly, the result of the postoperative electrophysiological study was a strong predictor of late outcome. The long-term survival was significantly lower (Figure 2), and the rate of VT return or sudden death significantly higher in patients with reinducible VT (Table 4). The most important factor that influenced the rate of postoperative VT reinducibility, the late return of spontaneous VT, and the rate of sudden death was the induction at the time of intraoperative mapping of at least one VT morphol-

Table 2
Overall Results

Early deaths	6
Late deaths	21
VT reinducible	13
Late sudden death	2
VT recurrence	6
5-year survival	72%
NYHA I/II	79
NYHA III/IV	13

VT = ventricular tachycardia.

Actuarial survival including operative mortality

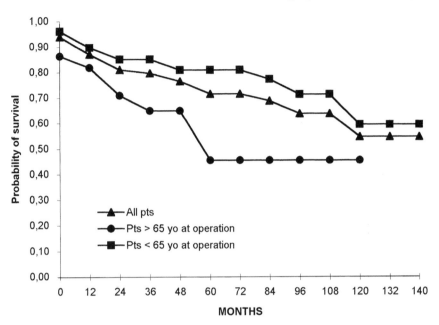

Figure 1. Actuarial survival in 100 patients operated for ventricular tachycardia (VT) with map-guided procedures at Sacré-Coeur Hospital in Montreal between September 1983 and October 1995. The 5-year survival rate was 72% overall, 81% for patients aged < 65 years at the time of operation and 46% for those older than 65 years.

ogy with the type 5 pattern (Figure 3).[10] We described this pattern in 1991 as a situation in which the epicardial breakthrough during VT occurs in the right ventricle, despite the absence of any scar tissue in this region, and precedes the left ventricular endocardial breakthrough. This pattern was found in 35 of the 84 patients mapped endocardially and epicardially with the computerized mapping system. Twelve patients in whom such a pattern was identified at mapping had reinducible VT and among them, one had sudden death and three presented recurrent VT (p < 0.001)(Table 4).

Septal Ventricular Tachycardias

The mapping data of 43 patients in whom at least one VT morphology was found to originate in the interventricular septum were reviewed. The patients were divided into two groups. Group I was comprised of 23 patients

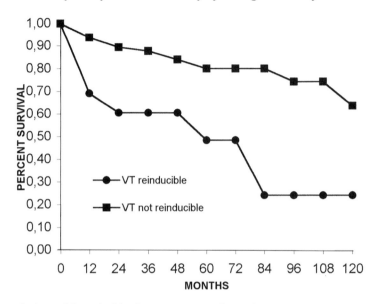

Figure 2. Actuarial survival in the 94 survivors who underwent postoperative electro-physiological testing. Note the marked difference in outcome depending on the results of the test (p < 0.001).

Table 3
Results as Per the Presence or Absence of a LV Aneurysm

Outcome	Aneurysm Present N = 66		Aneurysm Absent N = 34		P
	n (%)	(70% CL)	n (%)	(70% CL)	
Hospital deaths	3 (5)	(2–9)	3 (9)	(4–12)	NS
VT reinducible	7 (10)	(6–16)	6 (18)	(11–18)	NS
VT return	2 (3)	(1–7)	4 (12)	(6–21)	<0.05§
Sudden death	0	(0–4)	2 (6)	(2–4)	NS
Clinical events	2 (3)	(1–7)	5 (15)	(8–24)	NS
Arrhythmic events	8 (12)	(8–18)	9 (26)	(18–36)	0.01
5-year survival	72% (63–80)		72% (59–82)		NS
10-year survival	52% (44–59)		72% (58–81)		<0.05

CL = confidence interval; LV = left ventricle; NS = not significant.
§ χ^2 test.

Table 4
Analysis (Univariate) of Factors Associated With VT Return or Sudden Death

	Factor Present		Factor Absent		
Factor	n (%)	(70% CL)	n (%)	(70% CL)	P
VT reinducible	4 of 13 (31)	(16–49)	4 of 81 (5)	(3–9)	<0.01§
Type 5 VT	12* of 35 (34%)	(25–44)	2 of 47 (4)	(1–10)	<0.001§

CL = confidence intervals. Type 5 VT, VT activation pattern induced intraoperatively which displayed an epicardial breakthrough on the right ventricle preceding the onset of activation at the left ventricular endocardium.[10] This characteristic could be assessed in 82 patients. Factor was indicated as present when at least one of the VT morphologies induced and mapped intraoperatively fitted this pattern.
* Includes patients with inducible VT at postoperative electrophysical study.
§ χ^2 test.

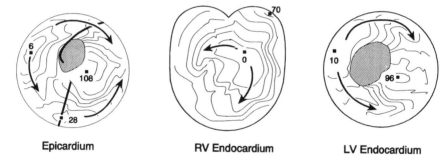

Epicardium   RV Endocardium   LV Endocardium

Figure 3. Diagrams showing epicardial and endocardial mapping of ventricular tachycardia (VT) originating in the *right* subendocardial layers of the septum in a patient with an anteroseptal infarct (shading). Mapping grids represent a polar view of the heart in which the base is at the periphery of the circle and the apex is at the center. The epicardial map **(left hand panel)** was obtained from data recorded with a shock electrode array. The center map was obtained from a specially designed balloon apparatus introduced in the right ventricle (RV) through the right atrium and the tricuspid valve. The right hand map was generated from data obtained with an oval shaped balloon electrode introduced in the left ventricle (LV) across the mitral valve. The endocardial grids display their corresponding septal and free-wall aspects. Semicircular upward extensions on the RV endocardial grid indicate the balloon prolongation into the right ventricular outflow tract. Activation sequence maps with isochrone lines drawn at 10-ms intervals. The right endocardial septal activation (0 activation time) preceded the left endocardial septal activation (10 ms). The epicardial breakthrough (six on the left hand map) occurred in the RV free-wall area and preceded the LV endocardial breakthrough, a typical feature of right or "deep" septal VT.

operated before the recognition of type 5 pattern as an indicator of deep septal VT. This group was compared to the next 23 consecutive patients in whom septal endocardial resection was combined to transmural cryosurgery (applied on the left ventricular aspect of the septum after the completion of endocardial resection), whenever a type 5 VT was identified. This type of VT was found at the retrospective analysis of mapping data in 11 group I patients and identified intraoperatively in 11 group II patients. All type 5 VTs were associated to a left bundle branch block morphology on the surface electrocardiogram. In the remaining patients, the mapping data showed that the epicardial breakthrough occurred in the anterior or inferior interventricular groove, and followed, rather than preceding the left ventricular endocardial breakthrough. Two patients died in each group. The results indicated that VT was reinducible in 7 patients in group I, and in only 1 patient in group II ($p < 0.05$, χ^2 test). Thus, we concluded from that study that type 5 activation pattern may correspond to a deep septal substratum and that its identification at the time of intraoperative mapping was mandatory.

Discussion

Although operative mortality averaged 23% in reports published prior to the nonthoracotomy ICD era (earlier than 1990),[11] most surgical series evaluated in the past 5 years indicate a mortality rate $< 5\%$.[12–16] There is strong evidence that recurrent symptomatic VT after acute MI is associated with a poor prognosis (1-year mortality varying from 12% to 54%).[17] Recent studies show that the 5-year actuarial survival varies from 33% to 71% depending on the degree of left ventricular structural damage existing preoperatively.[18] However, using the quality of the residual left ventricular function as a criterion for operability, van Hemel has reduced the in-hospital mortality to 1.3% and his 4-year actuarial survival was 85%.[18] Arrhythmia freedom without drugs after 5 years was 88% in our series, averaging about 75% in the current literature.[3,11,18] These figures show that surgery is a very acceptable alternative therapy in surgical candidates. In spite of a nonnegligible proportion of patients in whom VTs are still inducible after surgery (2% to 20%, but $< 15\%$ in most series, including ours) the long-term outcome of VT surgery is quite remarkable.[3,11,18] In many recent publications, the actuarial freedom of VT recurrence is 90% at 5 years, the overall 5-year survival rate is between 65% and 79% and the sudden death rate is 2.5% or less.[1,11,18]

A large number of preoperative clinical and laboratory factors influencing operative mortality have been evaluated in many reports. According to a review published by Cox in 1989,[11] the most frequently reported factors predisposing to an increased short-term mortality are age, history of congestive heart failure, emergency surgery, prior cardiac operation, the left ventricular ejection fraction, the functional status of nonaneurysmal segments, and the extent of coronary artery disease. However, the only consensus that appears throughout the literature is that operative mortality is increased: (1) if class III or IV congestive failure occurs preoperatively as the result of diffuse global left ventricular dysfunction; and (2) when intractable VT requires an emergency operation. More recently, it has been recognized that contraction of nonaneurysmal segments is a powerful determinant of early and late outcome. van Hemel et al have demonstrated that the presence of three or more left ventricular segments with a normal wall motion was associated with a good prognosis. Using a wall motion score derived from centerline chord motion analysis of the preoperative contrast right anterior oblique ventriculogram, Nath et al identified a score of 16% or more as the cut-off line for favorable outcome.[19] The preoperative use of amiodarone has been identified as a risk factor in some series,[20] but in our series it did not increase operative mortality. However, seven of our eight patients who have presented respiratory failure requiring several days of ventilatory support had received amiodarone for more than 6 months prior to surgery.

Postoperative VT Return

An impressive number of factors suspected of affecting the postoperative VT inducibility rate have also been evaluated.[11] Although no single factor has been identified as a powerful predictor of surgical failure, two seem to be associated with higher failure rates: (1) the preoperative occurrence of multiple, distinct VT morphologies or of polymorphic VT; and (2) localization of infarction in the inferior wall of the left ventricle. This has not been our experience and neither that of Nath et al.[21] Contradictory views are found in the literature concerning the need for intraoperative mapping. Some authors suggest that a wide, visually guided excision of endocardial scar may compensate for the unavailability or inadequacies of intraoperative mapping.[21] Detailed analysis of our mapping data has shown the following: (1) complete maps of one to five tachycardiac morphologies can be obtained intraoperatively in 100% of the patients; (2) a significant number of VTs have a subepicardial site of origin[10]; and (3) a specific pattern of activation during VT appears to be associated with a higher incidence of postoperative VT inducibility (designated as type 5). Careful examination of pace mapping data and activation patterns in canine preparations of septal infarcts has demonstrated that the type 5 pattern (as shown in Figure 3) corresponds to the involvement of intramural portions of the interventricular septum.[22] A modification of the surgical technique including a combination of septal endocardial resection and cryosurgery allowed a significant improvement of the surgical results.[23]

The preoperative identification of this type of VT with noninvasive methods[24] may thus help to assess the likelihood of VT suppression by surgery.

Indications

It is clear that an operation offered as a last resort is less likely to produce favorable results. Further analysis of the data accumulated in the literature and in our own series suggests that in patients < 65 years of age, without diffuse coronary artery disease, without unstable angina, with three or more left ventricular segments exhibiting normal contraction and without previous cardiac surgery, the risk of operative death is < 2%. In older patients in whom a reoperation is contemplated, particularly if nonaneurysmal segments are hypokinetic and/or ischemic, the operative mortality rate may be as high as 50%. In these patients, limited revascularization procedures combined with an implantable device appear to be the best strategy. When we evaluate a patient with sustained monomorphic VT, the first step is to carefully review the left ventricular angiogram. In Figure 4, a variety of angiographic patterns are shown. We do not hesitate to perform surgery for angiography patterns like those shown in panels A, B, D, E, F and G. However, when the infarcted area shows only a hypokinetic motion (panel C) or when the endocardial border shows an irregular aspect ("mottled," as in panel H), then surgery is not advisable. The presence of a discrete akinetic area is mandatory to allow direct surgery and the presence of an aneurysm, although not an absolute prerequisite, further supports the indication. Then the decision-making process depends on a number of other parameters that are difficult to incorporate into a rigid algorithm. These are listed in Table 5. Surgery may be offered as a first choice in low risk patients, in view of the extremely low incidence of recurrent arrhythmias over the long-term. However, in patients with intractable VT, direct surgery may be the only therapeutic alternative, in spite of the higher operative mortality that might be associated with the obligation to overlook other significant, albeit unavoidable risk factors. According to our results, the presence of threatening ischemia in nonscarred ventricular segments may increase the risk of perioperative death. In patients who have had previous cardiac surgery, a direct operation is contraindicated, except for patients with previous left ventricular aneurysmectomy, intractable arrhythmias, and no disease in the noninfarct-related coronary arteries. We fully agree with the recommendation of Breithardt and associates[3] that a cardioverter defibrillator should be implanted only if "curative" ablative procedures like catheter ablation or surgery are either not feasible or have failed. Recent studies indicate that analysis of the dynamic behavior of VT with new mathematical tools may provide insight in the mechanism of VT.[25] A new paradigm is emerging, whereby certain types of polymorphic VTs as well as the early

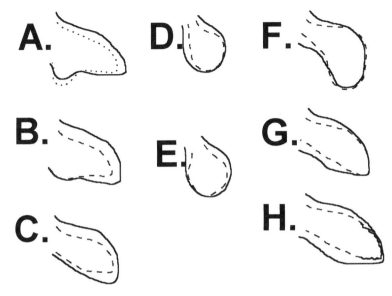

Figure 4. Left ventricular angiographic diagrams in the right anterior oblique projection (A, B, C, F, G, H) and left anterior oblique projection (D, E). Systolic (dashed line) and diastolic (solid line) endocardial contours are represented during two consecutive beats. Panels A through E are examples of inferior wall infarcts and panels F through H are examples of anterior wall infarcts. Left anterior oblique views of inferior infarcts may suggest left circumflex (D) or right (E) coronary artery-related scars. In patients with patterns similar to that shown in D, the mitral valve is more likely to be damaged during VT surgery, since the inferior papillary muscle (near the 6 o'clock point) is often involved in the VT site of origin, whereas the anterior papillary muscle (near the 2 o'clock point) is often fibrotic and dysfunctional. In patients with a pattern similar to that shown in E, scar tissue often involves the inferior septum leading to septal VT.

phase of ventricular fibrillation (VF) might be related to anatomical substrates which might be detectable with multielectrode mapping systems. Analyses of intraoperative records currently under way[25,26] suggest that: (1) in protracted episodes of polymorphic VTs, ventricular activation sequences of most individual beats correlate highly with a dominant activation pattern showing sites of origin in the scar region; and (2) likewise, the early beats in developing VF show activation sequences centered in the scar region. With these new tools, it may be possible to define the pathophysiological conditions under which patients with polymorphic VTs and/or VF may profit from the radical form of therapy provided by surgical ablation or modification of arrhythmia substrates.

Table 5
Weight of Clinical Factors Favoring Surgical Therapy in Patients with VT

	Weight		Weight
1. Sex	0	6. NYHA class I or II	+ + +
2. Age (years:		NYHA class III or IV	− −
<60	+ + + +	NYHA class III or IV	
60–64	+ +	due to correctable	
65–69	0	abnormality	+ +
>70	− −	7. No angina	+
3. Tolerated VT	+ +	Mild, stable angina	0
Syncopal VT	+ + +	Unstable angina	− − −
Incessant VT	+ + + +	8. Coronary artery disease:	
Frequent/intractable		Significant on 3 vessels	− −
VT > 1 week post MI	+ + + +	Significant on 2 vessels	+
4. Monomorphic VT		Significant on one vessel	+ + +
inducible	+ + + +	9. Drug failure	+ + +
Polymorphic VT,		Recurrence on amiodarone	+ + +
ventricular fibrillation	− − − −	Drug intolerance	+ + +
VT not inducible	− − − −	Chronic amiodarone	− −
5. LV angiogram:		10. Prior cardiac surgery:	
Discrete akinetic/		CABG	− − − −
diskinetic area	+ + + +	Aneurysmectomy alone	+
Hypokinetic area	− −	11. Patients preference	+ + + +
Irregular, "mottled"		Drug intolerance	+ + +
endocardial contour	− − −		
< 3 normally contracting			
segments	− − − −		

CABG = coronary artery bypass grafting.
+ to + + + +, favorable to very favorable to surgery.
− to − − − −, unfavorable to contraindication for surgery.

Summary

Fifteen years have passed since Harken, Josephson, and Horowitz have introduced the endocardial resection procedure in the management of patients with life-threatening VT. Despite the excellent results achieved with various modifications of this procedure throughout the world, most surgical electrophysiology teams have experienced a decline in the number of direct operations performed for life-threatening VT. This is probably due to the widespread use of thrombolytic therapy which has the potential to preserve the integrity of the myocardium during the acute phase of infarct formation. The other major reason for this decline is the advent of ICDs that are increasingly sophisticated, easy to use, and effective. Nevertheless, their use is still considered as a palliation rather than a cure. Their increased use over the past few years is related to the belief that direct operations for the eradication of VT foci bear a high operative mortality rate. Recent data indicate that these operations can now be performed with an operative mortality of < 5%, with a probability of long-term survival of up to 85% at 5 years, and an extremely low incidence of VT recurrence and sudden death. In our first 100 patients in whom VT surgical ablation was guided by computerized mapping of both the endocardium and epicardium, a particular type of VT activation pattern was found to be associated with a higher rate of arrhythmic failure due to a deep septal substratum. Appropriate management of this condition may further decrease the rate of VT reinducibility and long-term return of VT to a level yet unachieved by any other therapeutic modality. The results of catheter ablation are promising, but access to intramural substrates remains unresolved. In patients with sustained monomorphic VT associated with a discrete akinetic area of the left ventricle, the best surgical results will be obtained if the procedure is not offered as a last resort. The decision of its use should therefore be taken early before multiple drug trials go on.

References

1. Josephson ME, Harken AH, Horowitz LN. Endocardial excision: a new surgical technique for the treatment of recurrent ventricular tachycardia. *Circulation* 1979; 41:1035–1044.
2. Cox JL. Anatomic-electrophysiologic basis for the surgical treatment of refractory ischemic ventricular tachycardia. *Ann Surg* 1983;198:119–129.
3. Breithardt G, Borggrefe M, Wietholt D, et al. Role of ventricular tachycardia surgery and catheter ablation as complements or alternatives to the implantable cardioverter defibrillator in the 1990s. *PACE* 1992;15(4 Pt 3):681–689.
4. Selle JG. Presented at the Biennal International Arrhythmia Ablation Conference. In: Svenson RH (ed). Charlotte NC, May 26–28, 1994. Data from correspondence to Guiraudon JM, Fontaine G, Bolooki H, et al.
5. Bourke JP, Young AA, Richards DA, Uther JB. Reduction in incidence of inducible ventricular tachycardia after myocardial infarction by treatment with streptokinase during infarct evolution. *J Amer Coll Cardiol* 1990;16:1703–1710.
6. Hohnloser SH, Franck P, Klingenheben T, Zabel M, Just HIN. Open infarct artery, late potentials, and other prognostic factors in patients after acute myocardial infarction in the thrombolytic era. A prospective trial. *Circulation* 1994;90: 1747–1756.
7. Savard P, Rouleau JL, Davies RF, Dupuis R, Gardner M, Lauzon C, et al. Prediction of arrhythmic events after myocardial infarction using signal averaging ECG criteria specific for gender, age and myocardial infarction type. *Circulation* 1994; 90(4 Pt 2):I-389.
8. Leclercq JF, Coumel P, Denjoy I, et al. Long-term follow-up after sustained monomorphic ventricular tachycardia: causes, pump failure, and empiric antiarrhythmic therapy that modify survival. *Am Heart J* 1991;121(6 Pt 1):1685–1692.
9. Kirklin JW. The generation of knowledge from information, data, and analyses. In: Kirklin JW, Barratt-Boyes BG (eds). *Cardiac Surgery*, 2d edition. New York: Churchill Livingstone 1993, pp 249–284.
10. Kaltenbrunner W, Cardinal R, Dubuc M, et al. Epicardial and endocardial mapping of ventricular tachycardia in patients with myocardial infarction. Is the origin

of the tachycardia always subendocardially localized? *Circulation* 1991;84: 1058–1071.

11. Cox, JL. Patient selection criteria and results of surgery for refractory ischemic ventricular tachycardia. *Circulation* 1989;79(Suppl I):I-163–I-177.

12. McGiffin DC, Kirklin JK, Plumb VJ, et al: Relief of life-threatening ventricular tachycardia and survival after direct operations. *Circulation* 1987;76(Suppl V):V-93–V-103.

13. Swerdlow CD, Mason JW, Stinson EB, Oyer OE, Winckle RA, Derby GC. Results of operations for ventricular tachycardia in 105 patients. *J Thorac Cardiovasc Surg* 1986;92:105–113.

14. van Hemel NM, Kingma JH, Defauw JA, et al. Left ventricular segmental wall motion score as a criterion for selecting patients for direct surgery in the treatment of postinfarction ventricular tachycardia. *Eur Heart J* 1989;10(4):304–315.

15. Haines DE, Lerman BB, Kron IL, DiMarco JP. Surgical ablation of ventricular tachycardia with sequential mapguided subendocardial resection: electrophysiologic assessment and long-term follow-up. *Circulation* 1988;77:131–141.

16. Mickleborough LL, Mizuno S, Downar E, Gray GC. Late results of operation for ventricular tachycardia. *Ann Thorac Surg* 1992;54:832–838.

17. Willems AR, Tijssen JGP, van Capelle FJL, et al. Determinants of prognosis in symptomatic ventricular tachycardia or ventricular fibrillation late after myocardial infarction. *J Am Coll Cardiol* 1990;16:521–530.

18. van Hemel NM. Is surgery for ventricular tachycardia too risky? *Clin Cardiol* 1991;14:422–424.

19. Nath S, Haines DE, Kron IL, Barber MJ, DiMarco JP. Regional wall motion analysis predicts survival and functional outcome following subendocardial resection in patients with prior anterior myocardial infarction. *Circulation* 1993;88: 70–76.

20. Hargrove CW, Miller JM. Risk stratification and management of patients with recurrent ventricular tachycardia and other malignant ventricular arrhythmias. *Circulation* 1989;79(Suppl I):I-178–I-181.

21. Nath S, Haines DE, Kron IL, DiMarco JP. The long-term outcome of visually directed subendocardial resection in patients without inducible or mappable ventricular tachycardia at the time of surgery. *J Cardiovasc Electrocardiol* 1994;5: 399–407.

22. Kawamura Y, Pagé P, Cardinal R. Identification of deep septal ventricular tachycardia substrates from right ventricular epicardial breakthrough characteristics. *PACE* 1994;17(Pt 2):824.

23. Pagé PL, Cardinal R, Dubuc M, Cossette R, Nadeau R. Surgical approach of ventricular tachycardia with deep septal substratum. *Circulation* 1991;84(Suppl II): II-195.

24. SippensGroenewegen A, Spekhorst H, van Hemel NM, et al. Value of body surface mapping in localizing the site of origin of ventricular tachycardia in patients with previous myocardial infarction. *J Am Coll Cardiol* 1994;24:1708–1724.

25. Vinet A, Cardinal R, Rocque P, et al. Cycle length dynamics and spatial stability at the onset of induced monomorphic ventricular tachycardias induced in postinfarction canine preparations and in patients. *Circulation* (In press).

26. Cardinal R, Vinet A, Le Franc P, Hélie F, Pagé P. Beat-to-beat stability of spatial activation patterns during monomorphic and polymorphic ventricular tachycardias induced in human myocardial infarction. *Circulation* 1995;92(8):I-335.

Chapter 16

Surgical Approaches to Supraventricular Tachycardias

Gerard M. Guiraudon, MD,
George J. Klein, MD, Raymond Yee, MD,
Colette M. Guiraudon, MD

Introduction

July 1995 was the fifth anniversary of the dramatic advent of catheter ablation for supraventricular tachycardias. This chapter will review the current ebbing of surgery in the treatment of supraventricular tachycardias.

Supraventricular tachycardias are classified according to the site of their working mechanism, which is essentially a reentry mechanism.[1] Atrial tachycardias are associated with their electrocardiographic tachycardia pattern: focal atrial tachycardias; atrial flutter; and atrial fibrillation. Atrioventricular (AV) nodal tachycardias are reentrant tachycardias confined to the AV nodal region. The Wolff-Parkinson-White syndrome requires the entire heart and an obligatory accessory AV connection.

The rationale for interventions in supraventricular tachycardias is based on the arrhythmogenic target (arrhythmogenic anatomical substrate).

The identification of the arrhythmogenic anatomical substrate is achieved by electrophysiological studies, namely mapping of the cardiac activation sequence. The current rationale is to neutralize the arrhythmogenic anatomical substrate using various physical means: exclusion or "ablation" using various sources of energy: cryoablation,[2-4] DC shock[5-7] and radiofrequency (RF) electrical energy.[8-10] Radiofrequency is the currently preferred energy because it can be delivered on target by intracardiac catheters and is safe.

The ways the targeted tissues are approached and the therapy delivered define the type of intervention.

Surgery is defined by a transparietal approach (a median sternotomy)

From *Practical Management of Cardiac Arrhythmias* edited by Nabil El-Sherif, and Jean Lekieffre. Futura Publishing Co., Armonk, NY, © 1997.

which requires a general anesthetic with tracheal intubation and is associated with various adjunct maneuvers (i.e., cardiopulmonary bypass, cardiotomy, and aortic cross-clamping with cardioplegic myocardial preservation before the ablative therapy can be delivered). Each of the various steps used to approach the arrhythmogenic target are associated with inherent morbidity and mortality.[11,12] The "surgical" risk, consequently, is essentially associated with the delivery of the therapy and not the therapy itself.

Catheter techniques are a much less invasive delivery. After venous and/or arterial puncture, the catheter follows chartered natural routes to the heart and the arrhythmogenic target. Side effects and complications are currently very minimal, with dramatic progress in skill,[13] techniques, applied anatomy, and technology.

Electrophysiological intervention using surgical or catheter delivery are the only curative interventions. Other electrophysiological interventions using either drugs or antitachycardia devices are only palliative. His bundle ablation combined with permanent cardiac pacing may be used in selected patients.

Currently, catheter ablation using RF electrical energy is the preferred first therapy, when feasible. This principle implies that patients with the Wolff-Parkinson-White syndrome, and AV nodal reentrant tachycardias are effectively and safely cured by catheter ablation techniques.[14] Patients with atrial flutter also benefit from catheter ablation techniques.[15,16] Focal atrial tachycardias may be controlled using catheter ablation in selected patients.[17]

Atrial fibrillation is still approached surgically in a number of patients, while catheter or other ways of delivery are developing.[18–21]

In this chapter, we will review the "historical" contribution of surgical approaches to the Wolff-Parkinson-White syndrome, AV nodal reentrant tachycardia, atrial flutter, and focal tachycardias. The current surgical interventions used to control atrial fibrillation will be discussed. Their contribution to future catheter delivery contemplated.

However, because catheter ablation techniques may fail, patients should not be denied the benefit of a curative intervention and surgeons should stay current and readily available.

The Wolff-Parkinson-White Syndrome

The first successful surgical ablation of an accessory AV connection was performed by W.C. Sealy et al in 1968.[22] Along with the development of surgical practice came a better understanding of cardiac anatomy, accessory AV connection, anatomy, and electrophysiology. Better understanding paved the way to advanced surgical techniques with high efficacy and low morbidity and catheter techniques.[13]

The accessory AV connection, in the Wolff-Parkinson-White syndrome, is distinct to the normal AV nodal His bundle system and crosses over the AV attachment. Successful techniques for ablation of accessory connection requires in-depth knowledge of the complex anatomy of the AV attachment.[23,24] The AV attachment joins the atrial myocardium and the ventricular myocardium at the level of their AV orifices (Figure 1). The complexity of the attachment is determined by the anatomy of the left ventricle which presents with a single myocardial opening (the LV ostium) which accommodates the inflow (mitral valve) and outflow (aortic valve) orifices. Consequently, the AV attachment is composed of two segments: the annular; and the nonannu-

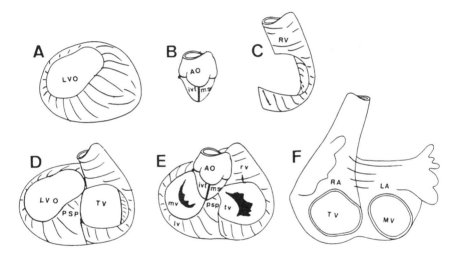

Figure 1. Construction of the atrioventricular attachment. The ventricles are viewed from behind whereas the atria are viewed from the front. **(A):** Left ventricle with its single orifice: the left ventricular ostium (LVO). **(B):** Aortic root with its appended membranous cuff: the aortoventricular membrane. Depicted are the aortic root, the inter-valvular trigone (IVT), and the membranous septum (MS). Between IVT and MS appended at the nadir of the noncoronary cusp is the right fibrous trigone, which is a cord-like structure and not a triangle-shaped structure. **(C):** The right ventricular free wall. **(D):** Attachment of the right ventricular free wall to the left ventricle. Formation of the tricuspid valve orifice (TV). The triangular segment of the left ventricular wall between the TV orifice and the LV ostium is the posterior superior process of the left ventricle. Covered by the right atrial wall, it will constitute the muscular AV septum in the anterior segment of the triangle of Koch (mid-septum of cardiological interventionists). **(E):** Addition of the aortic annuli and its aortoventricular membrane which attaches to the LVO and delineates the mitral valve orifice (MV). **(F):** Anterior view of the atria. The two AV orifices are widely separated as are the tricuspid and ventricular AV orifice. The segment in between will constitute the complex AV septum (triangle of Koch).

lar. The annular attachment is a simple fibrotic structure, the AV annulus (or lamina), which joins the adjacent atrial and ventricular rims of the AV orifices. The annular attachment is in close relationship with the coronary sulcus, which encircles the "base of the heart" around the annular AV attachment. The coronary sulcus is divided into four regions or segments: (1) the left free wall; (2) the posterior septal; (3) the right free wall; and (4) anterior septal (right coronary fossa) regions. These regions are arbitrarily defined and their limits are not materialized by specific anatomical landmarks and/or partitions. This absence of clear limits is the source of confusion, particularly for the anterior septal and posterior septal regions. The nonannular attachment is composed of the aortic annuli and their appended membraneous structures (i.e., the membranous septum, the right fibrous trigone, and the intervalvular trigone [subaortic curtain]). Part of the nonannular attachment is septal: the membranous septum. Another complex segment of the heart septum can be added to the AV attachment: the triangle of Koch which comprises two important features: the AV node; and the AV myocardial septum (posterior superior process of the left ventricle) covered by septal atrial myocardium. The AV myocardial septum is labeled mid-septum by the catheter interventionist.

The accessory AV connections are made of strands of working myocardium which bypass the AV attachment.[25,26] The typical accessory AV connections cross the annular attachment, most being para-annular.[27,28] The atypical accessory AV connections have been found in all parts of the nonannular attachment: within the AV myocardial septum (posterior septal, or midseptal pathways), adjacent to the membranous septum (para-Hisian anterior septal pathways), within the membranous pathway (membranous pathways with aberrant preexcitation) and over the intervalvular trigone (atypical posterior septal pathways). Two subvarieties of typical pathways deserve mentioning: the posterior septal pathway with slow decremental conduction associated with the permanent form of junctional reentrant tachycardia (Coumel's tachycardias),[29,30] and the right free wall pathway with anterograde decremental conduction (atriofascicular pathway associated with left bundle branch block pattern tachycardias).[31-34]

Surgical Techniques

The evolution of the surgical techniques for the Wolff-Parkinson-White syndrome exemplifies the new surgical philosophy: to attain efficacy with minimal side-effects (risk). Surgical risk is associated with every step used to approach the accessory AV connection (i.e., general anesthesia, median sternotomy, cardiopulmonary bypass, aortic cross-clamping, myocardial preservation, and cardiotomy).[11,12] Each step uses techniques which are associated with inherent morbidity and mortality. The actual ablation of the accessory

AV connection is the most benign part of the intervention. Based on these premises which advocate simplified approaches, we developed in 1983, a variant surgical technique (the epicardial approach)[35] aimed at decreasing risk, because the surgical ablation could be carried out without the need for aortic cross-clamping and cardiopulmonary bypass.

Two surgical approaches were described: the endocardial approach was pioneered and perfected by Sealy,[22,36–38] and Cox, et al[39] and Gallagher, et al.[40] This surgical success constitutes a landmark in the history of cardiac arrhythmias. The epicardial approach which combines epicardial exposure and cryoablation of the AV attachment.[35,41,42]

The heart is exposed via a medial sternotomy. After extensive examination of cardiac anatomy, epicardial mapping is carried out to confirm location of the accessory AV connection established during preoperative electrophysiological studies. Exploring electrodes are positioned along the atrial and ventricular side of the coronary sulcus at predetermined sites during atrial and/or ventricular pacing and AV reentrant tachycardias. Mapping the entire ventricles is used in rare, specific cases. The limitation of epicardial mapping is due to the anatomy of the sulcus and the location of the accessory AV connection. Because of the depth of the sulcus, the exploring electrode, is remote from the AV annulus and the accessory AV connection. Epicardial mapping cannot identify the very site of preexcitation as endocardial mapping does, but identifies a region. Cardiac mapping and electrophysiological testing using pacing techniques are repeated at each step of surgical ablation to confirm suppression of the conduction of the recognized accessory AV connection, and to potentially identify a second undiagnosed connection.

The Endocardial Approach

The endocardial approach combines an atrial incision along the AV annulus in the region of interest, and an extensive dissection of the entire region of the coronary sulcus.

The left free-wall connections are approached using a conventional exposure of the mitral valve similar to the one used for mitral valve surgery. The entire left free-wall region is dissected via a semicircular atrial incision along the mitral valve annulus from the right to the left trigone. The coronary sulcus dissection involves the identification of coronary artery and vein, and the separation of the atrial and ventricular wall from all attachments to divide all potential pathway insertions. The dissection is carried out under aortic cross-clamping and cardioplegic cardiac arrest.

The posterior septal, right free wall, and anterior septal regions are approached via a right atriotomy. Endocardial mapping and para-Hisian dissection can be carried out on the normothermic beating heart. However, most of the extensive dissection of the region of interest is performed under aortic cross-clamping and cold cardioplegic arrest.

The endocardial approach is associated with excellent efficacy. Surgical morbidity is still significantly associated with cold cardioplegic cardiac arrest and cardiopulmonary bypass.[39,40]

The Epicardial Approach

The epicardial approach combines epicardial dissection of the coronary sulcus, and exposure and cryoablation of the AV attachment (annulus).[41,42]

Typical accessory AV connection can be ablated using this approach on the beating heart without the need for cardiopulmonary bypass. The left free wall dissection is carried out by exposing the left coronary sulcus using a sling (Figure 2).[43] The AV attachment is exposed by dissection of the fat pad along the left ventricular wall. The obtuse cardiac vein is divided for better exposure, and the coronary arteries are carefully isolated. The posterior region is well exposed by deflecting the heart upwards using a rigid pledgetted suture. The right free wall and anterior septal regions are easily exposed. These typical

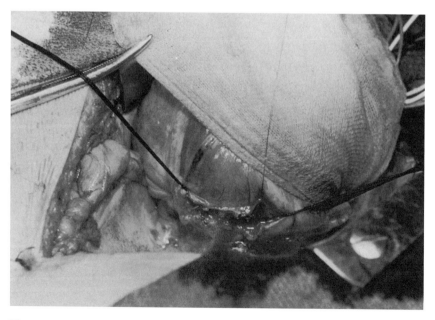

Figure 2. Dissection of the left atrioventricular sulcus on the normothermic beating heart without cardiopulonary bypass assist. The left ventricle is dislocated using a sling.

accessory AV connections located within the coronary sulcus are easily ablated with high efficacy and minimum morbidity associated with median sternotomy.[42]

Atypical accessory AV connections required an endocardial dissection carried out on the normothermic beating heart. Para-Hisian anterior septal connections are ablated using discrete dissection of the atrial myocardium overlying the atrial membranous septum.[44] We have ablated three atypical posterior pathways located over the intervalvular trigone region using discrete cryoablation.[45]

Atypical Intramembranous Pathways

We have operated on four patients with aberrant preexcitation and surgically documented intramembranous pathways. The aberrant preexcitation was over either the right ventricular infundibulum (3 patients) or the ventricular septum (1 patient).[46] The pathways were ablated by discrete cryoablation of the atrial membranous septum or of the ventricular attachment. These membranous accessory pathways are characteristically located within the membranous septum, with an atrial insertion in the atrial septum and a ventricular insertion at various sites in the septum along the membranous septum attachment to the ventricular septum. The membranous pathway differs from the so-called intermediate pathways,[47] which have normal anatomical features and function and are located in the mid-septal region.

Other Variant Preexcitation

Right Atriofascicular Fibers

In 1988, we documented in two patients that the anatomical substrate of the so-called Mahaim's fibers associated with left bundle branch block pattern tachycardias were a right ventricular free wall accessory pathway with antegrade decremental conduction and with a His bundle-like connection along the right ventricular free-wall (atriofascicular fiber).[31–34] Since then, both surgical and catheter ablation have revealed that almost all patients with the electrophysiologically documented Mahaim's entity have a right free-wall accessory pathway, the site of preexcitation being either close to the AV groove or at the right ventricular apex.[48] In five patients, findings from a biopsy specimen from the right atrium documented the presence of AV nodal cells at the atrial insertion of the pathway.[49] Our surgical experience comprises 13 patients. The surgical technique used in this setting is identical to that used for right free-wall accessory pathway dissection combined with endocardial cryoablation.

The Permanent Form of Junctional Reciprocating
Tachycardia (Coumel's Tachycardia)

Surgical dissection of the posterior septal region has documented that the permanent form of junctional reciprocating tachycardia is associated with a posterior septal accessory pathway, with only decremental retrograde conduction. A conventional posterior septal dissection using the epicardial approach uniformly ablates the pathway.[30]

The coronary sinus diverticulum is associated with posterior septal pathways that exhibit maximal preexcitation and a short antegrade refractory period. At surgery, the coronary sinus diverticulum is readily visible. The diverticulum is composed of a pouch and a neck which opens into the coronary sinus proximal to the mid-cardiac vein. The neck diameter ranges from 5 to 10 mm. Intramyocardial cardiac veins open into the coronary sinus diverticulum.[50] Accessory pathway conduction is usually interrupted when the neck of the diverticulum is divided. This represents evidence suggesting that the accessory pathway is part of the diverticulum. This anomaly is commonly associated with a very short antegrade refractory period: the pathway. Recent studies have documented the role of venous anomalies in posterior septal pathways.[51]

Multiple Accessory Pathways[52]

Because epicardial mapping is insufficiently discriminative within a region, we defined multiple accessory pathways as widely separated sites of preexcitation in distinct regions. Preoperative electrophysiological studies identify the presence of multiple pathways in about 7% of the patients.[53] A second pathway can become apparent only after ablation of the "dominant" accessory pathway. Most unexpected pathways detected intraoperatively are posterior septal pathways capable of only retrograde AV conduction. Multiple accessory pathways are ablated in sequence. If possible, the accessory pathway, which does not require cardiopulmonary bypass is ablated first.

Associated Cardiac Lesions

Two congenital cardiac abnormalities are associated with the preexcitation syndrome: Ebstein's anomaly; and the coronary sinus diverticulum. Symptomatic Wolff-Parkinson-White syndrome associated with the Ebstein's anomaly does not necessarily require anatomical repair, but all such surgical repairs of Ebstein's anomaly should be combined with ablation of the associated preexcitation syndrome.

Our current surgical strategy for concomitant cardiac procedures (coronary artery bypass grafting and valve replacement) is to ablate the accessory pathway first as an "independent procedure" and then to proceed with performing the associated cardiac surgical procedure.

Before closing the chest, four pairs of temporary pacing electrodes are attached to the cardiac chambers for postoperative electrophysiological testing.

Results

Before the era of catheter ablation, we reported on 502 patients operated on before August 1990. In all, 500 patients were cured without any mortality and low morbidity (mean follow-up, 4 years). These results were similar to those from other reported series.[28]

After the onset of catheter ablation, between August 1990 and August 1993, we operated on 51 patients (age 9 to 63 years; 35 men and 16 women) referred for surgical ablation from within our institution and elsewhere.[54] During the same period, 375 patients with problematic Wolff-Parkinson-White syndrome underwent catheter ablation procedures at our hospital. Surgical ablation was the initial therapy in 26 patients, because of physician preference in 23 and because of the need for concomitant cardiac surgical procedures in 3. Surgical treatment was carried out after attempted catheter ablation in 22 patients, three of whom had urgent surgical intervention.

Previous catheter ablation was not associated with added surgical difficulties and all pathways were ablated intraoperatively on the first attempt using the epicardial approach. Visible epicardial lesions produced by RF energy were observed in eight patients at the site of the accessory pathway (Figure 3).

Operative therapy gave some insights into the mechanism responsible for the failure of catheter ablation during the learning period: inadequate localization of the accessory pathway was suggested in four patients, in whom there were discrepancies between the intraoperative and preoperative localization of the pathway. Inadequate positioning of the catheter off the AV ring was observed in two patients (the catheter was in the obtuse marginal vein in one and in the left atrial appendage in the other). In most cases, adequate localization of the accessory pathway as well as the RF-induced lesions suggested inadequate contact of the catheter with the AV annulus or with an accessory pathway coursing at a distance from the annulus.

There was a significant preponderance of right free-wall pathways after catheter ablation, which suggests that a subepicardial location of the pathways may be a source of failed ablation, as we observed in one patient with a well-defined subepicardial AV myocardial bundle (Figure 4). Brodman and associates have reported similar observations in the setting of intraoperative right free-wall bundles.[55] Sealy reported that anterior right ventricular free-

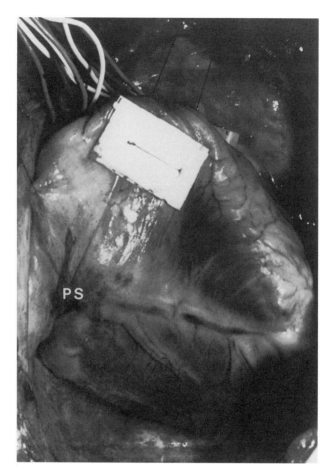

Figure 3. Operative view of the posterior septal region in a patient with attempted catheter ablation. Ecchymosis are seen in the posterior septal region (PS).

wall pathways can be subepicardial, as evidence by findings observed during AV fat pad dissection using the endocardial approach. We have previously reported that inferior right free-wall pathways are mostly "deep" para-annular or subendocardial in location, but anterior right ventricular free-wall pathways are epicardial because accessory pathway conduction is generally interrupted early during epicardial dissection. Rosenberg and colleagues noted a long subepicardial accessory pathway in the right ventricular position in a heart specimen.[56] This subepicardial location of right free-wall pathways makes them less amenable to catheter ablation. Nonetheless, catheter tech-

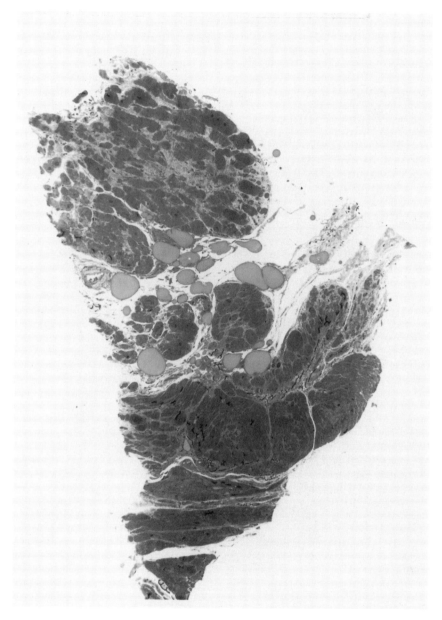

Figure 4. Histology of a right free-wall epicardial accessory pathway excised at surgery.

niques can be successful by ablating the atrial insertion of the accessory pathway, even if the pathway is situated at a distance from the AV annulus.

Conclusion

Surgical ablation laid the groundwork for catheter ablation by elucidating the anatomical characteristics of the AV attachments, as well as the "surgical anatomy of the accessory AV connection." With the advent of surgical ablation, nonpharmacological electrophysiological interventions became established as the primary choice for patients facing a life-long dependency on drug treatment.

Concerns about surgical morbidity encouraged the development of surgical techniques associated with minimal morbidity, by suppressing as many ancillary techniques as possible.

Now catheter ablation has eclipsed surgical ablation as the primary nonpharmacological therapy. Nonetheless, surgical ablation continues to have a limited role in the management of patients in whom catheter ablation has failed as the result of anatomical complexities or congenital heart lesions.

AV Nodal Reentrant Tachycardias

AV nodal reentrant tachycardias are a very common supraventricular tachycardia. For long, it was accepted knowledge that the reentrant mechanism was within the compact AV node.[57] Because this concept precluded direct surgical approach to disable the reentrant mechanism, His bundle ablation was the electrophysiological intervention used in severe resistant cases. However, an inadvertent cure of a patient with AV nodal reentrant tachycardia after attempted surgical ablation of the AV node suggested that discrete lesions of the AV node could interrupt the tachycardia.[58] Marquez-Montes et al[59] and Ross et al[60] were the first to report effective surgical approaches to the AV nodal region to interrupt AV nodal reentrant tachycardias.

The rationale of surgical approaches was consistent with AV nodal physiology as described by basic scientists,[61] and AV nodal anatomy.[62] To reconcile data from various disciplines, the concept of the greater AV nodal area which encompasses the AV node, as well as its atrial input was described (Figure 5).[63]

The reentrant mechanism, within the greater AV nodal area, uses atrial inputs as limbs or segments of the reentrant circuit.

Surgical approaches suggested that either modification or ablation of at least one atrial input was associated with the disabling of the reentrant mechanism. Johnson et al were the first to report two sites of atrial retrograde activation over the coronary sinus os, and at the apex of the triangle of Koch,

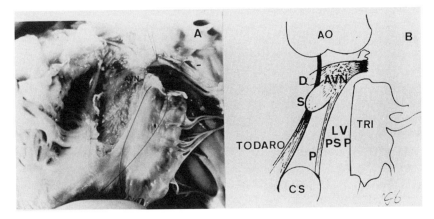

Figure 5. The atrioventricular (AV) nodal (AVN) region. **(A):** Dissection of the AV node in a heart specimen. The AVN and its atrial inputs span into the posterior segment of the triangle of Koch. **(B):** Schematic depiction of the specimen in A. The AVN is a macroscopic structure which can be modified by either surgical dissection or catheter ablation. AO = aortic root; AVN = atrioventricular node; D = deep atrial inputs; S = superficial (anterior) atrial inputs; P = posterior atrial inputs; CS = coronary sinus orifice; LV PSP = posterior superior process of the left ventricle; TRI = septal leaflet of the tricuspid valve; TODARO = tendon of Todaro.

consistent with respectively, the posterior (CS) atrial inputs and the superficial atrial input (currently labeled anterior, anterior referred to anterior septal position).

Direct surgical approaches to the AV node for AV nodal reentrant tachycardia use sharp dissection of the AV nodal atrial inputs guided by endocardial mapping[60] or not,[63] or cryomodification (perinodal cryoablation).[64]

Map-Guided Ablation of Atrial Inputs

On the normothermic heart, during AV nodal reentrant tachycardia, atrial mapping of the triangle of Koch is carried out. The earliest atrial activation is either near the apex (type A, common type) or near the coronary sinus os (type B, uncommon type). Most patients have only one type of tachycardia, some have two.

Cardiac dissection is then carried out on the cold arrested heart. In type A tachycardia, atrial inputs are divided superior (posterior) to the tendon of Todaro. In type B tachycardias, the posterior septal area around the coronary sinus os, inferior (anterior) to the tendon of Todaro is extensively dissected. Johnson et al[65] reported 72 patients. There was no mortality. Two patients had permanent complete heart block and three had early relapses of their tachycardia. During long-term follow-up (6 to 40 months) the clinical cure rate was 93% (90% in sinus rhythm).

Anatomically Guided Dissection of AV Nodal Atrial Inputs

The AV Nodal Skeletonization[66]

The dissection is carried out on the normothermic beating heart in two steps, while continuously monitoring the AV conduction. First using a similar technique as used for the Wolff-Parkinson-White syndrome, the anterior septal and posterior septal regions are dissected using an epicardial approach.

Then, cardiopulmonary bypass is instituted, using double venous cannulae combined with snaring of the venae cavae. The heart is electrically fibrillated before the right atriotomy is performed along the exposed tricuspid valve annulus in the anterior septal region and the AV fat pad in the right free-wall region. The atrial septum is inspected for defect and a patent foramen ovale is closed. The heart is then defibrillated.

The skeletonization of the AV node is then carried out. The right atriotomy is extended up to the atrial membranous septum. The tendon of Todaro is identified. The inferior medial (septal) wall of the right atrium is incised along the septal segment of the tricuspid valve anulus below the atrial membranous septum. A plane of dissection is found between the septal right atrial wall and the subjacent intermediate AV node. The septal atrial wall is then opened and the intermediate AV node is exposed. The AV node is identified by its oblique pale myocardial fibers mixed with yellowish fatty streaks. It is dissected from surrounding tissue to separate posterior (CS) and superficial (anterior) atrial inputs, while the deep (left) atrial input is spared.

Forty-six patients were reported.[63] There were 38 women and 8 men. Age ranging from 9 to 71 (mean 36 years). Five patients had associated arrhythmias which were concomitantly, surgically ablated (3 Wolff-Parkinson-White, and 2 Mahaim's fibers). There were no surgical complications. Three patients had second degree heart block with adequate ventricular heart rate during treadmill testing. Dual AV nodal pathway physiology was present in four patients postoperatively, two having inducible tachycardias. During long-term follow-up, three patients had clinical recurrences of their tachycardias. The three patients underwent a successful repeat dissection. After a mean follow-up of 17 months (1–45 months) all patients were free of arrhythmias and off antiarrhythmic drugs.

Perinodal Cryoablation[64]

The surgery is carried out on the normothermic heart and exposure of the triangle of Koch. AV conduction is continuously monitored. Cryoablation used a cryoprobe 3 mm in diameter, cooled at $-60°C$ during 2 minutes or less until transient heart block occurs. Three cryolesions are placed along the tendon of Todaro between the coronary sinus orifice and the apex of the triangle of Koch. Then three cryolesions are placed along the septal segment of the tricuspid annulus. Two more cryolesions are placed at the base of the triangle above the coronary sinus ostium to connect the previous application and circumscribe the AV nodal area.

Twenty patients were reported with all patients free of tachyarrhythmia in the short- and long-term.

Comments

Currently, surgical techniques for AV nodal reentrant tachycardias are no longer used. Ablation using catheter delivery is associated with excellent control of the tachycardia and with more discrete electrophysiological changes.[67]

Atrial Tachycardias

Focal atrial tachycardias are classified into two subgroups: ectopic atrial tachycardias originate from outside the sinus node area; and sinus node tachycardias originate from within the sinus node area.

Ectopic atrial tachycardias are rare in the adult population (0.5% to 1%) and most frequent in children (10% of supraventricular tachycardias).[68] At electrophysiological studies, they have the characteristics of automatic focus tachycardias. During tachycardia, the P wave morphology significantly differ from sinus node P waves. The site of origin is mostly within the right atrial wall (68%) along the crista terminalis, the left atrial free wall (26%), and the interatrial septum (6%). The tachycardia is frequently incessant. These characteristics explain why tachycardia-induced dilated cardiomyopathy is frequently present (60% of cases).

Ectopic atrial tachycardias are potentially severe arrhythmias and should be controlled using electrophysiological intervention. Surgical techniques are currently considered only after attempted catheter ablation.

Because ectopic atrial tachycardias are not inducible, preoperative catheter mapping must be obtained to precisely localize the site of origin.

Surgical techniques use resection, cryoablation, and exclusion singly or in combination. Resection applies to right atrial free wall, and right and left appendage locations. Appendectomies may not require cardiopulmonary bypass. Right atrial excision is repaired using autologous pericardial patch. Cryoablation can be combined with resection, but is particularly convenient for septal locations. Exclusion is used essentially for the left atrial locations.

Our experience comprises five patients, none of them had incessant tachycardia associated with tachycardia-induced dilated cardiomyopathy.[69] Three patients had a right free-wall tachycardia localized over the inferior segment of the crista terminalis, and underwent extensive right free-wall resection combined with autologous pericardial patch reconstruction. One patient had a right atrial appendage tachycardia. The right atrial appendage was resected without using cardiopulmonary bypass. One patient had a left atrial tachycardia. Because the location of the tachycardia was not accurately determined, a left atrial exclusion was carried out.

There were no surgical complications. No patient had a recurrence of tachycardia. The patient with left atrial exclusion developed AV nodal conduction disturbances associated with syncopal ventricular pauses during long-term follow-up. A permanent pacemaker was implanted.

Lowe et al[68] published a review of the literature. He collected 125 patients with ectopic atrial tachycardias. Fifty-two patients were treated using antiarrhythmic drugs, 46 (89%) of whom were controlled. Seventy-three patients were treated using surgical techniques. Fifty-six (89%) were cured.

Currently, surgical techniques are only indicated after attempted catheter ablation.

Sinus node tachycardias comprise "inappropriate" sinus node tachycardias and reentrant sinus node tachycardias. Surgical experience with inappropriate sinus tachycardias documented that surgical ablation was associated with good short-term results,[69] but poor long-term results[70] complicated with atrial fibrillation and AV conduction disturbances. These surgical results suggest that catheter ablation[71] or other ablative techniques[72] are only palliative. Catheter ablation in patients with reentrant sinus node tachycardias[73] attain good results, consistent with those obtained by surgical ablation.

Atrial Flutter

Atrial flutter was first characterized by its electrocardiographic pattern[74] as a rapid regular atrial tachycardia associated with a typical saw-toothed configuration of the atrial electrogram on the surface electrocardiogram. Atrial flutter, in humans, has been classified as "common" if negative flutter waves are present in leads II, III, and aVF, and "uncommon" if flutter waves are positive in same leads.[75] More recently, the common flutter was labeled type 1, and uncommon type 2.[76]

Currently, there is a large body of experimental[77-80] and clinical[81-87] evidence which documents that atrial flutter is associated with a macroreentry mechanism associated with a large excitable gap in the right atrium and an area of slow conduction in the triangle of Koch. Recent studies showed that common and uncommon types share the same mechanism on location.[88,89]

The reentry circuit is determined by the functional anatomy of the right atrium. The area of slow conduction at the base of the triangle of Koch in the area of the coronary sinus os occupies a narrow segment (isthmus) between the inferior vena cava and the tricuspid valve orifices. The reentrant activation exits the area of slow conduction, and propagates rapidly via the anterior and middle internodal pathways, which are anterior to the fossa ovalis. The reentrant activation then circulates through the sinus node area, travels caudally within the crista terminalis and returns to the base of the triangle of Koch where the slow conducting isthmus channels, and slows down the activation before it exits again. In addition, the fossa ovale and transversal relative slow conduction (anisotrope) contribute to the presence of a zone of septal block.[90]

Cardiac mapping, during electrophysiological studies and before surgical ablation, confirm the functional anatomy of the reentrant circuit. The area of slow conduction within the isthmus at the base of the triangle of Koch is identified as the arrhythmogenic anatomical substrate, albeit the open circuit circulating along the rapidly conducting bundle may also be obligatory for the perpetuation of the flutter, and could be considered as a second "arrhythmogenic anatomical substrate."

Surgical Rationale

The current accepted rationale is to ablate the slow conducting isthmus between the inferior vena cava orifice and the tricuspid valve annulus at the base of the triangle of Koch, using cryoablation. We used a different rationale in our first case. A right atrial transection was carried out to interrupt the two limbs of the circuit (internodal pathways and crista terminalis).

Intraoperative Cardiac Mapping

We obtained four intraoperative mappings at surgery. Epicardial maps in two patients confirmed the slow conduction over the isthmus and circular activation of the right atrium, while the left atrium received collateral activation from the circuit (Figure 6). Endocardial cardiac mapping was obtained in two patients, and documented circular activation in one patient around the tricuspid annulus, and an area of slow conduction in the isthmus with apparent circular activation within the isthmus, in another patient.

Surgical technique used epicardial extensive cryoablation of the area be-

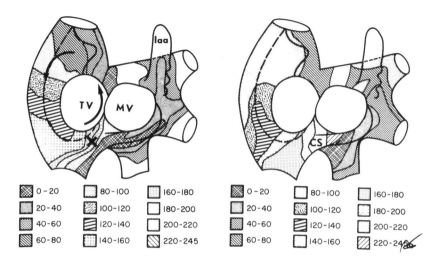

▨ 0 - 20	☐ 80-100	☐ 160-180
▦ 20-40	▨ 100-120	☐ 180-200
▤ 40-60	▱ 120-140	☐ 200-220
▧ 60-80	⋮ 140-160	▨ 220-245

▨ 0 - 20	☐ 80-100	☐ 160-180
▦ 20-40	▨ 100-120	⋮ 180-200
▨ 40-60	▱ 120-140	☐ 200-220
▧ 60-80	☐ 140-160	▱ 220-245

Figure 6. Epicardial map in two patients during the common form of atrial flutter. Slow conduction is present in the coronary sinus ostium (CS os) region. The right atrial activation circumscribes the tricuspid valve annulus.

tween the tricuspid annulus, the coronary sinus os, and the orifice of the inferior vena cava (Figure 7). In four patients, endocardial cryoablation was used with extensive ablation of the base of the triangle of Koch.

Results

Our experience comprises seven male patients (ages 33 to 63) with problematic symptoms (duration 4 to 20 years). No patient had associated structural heart disease. All patients had the common form. Preoperative electrophysiological studies confirmed the typical characteristics of the flutter with an area of slow fragmented conduction in the coronary sinus os region and a large excitable gap within the right atrium.

Postoperatively, there were no complications. At predischarged electrophysiological studies, atrial flutter was not inducible. During long-term follow-up, one patient had recurrence of atrial fibrillation and underwent a corridor operation 1 year later. The six other patients were free of arrhythmia without taking antiarrhythmic drugs with a follow-up of 16, 9, 3, 2, and 2 years respectively.

Comments

Successful surgical ablation combined with intraoperative mapping confirmed the mechanism of the atrial flutter.

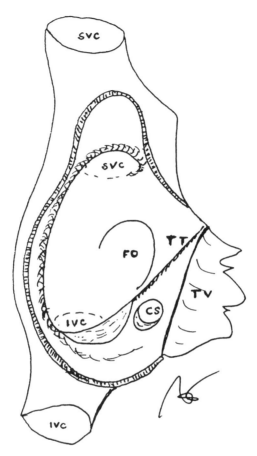

Figure 7. Schematic depiction of the right atrium. The anatomical isthmus between the inferior vena cava orifice and the tricuspid orifice is depicted. The isthmus is divided further by the coronary sinus ostium (CS os).

Atrial Fibrillation

Atrial fibrillation is the most common supraventricular arrhythmia, but has only recently been approached surgically. Atrial fibrillation is a complex arrhythmia without discrete anatomical substrate. Surgical rationales used for other supraventricular tachycardias do not apply, new surgical concept and rationales had to be developed.

Atrial Functional Anatomy

Atrial fibrillation alters dramatically, atrial functional anatomy.[91] The atria are two compliant pouches between the venous return and the ventricles.

They harbor two critical structures: the sinus node; and the AV node. The atria are of small size (60 ml) and cannot function as a reservoir. The role of atrial contraction is defined by the Frank Starling Law which applies to the failing heart. The normal ventricle is a sucking pump with active diastole and does not require atrial contraction to enhance its function.[92] Chronotropic function is the primary determinant of increased cardiac output during exercise, with increased contractility (humeral regulation). Atrial contraction is critical to sustain cardiac function of the failing heart.[93] However, the respective role of chronotropic function with regular rhythm and atrial contraction has not been elucidated.

Prevention of intracavitary thrombus is a major function of the atria. Alterations of atrial geometry (dilatation), pathology alteration of atrial wall (endothelium), and contraction (left atrial appendage washout) are the accepted causes of intracavitary thrombus and systemic emboli in atrial fibrillation. The left atrial appendage with its special morphology and physiology is the primary culprit.[94]

Atrial Pathology

Atrial fibrillation is commonly associated with primary structural heart disease. Atrial pathology in this setting has been well-reported.[95,96] Recent works have focused on myocardial pathology associated with "lone" atrial fibrillation, which seems to develop in the absence of clinically detectable structural heart disease.[97,98] We have reported atrial myocardial pathology in 12 patients with lone atrial fibrillation who underwent a "corridor operation."[99,100] There was a dramatic decrease in nerve endings and ganglion cells in all heart specimens which is consistent with the concept of cardioneuropathy or the role of the autonomous nervous system in atrial fibrillation. Myocardial pathology was present in all but one patient. Myocardial hypertrophy was observed in four patients, suggesting a tachycardia-related mechanism. Atrial myocardiopathy was present in six patients: adiposis and/or fibrosis was associated with moderate myocardial hypertrophy. Because biopsies were obtained from the high right atrium, sinus node tissue was present in four heart specimens. The sinus node was abnormal in three, with hypocellularity and fatty infiltration. In two, the sinus node artery presented with fibromuscular hyperplasia. None of the patients with sinus node pathology presented with sinus node dysfunction.

Mechanism

Atrial fibrillation is characterized by its electrocardiographic pattern of rapid irregular atrial activation associated with irregular ventricular contractions. Moe speculated, on a computer model, that atrial fibrillation was associated with simultaneous multiple wavelets of activation.[101] Allessie et al confirmed similar findings on animal experiments.[102] Common atrial fibrillation is of the "random reentry type." Four to six wavelets are moving randomly. Their activation front is generally narrow. Wavelets are short-lasting, but new wavelets are generated by division of existing wavelets. Atrial vulnerability, or atrial propensity to sustain atrial fibrillation are determined by atrial surface area (size), morphology, anatomical obstacle and spatial distribution of non-homogeneous electrophysiological characteristics (dispersion).[103] These characteristics may vary over time according to underlying pathology and duration of atrial fibrillation: self-aggravating; and perpetuating mechanism. Atrial fibrillation begets atrial fibrillation by modifying electrophysiological characteristics (atrial remodeling).[104]

This currently accepted mechanism may not be the only mechanism observed in clinical fibrillation. Atrial flutter with chaotic left atrial activation and/or multiple atrial foci or else may be present.

Although established atrial fibrillation is not focal in nature, there are experimental suggestions that the presence of a critical segment of atrial tissue with a very short refractory period may be mandatory for the perpetuation of fibrillation. Morillo, et al were able to interrupt and prevent atrial fibrillation by focal cryoablation in an animal model.[105] These studies and their potential development may dramatically modify the future of interventional approaches.

Clinical Presentations and Problematic Symptoms

Patients with atrial fibrillation present with three orders of symptoms: (1) those associated with the arrhythmia itself; (2) those related to associated structural heart disease; and (3) those associated with intracavitary thrombosis.

Symptoms associated with atrial fibrillation are well-identified in patients with lone atrial fibrillation. Many patients with lone atrial fibrillation are asymptomatic, with a stroke as the initial presentation in 25%. Other patients have palpitations associated or not with panic syndrome and/or posttachycardia syndrome. Exercise capacity may be altered during the attacks.

Symptoms related to associated structural heart disease may be predominant and obscure symptoms associated with atrial fibrillation, which is an aggravating factor.

Risk of stroke has been recently well-studied as well as its prevention.[106]

Surgical Rationales

Surgical rationales are based on the random intra-atrial reentry mechanism, although this mechanism may not be present in all patients with atrial fibrillation. Three elementary concepts are used: exclusion; fragmentation; and channeling (Figure 8).

Exclusion is used to isolate the fibrillating atrium (left atrial exclusion in patients with mitral valve disease), and to protect critical function (corridor operation, which isolates sinus node and AV node from the rest of fibrillating atria).

Fragmentation used atriotomies to produce semiexcluded atrial segments. Random reentry cannot be sustained in each semi-isolated segment because of reduced size (critical surface area), but all segments can contract sequentially in harmony.

Channeling is aimed at modifying the geometry of atrial tissue. A two-dimensional surface area is transformed into a unidimensional surface (strips of atrial tissue). It is speculated that a unidimensional strip of atria cannot sustain reentry.

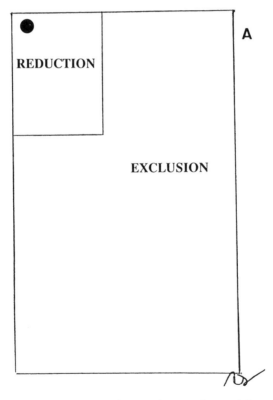

Figure 8. Diagrammatic depiction of surgical rationales used for atrial fibrillation. **(A):** Reduction/exclusion.

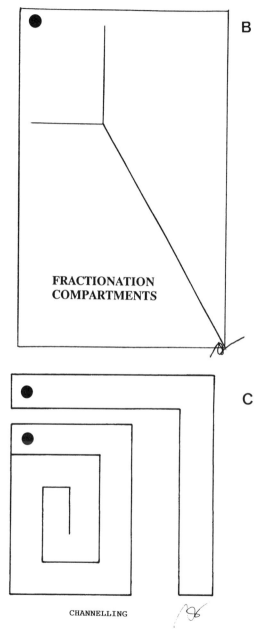

Figure 8. *(continued)* **(B):** Fragmentation. **(C):** Channeling. (See text for explanation.)

Surgical techniques have been described: (1) the left atrial exclusion; (2) the corridor operation, based on an excluded channel, which harbors the sinus node and the AV node; (3) the Maze operation, which combines subtotal exclusion of the left atrium with channeling and fragmentation; (4) the compartment operation; and (5) recently we have used the spiral operation, which "channels" the entire left atrium and fragments the right atrium.

All surgical techniques are associated with resection of the left atrial appendage, which is documented as the main site of intracavitary thrombus. Each technique is aimed at restoring sinus node chronotropic function, whereas the other atrial functions are restored to various degrees. An inherent limitation to all surgical techniques is the potential for sinus node dysfunction, which may require permanent pacing after surgery.

Surgical Techniques

Corridor Operation

A strip (channel) of atrial tissue (corridor) is isolated to restore sinus node function (Figure 9).[107-109] The strip of atrial tissue has a small surface

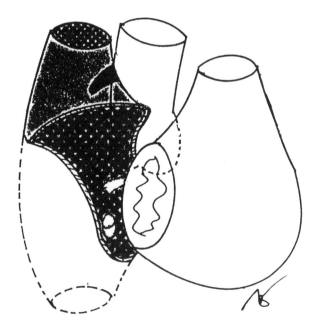

Figure 9. Schematic depiction of the corridor operation. The corridor constructs a strip (channeling) of atrial tissue harboring the sinus node and atrioventricular (AV) node (exclusion-reduction).

area and should be able to sustain atrial fibrillation. The corridor operation is performed under cardiopulmonary bypass and cold cardioplegic cardiac arrest. The surgical technique comprised exclusion of the left atrial free wall by using a horseshoe incision along the attachment of the left atrial wall onto the atrial septum. The ends of the left atrial incision attach onto the mitral valve annulus in the anterior and posterior commissure regions. The posterior commissure area (posterior septal region) must be carefully dissected, including the coronary sinus to attain uniform exclusion of the left atrium. Cryosurgical ablation at the mitral valve annulus ensures complete exclusion; construction of the corridor using a horseshoe incision attaching onto the tricuspid annulus circumscribing the corridor, which includes a cuff of right atrium that harbors the sinus node region, the AV node region, and a strip of atrial septum bridging the two nodes.

We have reported our experience with nine patients. Nine patients with drug refractory atrial fibrillation underwent this operation; four patients had chronic atrial fibrillation and five had paroxysmal atrial fibrillation; the mean duration of symptoms was 12 ± 8 years. Patients ages ranged from 25 to 68 years (mean 48 ± 12). At preoperative electrophysiological study, no patient had evidence of an accessory AV pathway or AV node reentry. Sinus node recovery time could not be determined in five patients because of recurrent atrial fibrillation during or before programmed stimulation.

At operation, the corridor of atrial tissue connecting the sinus and AV nodes was successfully isolated from the remaining left and right atrial tissue in all patients (Figure 10). There were no perioperative complications. One patient required early reoperation for recurrent atrial fibrillation before hospital discharge. At the predischarge electrophysiological study, the corridor operation remained isolated in all patients except for one patient who had intermittent conduction between the corridor and excluded right atrium. One patient had nonsustained atrial fibrillation and one had atrial tachycardia evidence in the corridor. Atypical AV node reentry of uncertain significance was induced in one other patient.

At exercise testing before discharge, the heart rate in the nine patients increased from a mean of 78 ± 20 to 114 ± 17 beats per minute, the maximal heart rate achieved ranged from 41% to 84% (mean 68% ± 17%) of the predicted maximal heart rate based on age and gender criteria.

The total follow-up time was 191 patient months (mean, 21 months; range, 3 to 52 months). Seven patients remain free of symptomatic supraventricular tachycardia. Two patients (cases 6 and 7) have had recurrences of atrial fibrillation during follow-up. The arrhythmia in one of these patients has been well-controlled with propafenone (no recurrence in the last 36 months); the other patient has experienced paroxysmal episodes of atrial fibrillation (approximately weekly) while taking quinidine and verapamil.

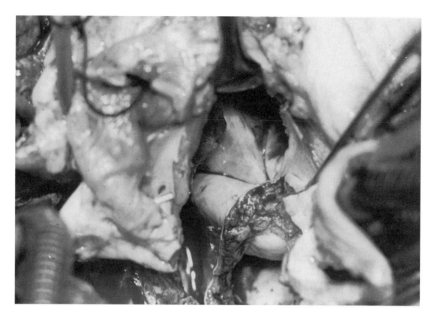

Figure 10. Operative view of the corridor operation.

A permanent ventricular pacemaker was implanted in three patients after surgery. In two patients, a pacemaker was implanted after symptomatic sinus pauses and a pacemaker was implanted prophylactically when prolonged sinus pauses were demonstrated at the postoperative electrophysiological study. A patient who had undergone previous cardiac surgery and pacemaker implantation had an atrial pacemaker reimplanted postoperatively, because of prolonged sinus pauses associated with bradycardia-dependent atrial arrhythmias.

These initial results demonstrate that the corridor operation can maintain sinus rhythm in patients with atrial fibrillation.

Since then, four additional patients have had a corridor operation. Improved selection criteria allowed normal sinus node function after surgery.

Gursoy et al,[110] reported five patients with the corridor operation for "lone atrial fibrillation." Sinus node chronotropic function was normal postoperatively with good exercise tolerance.[110]

Vigano et al recently reported 13 patients (9 males and 4 females) with the corridor operation for paroxysmal lone atrial fibrillation (10 patients), and 3 atrial flutter (3 patients).[111] The follow-up ranged from 9 to 47 months. There were no surgical complications. All patients were in sinus rhythm with adequate exercise capacity. No patients were on antiarrhythmic drugs or had a pacemaker implanted.

van Hemel et al reported 36 patients with the corridor operation for paroxysmal lone atrial fibrillation.[112] The follow-up was 41 ± 16 months. Thirty-one patients had successful construction of the corridor. Twenty-five patients were arrhythmia-free without medication (4-year actuarial freedom, 72% ± 9%). Twenty-six patients had normal sinus node function at rest and during exercise (4-year actuarial freedom of sinus node dysfunction, 81% ± 7%). Five patients had pacemaker implantation.

Overall, the corridor operation gave good control of the arrhythmia, restored sinus rhythm, with a good functional capacity. One patient from Utrecht (The Netherlands) ran a marathon.

Maze Operation

Since the first report,[113] the Maze operation has undergone many modifications and alterations by its designer and others. The master plan comprises a subtotal left atrial exclusion and multiple atriotomies combined with cryoablation. One left atriotomy divides the circular cuff of the left atrium around the mitral valve. Multiple right and septal atriotomies fragment and channel the right atrium and septum (Figure 11).

Cox et al[114–118] reported 87 patients with the Maze procedure for the treatment of atrial flutter and/or fibrillation. There were 64 males and 23 females with an average age of 54 years. The presenting arrhythmia was paroxysmal atrial flutter in six patients, paroxysmal atrial fibrillation in 37 patients, and chronic atrial fibrillation in 44 patients. All patients had failed extensive medical therapy with an average of five drugs per patient (36% had failed amiodarone).

Forty-three patients had paroxysmal atrial flutter or fibrillation (49%) and 44 patients chronic atrial fibrillation (51%). The first 33 patients had the standard Maze procedure, whereas the remainder had variants that did not differ significantly from the original technique, but were aimed at better preservation of the sinus node function. Twenty-four patients had concomitant cardiac repair, and seven had previous cardiac surgery.

Three patients died during surgery. Two patients had postoperative transient ischemic attacks. Early in the series, patients had postoperative fluid retention and pulmonary edema. This was caused by atrial natriuretic factor and was treated by spirolactone, which is now routinely prescribed. In the first 3 months after surgery, 47% of patients had recurrence of atrial fibrillation or flutter. Of the 78 patients with more than 3 months of follow-up, 32 required permanent pacing (AAI). Some patients had sinus node dysfunction before surgery. All patients were assessed in terms of exercise tolerance, arrhythmia (Holter), and cardiac function (atrial contraction). Overall, atrial fibrillation/flutter has been controlled by surgery alone in 71 of 78 patients, whereas 32 patients (41%) required a pacemaker implantation.

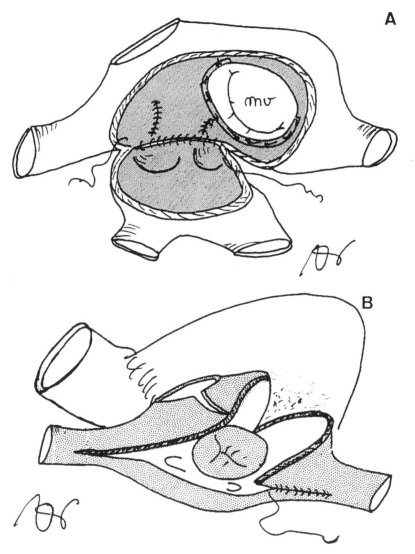

Figure 11. Maze operation. **(A):** Left atrial incisions; **(B):** right atrial incisions.

Left Atrial Isolation

Graffigna et al have reported left atrial isolation in 184 patients with concomitant mitral valve surgery.[119] Seventy-one percent of patients returned to sinus rhythm after surgery, whereas 19% of patients with only mitral valve surgery returned to sinus rhythm (no controlled trial; p < 0.001). Patients with restored sinus rhythm had significant improvement of their exercise capacity.

Fragmentation or Compartment Operation
(Open Corridor)

Shyu et al[120] reported their experience with the compartment operation in 22 patients. All patients had concomitant mitral valve surgery. The compartment operation is best described as an open corridor operation, the atriotomy which "normally" isolates the left atrium and the corridor itself are left incomplete and allow persistent connections between the three constructed segments of atria.

The compartment operation was not associated with increased surgical morbidity. Fourteen patients (64%) were in sinus rhythm at 6 months of follow-up. Atrial mechanical function, as assessed by echo-Doppler studies, was not always present after restoration of sinus rhythm.

The Spiral Operation

We have designed a new surgical technique to control atrial fibrillation, based on channeling of the right and left atria, with special concern for patients with mitral valve dysfunction associated with chronic atrial fibrillation. Cardiac physiology and recent clinical studies emphasize the critical additional benefit of restored sinus rhythm after surgical correction of mitral valve disease. Atrial pathology and its problematic symptoms (atrial fibrillation) and mitral valve disease are two sides of the same coin and should be addressed routinely in a two-pronged operation.

We wanted to design adjunct atriotomies aimed at disabling atrial fibrillation as a simple "extension" of the atriotomies used to explore the mitral valve. For mitral exposure we selected the vertical trans-septal approach or "transplant incision" (as coined by Duran) because it has become the exposure of choice for mitral valve surgery. The spiral combines channeling of the right atria by using the trans-septal approach and the left atrium by transforming the left atrium into a circumvoluted (spiral) strip like an orange peel, of atrial tissue (Figure 12). We anticipate that the spiral operation will restore sinus rhythm, as well as contraction of the entire left atrium including the posterior wall, which, along with the left atrial appendage, is recognized as a site of thrombosis.

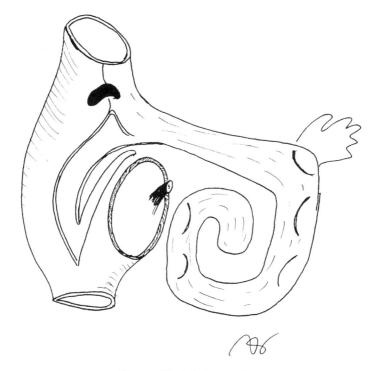

Figure 12. Spiral operation.

The heart is exposed via a median sternotomy. Cardiopulmonary bypass is attached to the patient using double venous cannulation (the superior vena cava can be directly cannulated according to the surgeon's preference and/or cardiac anatomy). Cardioplegic solution is easily delivered by means of the exposed coronary sinus ostium. At that point, the surgery is performed in three steps: modified extended trans-septal approach; mitral valve surgery if indicated); and spiraling of the left atrium combined with left atrial appendage exclusion.

Modified Vertical Trans-septal Approach[121]

A quasi-circumferential incision of the right atrium is performed (transplant incision). The right atrial free wall is incised along the right AV sulcus and is prolonged by the vertical septal incision through the fossa ovale. The incision of the superior wall (roof) of the left atrium extends from the septal incision and curves to reach the mitral valve annulus. The mitral valve is exposed using essentially stay sutures, and mitral valve surgery is performed.

Spiraling of the left atrium is performed using a left atrial incision that is started at the mitral valve annulus in the left posterior septal region. The incision circumscribes the right pulmonary veins and proceeds transversely to circumscribe the left pulmonary veins, traveling at the inferior pole of the left atrial appendage orifice. At that point, the incision involves the left atrial posterior wall. The extent of the spiraling incision depends on the posterior wall. The spiral incision can be done using conventional RF cauterization. The incision is not transmural with coagulation of the deeper layer by heart energy. The spiral incision is easy and rapidly repaired by running sutures for safety, as well as other atriotomies.

Our initial experience comprised six patients (three with lone atrial fibrillation and three with mitral valve disease). Early, good results need longer follow-up to be reliably assessed.

Comments

Current surgical techniques may interrupt atrial fibrillation. The surgical rationales are based either on the "site of the origin" of atrial fibrillation as in left atrial exclusion or based on neutralizing the reentrant mechanism of atrial fibrillation (i.e., random reentry). However, surgical successes are not irrefutable evidence that the surgical rationales are true, and that other underlying mechanisms are not present.

Surgical failures can be classified in four groups: failure to interrupt atrial fibrillation; failure to reestablish sinus node function with adequate chronotropic response to exercise; failure to restore atrial contraction; and failure to prevent intra-atrial thrombus formation and its associated systemic embolic events.

Failure to Interrupt Atrial Fibrillation

The identical atrial fibrillation mechanism could be presented postoperatively, because the surgical rationale is inappropriate, because the working mechanism is a variant of the one currently accepted (focal mechanism?), or because the surgery was not adequately executed. Failure to interrupt atrial fibrillation may be an illusion because new atrial tachycardia, such as multifocal atrial tachycardia, which can mimic the clinical presentation of atrial fibrillation are present after surgery. Current catheter electrophysiological studies have limited power to distinguish among these various mechanisms. These postoperative arrhythmias may be transitory, but are disturbing evidence that our understanding of atrial fibrillation is rudimentary and that there might be more than one working mechanism.

Failure to Restore Sinus Node Function

Sinus node dysfunction may be present before surgery and is part of atrial fibrillation pathophysiology. It can be induced surgically because of the site of atriotomies and/or associated ischemic changes. Although AAI pacemaker implantation can restore atrial contraction and chronotropic function, sinus dysfunction is a significant setback.

Atrial Contraction

Loss of atrial contraction can be part of surgical design (corridor or left atrial exclusion) or may be present because of evidence of electromechanical dissociation. Atria may not contract because of irreversible myocardial damage.[99,100,120,122]

Myocardial Pathology

Severe cardiac pathology including the sinus node, was present in all our patients, and some had primary atrial cardiomyopathy. Some patients might have irreversible tachycardia-induced cardiomyopathy. Underlying cardiac pathology has been overlooked in most studies.

Surgical Indication

Surgical indication is controversial. Other nonpharmacological electrophysiological intervention provides excellent control of arrhythmia with fewer side-effects and risk. Patients with mitral valve disease, who require concomitant mitral valve surgery, seem to be the indication of choice.

It is currently used extensively by some surgical teams.[123–127] Concomitant surgery for atrial fibrillation seems a benign adjunct to mitral valve surgery, although it may increase surgical risk in various ways: atriotomies; prolongation of aortic cross-clamping time; and prolongation of cardiopulmonary bypass time. Mitral valve disease associated with atrial fibrillation is a complex entity with multiple components: valvular anatomy; left ventricular function; left atrial dimension; duration of symptoms; age; and sex, etc. Recent studies show that left ventricular function is the main independent prognostic marker. A recent review[128] of long-term follow-up of patients after mitral valve repair shows no difference between patients with or without atrial fibrillation in terms of survival and even morbidity. Despite the large number of reported patients with combined surgery for atrial fibrillation, no comparative randomized series has been published. Atrial fibrillation might share the same value as ventricular arrhythmia in patients with coronary artery disease. The premier marker of survival is cardiac function.

Further Directions

If electrophysiological assessment of atrial fibrillation becomes more precise, new rationales may develop guided by atrial mapping. Some atrial fibrillations may be associated with a focal, perpetuating site which could be ablated.

However, it should be expected that surgery for atrial fibrillation shares the fate of other surgical approaches to supraventricular arrhythmias. Surgical techniques are associated with significant morbidity and should be only temporarily necessary. Surgical approaches should be the opportunity to collect data, and assess new rationales and techniques which would be delivered by less invasive approaches.

Recently, catheter ablation techniques have been used to control atrial fibrillation. First, Haissaguerre et al used catheter ablation techniques for unusual forms of atrial fibrillation.[18] Common forms of lone atrial fibrillation have been successfully approached using catheter techniques.[19-21] These developments suggest that catheterization of atrial fibrillation will be a common practice in the foreseeable future.

References

1. Guiraudon GM, Klein GJ, Yee R. Surgery for cardiac tachyarrhythmias. *ACC Educational Highlights* 1990;6:5–10.
2. Guiraudon GM. Cryoablation, a versatile tool in arrhythmia Surgery. *Ann Thorac Surg* 1987;43:129–130 (Editorial).
3. Harrison L, Gallagher JJ, Kasell J, et al. Cryosurgical ablation of the AV node-His bundle: a new method for producing AV block. *Circulation* 1977;55:463.
4. Klein GJ, Harrison L, Ideker RF, et al. Reaction of the myocardium to cryosurgery: electrophysiology and arrhythmogenic potential. *Circulation* 1979;59:364.
5. Warin JF. Catheter ablation of accessory atrioventricular connections. In: Touboul P, Waldo AL (eds): *Atrial Arrhythmias. Current Concepts and Management.* St. Louis: Mosby-Year Book, 1990, pp 476–487.
6. Warin JF, Haissaguerre M, Lemetayer P, et al. Catheter ablation of accessory pathways with a direct approach: results in 35 patients. Circulation 1988;78:800–815.
7. Brugada P, Wellens HJJ. Where to fulgurate in supraventricular tachycardia. In: Fontaine G, Scheinman MM (eds): *Ablation in Cardiac Arrhythmias.* Mount Kisco, NY: Futura Publishing Co., Inc., 1987, pp 141–149.
8. Jackman WM, Wang X, Friday KJ, et al: Catheter ablation of accessory atrioventricular pathways (Wolff-Parkinson-White syndrome) by radiofrequency current. *N Engl J Med* 1991;324:1605–1611.
9. Calkins H, Sousa J, El-Atassi El, et al. Diagnosis and cure of the Wolff-Parkinson-White syndrome or paroxysmal supraventricular tachycardias during a single electrophysiologic test. *N Engl J Med* 1991;324:1612–1662.
10. Leather RA, Leitch JW, Klein GJ, et al. Radiofrequency catheter ablation of accessory pathways: a learning experience. *Am J Cardiol* 1991;68:1651–1655.

11. Kirklin JW. The science of cardiac surgery. *Eur J Cardiothorac Surg* 1990;4: 63–71.
12. Buckberg GD. Myocardial protection: an overview. *Semin Thorac Cardiovasc Surg* 1993;5:98–106.
13. Scheinman MM. North American Society of Pacing and Electrophysiology (NASPE) Survey on radiofrequency catheter ablation: implications for clinicians, third party insurers, and government regulatory agencies. PACE 1992;15: 2228–2231.
14. Scheinman MM. Catheter ablation. Present role and projected impact on healthcare for patients with cardiac arrhythmia. *Circulation* 1991;83:1489–1498.
15. Kirkorian G, Moncada E, Chevalier P, et al. Radiofrequency ablation of atrial flutter. Efficacy of an anatomically guided approach. *Circulation* 1994;90: 2804–2814.
16. Olshansky B, Okumura K, Henthorn R, et al. Atrial mapping of human atrial flutter demonstrates reentry in the right atrium. *J Am Coll Cardiol* 1988;7:194A.
17. Chen SA, Chiang CE, Yang CJ, et al. Radiofrequency catheter ablation of sustained intra-atrial reentrant tachycardia in adult patients. *Circulation* 1993;88: 578–587.
18. Haissaguerre M, Marcus FI, Fischer B, et al. Radiofrequency catheter ablation in unusual mechanisms of atrial fibrillation: report of 3 cases. *J Cardiovasc Electrophysiol* 1994;5:743–751.
19. Haissaguerre M, Gencel L, Fischer B, et al. Successful catheter ablation of atrial fibrillation. *J Cardiovasc Electrophysiol* 1994;5:1045–1052.
20. Elvan A, Pride HP, Eble JN, et al. Radiofrequency catheter ablation of the atria reduces the inducibility and duration of atrial fibrillation in dogs. *Circulation* 1995;91:2235–2244.
21. Swarz J, Pellersels G, Silvers J, et al. A catheter-based approach to atrial fibrillation in humans. *Circulation* 1994;90(Suppl 4):I-335 (Abstract).
22. Sealy WC, Hattler BG, Blumennschein SD, et al. Surgical treatment of Wolff-Parkinson-White Syndrome. *Ann Thorac Surg* 1969;8:1–11.
23. Guiraudon GM. Anatomy of atrioventricular attachments, connections and junction: in medio stat virtus. *JACC* 1994;24:1732–1734 (Editorial Comment.
24. McAlpine WA. Heart and coronary arteries. In: An Anatomical Atlas for *Clinical Diagnosis, Radiological Investigation, and Surgical Treatment*. New York: Springer-Verlag, 1975.
25. Wood FC, Wolferth CC, Geckeler GD. Histologic demonstration of accessory muscular connections between auricle and ventricle in a case of short PR interval and prolonged QRS complex. *Am Heart J* 1943;25:454–462.
26. Hackel DB. Anatomic basis for preexcitation syndromes. In: Benditt DG, Benson DW (eds): *Cardiac Preexcitation Syndromes: Origins, Evaluation and Treatment*. Boston: Martinus Nijhoff, 1996, pp 31–40.
27. Guiraudon G, Klein G, Sharma A, et al. Regional subclassification of accessory pathways in the Wolff-Parkinson-White syndrome based on dissection and electrophysiology. *PACE* 1989;12(Suppl 1):653 (Abstract).
28. Guiraudon GM, Klein GJ, Yee R. Surgery for Wolff-Parkinson-White syndrome and supraventricular tachycardias. In: Josephson ME, Wellens HJJ (eds): *Tachycardias: Mechanisms and Management*. Mount Kisco: NY, Futura Publishing Co, 1993, pp 479–504.
29. Coumel P, Cabrol C, Fabiato A, et al. Tachycardie permanent par rhythm reci-

proc ae. 1. Preuves du diagnostic par stimulation auriculaire et ventriculaire. *Arch Mal Coeur* 1967;60:18130.

30. O'Neill BJ, Klein GJ, Guiraudon GM, et al. Results of operative therapy in the permanent form of junctional reciprocating tachycardia. *Am J Cardiol* 1989;63: 1074–1079.

31. Klein GJ, Guiraudon GM, Kerr CR, et al. "Nodoventricular" accessory pathway: evidence for a distinct accessory atrioventricular pathway with atrioventricular node-like properties. *J Am Coll Cardiol* 1988;11:1035–1040.

32. Gallagher JJ. Variants of preexcitation: update 1984. In: Zipes DP, Jalife J (eds): *Cardiac Electrophysiology and Arrhythmias*. Orlando, FL: Grune & Stratton, 1985, pp 419–433.

33. Cappato R, Schluter M, Weib C, et al. Catheter-induced mechanical conduction block of right-sided accessory fibers with Mahaim-type preexcitation to guide radiofrequency ablation. *Circulation* 1994;90:282–290.

34. Grogin HR, Lee RJ, Kwasman M, et al. Radiofrequency catheter ablation of atriofascicular and nodoventricular Mahaim tracts. *Circulation* 1994;90:272–281.

35. Guiraudon GM, Klein GJ, Gulamhusein S, et al. Surgical repair of Wolff-Parkinson-White syndrome: a new closed-heart technique. *Ann Thorac Surg* 1984;37: 67–71.

36. Sealy WC. Kent bundles in the anterior septal space. *Ann Thorac Surg* 1983;36: 180–186.

37. Sealy WC. The evolution of the surgical methods for interruption of right free wall Kent bundles. *Ann Thorac Surg* 1983;36:29–36.

38. Sealy WC, Gallagher JJ. The surgical approach to the septal area of the heart based on experiences with 45 patients with Kent bundles. *J Thorac Cardiovasc Surg* 1980;79:542–551.

39. Cox JL, Gallagher JJ, Cain ME. Experience with 118 consecutive patients undergoing operation for the Wolff-Parkinson-White syndrome. *J Thorac Cardiovasc Surg* 1985;90:490–501.

40. Gallagher JJ, Sealy WC, Cox JL, et al. Results of surgery for preexcitation in 200 cases. *Circulation* 1981;64(Suppl IV):146 (Abstract).

41. Guiraudon GM, Klein GJ, Sharma AD, et al. Closed heart technique for Wolff-Parkinson-White syndrome: further experience and potential limitations. *Ann Thorac Surg* 1986;42:651–657.

42. Guiraudon GM, Klein GJ, Sharma AD, et al. Surgery for the Wolff-Parkinson-White syndrome: the epicardial approach. *Semin Thorac Cardiovasc Surg* 1989; 1:21–33.

43. Guiraudon GM, Klein GJ, Yee R, et al. Surgical epicardial ablation of left ventricular pathway using sling exposure. *Ann Thorac Surg* 1990;50:968–971.

44. Guiraudon GM, Klein GJ, Sharma AD, et al. Surgical approach to anterior septal accessory pathways in 20 patients with the Wolff-Parkinson-White syndrome. *Eur J Cardiothorac Surg* 1988;2:201–206.

45. Guiraudon GM, Klein GJ, Sharma AD, et al. "Atypical" posterior septal accessory pathway in the Wolff-Parkinson-White syndrome. *J Am Coll Cardiol* 1988; 12:1605–1608.

46. Teo WS, Guiraudon GM, Klein GJ, et al. A unique preexcitation pattern related to an atypical anteroseptal accessory pathway. *PACE* 1992;15 (Pt 1):1696–1701.

47. Gallagher JJ, Selle JG, Sealy WC, et al. Intermediate septal accessory pathways (IS-AP): a subset of preexcitation at risk for complete heart block/failure during WPW surgery. *Circulation* 1986;74(Suppl 2):387 (Abstract).

48. Murdock CJ, Klein GJ, Guiraudon GM, et al. Epicardial mapping in patients with "nodoventricular" accessory pathways. *Am J Cardiol* 1991;68:208–214.
49. Guiraudon CM, Guiraudon GM, Klein GJ, et al. "Nodal ventricular" Mahaim pathway: histologic evidence for an accessory atrioventricular pathway with AV node-like morphology. *Circulation* 1988;78(Suppl II):II-40 (Abstract).
50. Guiraudon GM, Guiraudon CM, Klein GJ, et al. The coronary sinus diverticulum: a pathological entity associated with the Wolff-Parkinson- White syndrome. *Am J Cardiol* 1988;62:733–735.
51. Arruda MS, Beckman KJ, McClelland JH, et al. Coronary sinus anatomy and anomalies in patients with posteroseptal accessory pathway requiring ablation within a venous branch of the coronary sinus. *J Am Coll Cardiol* 1994;23:224A (Abstract).
52. Guiraudon GM, Klein GJ, Sharma AD, et al. Multiple accessory pathways—the elusive posterior septal pathways. Experience with 17 patients. *PACE* 1988; 11(Suppl):935 (Abstract).
53. Gallagher JJ, Sealy WC, Kasell J, et al. Multiple accessory pathways in patients with the preexcitation syndrome. *Circulation* 1976;54:571–590.
54. Guiraudon GM, Guiraudon CM, Klein GJ, et al. Operation for the Wolff-Parkinson-White syndrome in the catheter ablation era. *Ann Thorac Surg* 1994; 57:1084–1048.
55. Brodman R, Fisher J, Mitsudo S, et al. Kent pathways visualized in situ and removed at operation. *Am J Cardiol* 1983;51:1457–1458.
56. Rosenberg HS, Klima T, McNamara DG, et al. Atrioventricular communication in the Wolff-Parkinson-White syndrome. *Am J Clin Pathol* 1971;56:79–90.
57. Sharma AD, Yee R, Guiraudon GM, et al. AV Nodal Reentry—Current concepts and surgical treatment. In: Zipes DP, Rowlands DJ (eds): *Progress In Cardiology*. Pennsylvania: Lea & Febiger, 1988, pp 129–145.
58. Pritchett ELC, Anderson RW, Benditt DG, et al. Reentry within the atrioventricular node: surgical cure with preservation of atrioventricular conduction. *Circulation* 1979;60:440–446.
59. Marquez-Montes J, Rufilanchas JJ, Esteve JJ, et al. Paroxysmal nodal reentrant tachycardia, surgical cure with preservation of atrioventricular conduction. *Chest* 1983;83:690–694.
60. Ross DL, Johnson DC, Denniss AR, et al. Curative surgery for atrio ventricular junctional ("AV Nodal") reentrant tachycardia. *J Am Coll Cardiol* 1985;6: 1282–1392.
61. Meijler FL, Janse MJ. Morphology and electrophysiology of the mammalian atrioventricular node. *Physiol Rev* 1988;68:608–647.
62. Anderson RH, Becker AE, Brechenmacher C, et al. The human atrioventricular junctional area. A morphological study of the A-V node and bundle. *Eur J Cardiol* 1975;3:11–25.
63. Guiraudon GM, Klein GJ, van Hemel N, et al. Anatomically guided surgery to the AV node. Av nodal skeletonization: experience in 46 patients with AV nodal reentrant tachycardia. *Eur J Cardiothorac Surg* 1990;4:461–465.
64. Cox JL, Holman WL, Cain ME. Cryosurgical treatment of atrioventricular node reentrant tachycardia. *Circulation* 1987;76:1329–1336.
65. Johnson DC, Nunn GR, Meldrum-Hanna W, et al. Surgery for atrioventricular node reentry tachycardia: the surgical dissection technique. *Semin Thorac Cardiovasc Surg* 1989;1:53–57.
66. Guiraudon GM, Klein GJ, Sharma AD, et al. Skeletonization of the atrioventric-

ular node surgical alternative for AV nodal reentrant tachycardia. Experience with 32 patients. *Ann Thorac Surg* 1990;49:565.

67. Natale A, Wathen M, Wolfe K, et al. Comparative atrioventricular node properties after radiofrequency ablation and operative therapy of AV node reentry. *PACE* 1993;16(PartI):971–977.

68. Lowe JE, Hendry PJ, Packer DL, et al. Surgical management of chronic ectopic atrial tachycardia. *Semin Thorac Cardiovasc Surg* 1989;1:58–66.

69. Guiraudon GM, Klein GJ, Yee R, et al. Supraventricular tachycardias: the role of surgery. *PACE* 1993:16(Part II):658–670.

70. Sharma AD, Klein GJ, Guiraudon GM, et al. Paroxysmal sinus tachycardia: further experience with subtotal right atrial exclusion suggesting diffuse atrial disease. *J Am Coll Cardiol* 1986;7:128 (Abstract).

71. Morillo CA, Klein GJ, Thakur RK, et al. Mechanism of "inappropriate" sinus tachycardia. Role of sympathovagal balance. *Circulation* 1994;90:873–877.

72. Gomes A, Mehta D, Langan MN, et al. Sinus node reentrant tachycardia. *PACE* 1995;18(Pt I):1045–1057.

73. Sanders WE, Sorrentino RA, Greenfield RA, et al. Catheter ablation of sinoatrial node reentrant tachycardia. *J Am Coll Cardiol* 1994;23:926–934.

74. Jolly WA, Ritchie WT. Auricular flutter and fibrillation. *Heart* 1910;2:177.

75. Prinzmetal M, et al. The Auricular Arrhythmias. Springfield, Ill: Charles C. Thomas, Publisher, 1952.

76. Wells JL, James L, MacLean WAH, et al. Characterization of atrial flutter: studies in man after open heart surgery using fixed atrial electrodes. *Circulation* 1979;60:665–673.

77. Lewis T, Freil HS, Stroud WD. Observations upon flutter and fibrillation. II. The nature of auricular flutter. *Heart* 1920;7:191.

78. Boineau JP, Schuessler RB, Mooney CR, et al. Natural and evoked atrial flutter due to circus movement in dogs. *Am J Cardiol* 1980;45:1167–1181.

79. Allessie MA, Lammers WJEP, Bonke IM, et al. Intraatrial reentry as a mechanism for atrial flutter induced by acetylcholine in rapid pacing in the dog. *Circulation* 1984;70:123.

80. Page P, Plumb VJ, Okumura K, et al. A new model of atrial flutter. *J Am Coll Cardiol* 1986;8:872.

81. Puech P, Latour H, Grolleau R. Le flutter et ses limites. *Arch Mal Coeur* 1970; 63:116.

82. Klein GJ, Guiraudon GM, Sharma AD, et al: Demonstration of macro-reentry and feasibility of operative therapy in the common type of atrial flutter. *Am J Cardiol* 1986;57:587.

83. Disertori M, Inama G, Vergara G, et al. Evidence of a reentry circuit in the common type of atrial flutter in man. *Circulation* 1983;67:434.

84. Waldo AL, MacLean WAH, Karp RB, et al. Entrainment and interruption of atrial flutter with atrial pacing: studies in man following open heart surgery. *Circulation* 1977;56:737–745.

85. Waldo AL, Carlson MD, Biblo LA, et al. The role of transient entrainment in atrial flutter. In: Touboul P, Waldo AL(eds): *Atrial Arrhythmias—Current Concepts and Management.* St. Louis, Missouri: Mosby Year Book, 1990, p 210.

86. Cosio FG. Endocardial Mapping of Atrial Flutter. In: Touboul P, Waldo AL (eds): *Atrial Arrhythmias—Current Concepts and Management.* St. Louis, Missouri: Mosby Year Book, 1990, p 229.

87. Chauvin M, Brechenmacher C, Voegltin JR. Applications de la cartographie endocavitaire a l'etude du flutter auriculaire. *Arch Mal Coeur* 1983;76:1020.
88. Cosio FG, Goicolea A, Lopez-Gil M, et al. Atrial endocardial mapping in the rare form of atrial flutter. *Am J Cardiol* 1990;66:715.
89. Puech P, Gallay P, Grolleau R. Mechanism of atrial flutter in humans. In: Touboul P, Waldo AL (eds): *Atrial Arrhythmias—Current Concepts and Management.* St. Louis, Missouri: Mosby Year Book, 1990, p 190.
90. Allessie MA, Rensma W. Brugada J, et al. In: Touboul P, Waldo AL, (eds): *Atrial Arrhythmias—Current Concepts and Management.* St. Louis, Missouri: Mosby Year Book, 1990, pp 112.
91. Guiraudon GM, Guiraudon CM. Atrial functional anatomy. In: Kingma JH, van Hemel NM, Lie KI (eds): *Atrial Fibrillation: A Treatable Disease?* Boston, Massachusetts: Kluwer Academic Publisher, 1992, pp 23.
92. Robinson TF, Factor SM, Sonnenblick EH. The heart as a suction pump. *Sci American* 1986;254:84.
93. Lamas GA. Physiological consequences of normal atrioventricular conduction: applicability to modern cardiac pacing. *J Cardiac Surg* 1989;4:89.
94. Gosselink AT, Crijns HJGM, Lie KI. Risk and prevention of embolism in atrial fibrillation. In: Kingma JH, van Hemel NM, Lie KI (eds): *Atrial Fibrillation: A Treatable Disease?* Boston, Massachussetts: Kluwer Academic Publishers, 1992, p 237.
95. James TN. Diversity of histopathologic correlates of atrial fibrillation. In: Kulbertus HE, Olson SB, Schlepper M (eds): *Atrial Fibrillation.* Modudal, Sweden: Astra Publishers, 1982, p 13.
96. Bharati S, Lev MJ. Histology of the normal and diseased atrium. In: Falk RH, Podrid PJ (eds): *Atrial Fibrillation, Mechanisms and Management.* New York: Raven Press Publishers, 1992, p 15.
97. Frustaci A, Caldarulo M, Buffon A, et al. Cardiac biopsy in patients with "primary" atrial fibrillation; histologic evidence of occult myocardial diseases. *Chest* 1991;2:303.
98. Sekiguchi M, Hiroe M, Kasanuki H, et al. Experience of 100 atrial endomyocardial biopsies and the concept of atrial cardiomyopathy. *Circulation* 1984;70(Suppl 2):118 (Abstract).
99. Guiraudon CM, Ernst NM, Guiraudon GM, et al. The pathology of drug resistant lone atrial fibrillation in eleven surgically treated patients. In: Kingma JH, van Hemel NM, Lie KI (eds). *Atrial Fibrillation: A Treatable Disease?* Boston, Massachusetts: Kluwer Academic Publishers, 1992, p 41.
100. Guiraudon CM, Ernst NM, Klein GJ, et al. The pathology of intractable "primary" atrial fibrillation. *Circulation* 1992;86(Suppl 1):I-662 (Abstract).
101. Moe GK. On the multiple wavelet hypothesis of atrial fibrillation. *Arch Int Pharmacodyn* 1962;140:183.
102. Allessie MA, Lammers WJEP, Bonke FIM. Experimental evaluation of Moe's multiple wavelet hypothesis of atrial fibrillation. In: Zipes DP, Jalife J (eds): *Cardiac Electrophysiology and Arrhythmias.* New York: Grune & Stratton, Inc., 1985, p 265.
103. Allessie M, Kirchhof C. Termination of atrial fibrillation by class IC antiarrhythmic drugs, a paradox? In: Kingma JH, van Hemel NM, Lie KI (eds): *Atrial Fibrillation: A Treatable Disease?* Boston, Massachusetts: Kluwer Academic Publishers, 1992, p 265.

104. Wijffels M, Kirchhof C, Frederiks J, et al. Atrial fibrillation begets atrial fibrillation. *Circulation* 1993;86(Suppl 1):I-18 (Abstract).
105. Morillo CA, Klein GJ, Jones DL, et al. Experimental atrial fibrillation: evidence for a focal mechanism. *J Am Coll Cardiol* 1993;21,2:183A (Abstract).
106. Stroke Prevention in Atrial Fibrillation Study Group Investigators. Preliminary report of the Stroke Prevention in Atrial Fibrillation study. *N Engl J Med* 1990; 322:863.
107. Guiraudon GM, Campbell CS, Jones DL, et al. Combined sino-atrial node atrioventricular isolation: a surgical alternative to His bundle ablation in patients with atrial fibrillation. *Circulation* 1985;72(Suppl 2):III-220 (Abstract).
108. Leitch JW, Klein G, Yee R, et al. Sinus node-atrioventricular node isolation. Long term results with the corridor operation for atrial fibrillation. *J Am Coll Cardiol* 1991;17:970.
109. Guiraudon GM, Klein GJ, Guiraudon CM, et al. Treatment of atrial fibrillation: preservation of sinoventricular impulse conduction (the corridor operation). In: Olsson SB, Allessie MA, Campbell RWF, (eds): *Atrial Fibrillation—Mechanisms and Therapeutic Strategies*. Armonk, NY: Futura Publishing, 1994, p 349.
110. Gursoy S, de Bruyne B, Atie J, et al. Interatrial dissociation following the corridor operation: role of atrial contraction in thrombogenesis. *Eur Heart J* 1991; 12(Suppl):337 (Abstract).
111. Vigano M, Graffigna A, Pagnani F, et al. The surgical treatment for supraventricular arrhythmias. In: D'Alessandro LC (ed): *Heart Surgery*. Rome, Italy: Casa Editrice Scientifica Internazionale, 1993, p 403.
112. van Hemel NM, Defaux JJAMT, Kingma JH, et al. Longterm results of the "corridor" operation for atrial fibrillation. *Br Heart J* 1994;71:170.
113. Cox JL, Canavan TE, Schuessler RB. The surgical treatment of atrial fibrillation: II. Intra-operative electrophysiologic mapping and description of the electrophysiologic basis of atrial flutter and atrial fibrillation. *J Thorac Cardiovasc Surg* 1991;101:406.
114. Cox JL. Evolving applications of the maze procedure for atrial fibrillation. *Ann Thorac Surg* 1993;55:578–580.
115. Cox JL, Boineau JP, Schuessler RB, et al. Successful surgical treatment of atrial fibrillation: review and clinical update. *JAMA* 1991;266:1976–1980.
116. Cox JL, Boineau JP, Schuessler RB, et al. Five-year experience with the maze procedure for atrial fibrillation. *Ann Thorac Surg* 1993;56:814–824.
117. Cox JL, Boineau JP, Schuessler RB, et al. In: Olsson SB, Allessie MA, Campbell RWF (eds): *Atrial Fibrillation: Mechanisms and Therapeutic* Strategies. Armonk, NY: Futura Publishing Company, Inc., 1994, pp 373–404.
118. Cox JL, Schuessler RB, Cain ME, et al. Surgery for atrial fibrillation. *Semin Thorac Cardiovasc Surg* 1989;1:67–73.
119. Graffigna A, Ressia L, Pagnani F, et al. Left atrial isolation for the treatment of atrial fibrillation due to mitral valve disease: hemodynamic evaluation. *N Trend Arrhyth*, 1993;ix:1069.
120. Shyu KG, Cheng JJ, Chen JJ, et al. Recovery of atrial function after atrial compartment operation for chronic atrial fibrillation in mitral valve disease. *JACC* 24:392–398.
121. Guiraudon GM, Ofiesh JG, Kaushik R. Extended vertical trans-septal approach to the mitral valve. *Ann Thorac Surg* 1991;52:1058.
122. Feinberg MS, Waggoner AD, Kater KM, et al. Restoration of atrial function after

the maze procedure for patients with atrial fibrillation: assessment by Doppler echocardiography. *Circulation* 1994;90(Suppl 12):II-285.

123. Brodman RF, Frame R, Fisher JD, et al. Combined treatment of mitral stenosis and atrial fibrillation with valvuloplasty and left atrial maze procedure. *J Thorac Cardiovasc Surg* 1994;107:622 (Letter).

124. Hioki M, Ikeshita M, Iedokoro Y, et al. Successful combined operation for mitral stenosis and atrial fibrillation. *Ann Thorac Surg* 1993;55:776–778.

125. Bonchek LI, Burlingame MW, Worley SJ, et al. Cox/maze procedure for atrial septal defect with atrial fibrillation: management strategies. *Ann Thorac Surg* 1993;55:607–610.

126. McCarthy PM, Cosgrove DM, Castle LW, et al. Combined treatment of mitral regurgitation and atrial fibrillation with valvuloplasty and the maze procedure. *Am J Cardiol* 1993;71:483–486.

127. Kosakai Y, Kawaguchi AT, Isobe F, et al. Cox maze procedure for chronic atrial fibrillation associated with mitral valve disease. *J Thorac Cardiovasc Surg* 1994; 108:1049–1055.

128. Chua YL, Schaff HV, Orszulak TA, et al. Outcome of mitral valve repair in patients with preoperative atrial fibrillation. *J Thorac Cardiovasc Surg* 1994;107: 408–415.

Chapter 17

The Implantable Cardioverter Defibrillator:
Modern Implantation Techniques and Their Impact on Outcomes

Richard M. Luceri, MD, Philip Zilo, MD,
Daniel N. Weiss, MD

Introduction

Since the first human implantation of the automatic implantable cardioverter defibrillator (ICD) in 1980, by Mirowski and colleagues,[1] this rather revolutionary therapy has been introduced throughout the world and has been implanted in more than 150,000 patients. As a consequence of both medical acceptance of this therapy and progress in technology, the ICD is now considered a reliable option for the termination of lethal ventricular arrhythmias. In 15 years, both of these factors have resulted in widespread acceptance of the ICD as both a primary and adjunct therapy for the prevention of sudden arrhythmic death in susceptible patients. While the definitive indications for implantation of the ICD are currently the subject of several randomized trials versus other types of therapy,[2,3] most physicians will agree that the ICD represents a dramatic solution to a problem that has figured prominently as the leading cause of cardiac mortality in the western world.

This chapter will focus on the techniques of ICD implantation and their results, with particular emphasis on modern ICD enhancements and their effects on outcomes.

Historical Perspective on ICD Implantation

Soon after the first human implant in 1980 in Baltimore, the US Food and Drug Administration (FDA) allowed expansion of the clinical trial to

From *Practical Management of Cardiac Arrhythmias* edited by Nabil El-Sherif, and Jean Lekieffre. Futura Publishing Co., Armonk, NY, © 1997.

other US centers in 1982. Concomitantly, the technology was brought to Europe as well. In 1985, the FDA released the device in the United States for patients who survived a cardiac arrest and in whom the ICD represented the best option for therapy. All of these devices were of the "shock only" variety, and required epicardial placement of one or two defibrillator patches, with separate sensing leads (epicardial or endocardial). Most of the experience of the first decade of ICD therapy was with this type of device.[4,5]

The second decade of ICD therapy was heralded by significant technological advances. These included the introduction of multiprogrammability, biphasic energy, antitachycardia pacing, and antibradycardia pacing to the cardioverting-defibrillating capability of the ICD. Equally important was the introduction of transvenous lead systems which resulted in the abandonment of the thoracotomy technique (or its variants) in favor of a significantly less burdensome operative procedure.[6]

Today, the ICD of choice is implanted pectorally, with little or no operative morbidity and mortality, with a variety of transvenous lead systems. The devices are fully programmable and have a battery longevity approaching 4 to 5 years.

Implantation Techniques

Current primary implantation techniques for ICDs depend upon the choice of ICD model and the type of lead system selected. The operative approach to device replacements or upgrades is a function of the clinical requirements and the integrity of the chronic lead system.

Device Selection

At the time of this writing there are several models of ICDs that can be considered for pectoral implantation (Table 1). Although earlier (larger)

Table 1
Pectoral-Size Implantable Cardioverter Defibrillators Currently Available
(November 1995)

Manufacturer	Name	Model	Volume (cc)	Max Stored Energy (joules)
Medtronic	Jewel	7219 B, D, E	83–89	34
Ventritex	Cadet	V-115	73	42
CPI	Mini	1740	68	33
CPI	Mini +	1741	73	33
Telectronics	Sentry	4310	78	34
Biotronik	Phylax	06	72	30

models from several manufacturers have been implanted in the pectoral position, we tend to consider those as anecdotes to what is generally accepted as a pectoral size device. These currently available devices vary in volume from 68 to 89 cubic centimeters (cc), and are all capable of delivering biphasic shocks. Maximum stored energy varies from 30 to 42 Joules depending upon the model selected. In the large majority of patients, however, all provide adequate safety margins of energy when used with the lead system options that are currently available. For some, issues such as device longevity, energy output, and costs remain factors which influence the selection of one of these devices over another.

Lead Configurations

Several types of lead configurations have evolved along with the ICDs themselves. The initial worldwide experience with the Endotak™ single pass lead system (Cardiac Pacemaker, Inc., St. Paul, MN, USA) provided the bulk of clinical data in regard to the feasibility and initial efficacy of transvenous defibrillation.[7] When biphasic waveforms were introduced in ICDs, the data showed a better performance of these leads, often without the addition of a subcutaneous patch electrode.[8] Subsequently, several other types of lead systems were implanted with overall similar success.

The "Unipolar" ICD Lead System

In 1994, Bardy and coworkers described a nonthoracotomy lead system using a single apical right ventricular pace/sense electrode and the active shell or "can" of the ICD itself as a second shock electrode.[9] Prospective and randomly obtained data confirmed the success of this approach vis-à-vis defibrillation thresholds (DFTs) and overall efficacy. The mean stored energy DFT reported from this study was 7.4 Joules, and compared favorably to traditional two and three lead systems. In fact, Bardy additionally reported that the addition of a second superior vena cava (SVC) electrode added little to reduce the DFT. This system became known as the "unipolar" ICD systems, with the can serving as the cathode, while the right ventricular (RV) lead was used as the anode.

A variant of this technique is referred to as the patch-in-pocket approach. In this case, a standard patch electrode is placed in the ICD pocket (the can itself not being electrically active), with an RV apical electrode similarly serving as the second pole of the circuit. Initial unpublished data with the Sentry 4310™ (Telectronics Pacing Systems, Englewood, CO, USA) suggests comparable efficacy with this modified version of the unipolar defibrillator.

Advantages of using the pectoral pocket as the location for one of the electrodes include: ease of implantation (single transvenous electrode placement); and utilization of a single incision for the entire system. Also, this method may obviate the need for placing subcutaneous patch electrodes in other axillary positions which tend to be somewhat uncomfortable for the patients. Long-term performance of the "unipolar" ICD system is currently unknown, particularly in regard to stability of DFTs and integrity of the lead, patch and can material in these positions.

The Dual Lead Dual-Chamber ICDs

As of this writing, the Defender 9001™ (ELA Medical, Montrouge, France), the world's first dual-chamber pacing defibrillator, has been successfully implanted in ten patients in Europe. Two lead configurations were utilized: the Enguard system from Telectronics; and an Endotak from CPI plus an atrial bipolar active fixation lead from ELA Medical.[10] This ICD with DDD pacing capability, although not of pectoral size, is expected to particularly serve the needs of a growing number of ICD patients who require dual-chamber pacing as well. This may be particularly advantageous in patients with concomitant heart failure.

Enhancements of the Single-Pass Lead

A recent publication by Kall and coworkers[11] described the benefits of a subcutaneous lead array in combination with a transvenous defibrillation electrode via a single infraclavicular incision. Although reporting on only two patients, the authors suggested that the placement of the array lead using the same incision as the can resulted in lower DFTs in these patients. While the subcutaneous array has traditionally been implanted in a separate left chest position, the potential benefits of using this lead in a single incision merit further investigation.

Other Transvenous Lead Configurations

The ICD recipient may also benefit from a variety of other lead configurations that have all been reported with success. These include dual lead (right atrial-right ventricular) configurations such as the Telectronics Enguard system[12]; triple lead configurations (RV + coronary sinus + SVC) or variations thereof such as the Transvene system™[13] (Medtronic, Inc., Minneapolis, MN, USA). Each of these potential configurations may add or eliminate one lead by the use of an optional subcutaneous patch electrode.

Morbidity and Mortality with Nonthoracotomy Lead Systems

Significant reductions in operative morbidity and mortality have been anticipated with the widespread use of nonthoracotomy lead systems in ICDs.

Table 2

Operative Mortality With Nonthoracotomy ICD Lead Systems

Author	Year	n =	Operative Deaths (%)
Bocker[17]	1993	99	1
Hauser[18]	1993	414	1.3
Sra[19]	1994	144	0
Raviele[20]	1995	307	0

The mean 30-day operative mortality for the group = <0.5%.

Several recent reports have examined 30-day operative mortality in patients undergoing initial implantation of an ICD system. The results are significantly lower than those with traditional thoracotomy systems, with mortality ranging from 0% to 1.3% from large series. Table 2 depicts the results of four recently published studies accounting for a total of 964 patients having a mean operative mortality of < 0.5%. In addition, a recent report by Ong et al[14] contrasts the proarrhythmic effect of implantation between epicardial and nonthoracotomy systems. In similar cohorts, postoperative VT occurrence was 5% for nonthoracotomy leads versus 14% for epicardial systems. Similarly, postoperative occurrences of atrial fibrillation were reduced from 15% for epicardial to 1% for endocardial leads.

While the low operative mortality of nonthoracotomy ICD systems appears to fulfill expectations, the same is not exactly true for implant morbidity, particularly in regard to complications due to system components. In a revealing recent publication, Schwartzman and colleagues[15] reported a complication rate of 16% in 27 of 170 nonthoracotomy implants followed for a mean of 17 months postoperatively (Table 3). Of these, 17 out of 27 (63%), required

Table 3

Complications of Nonthoracotomy Lead Systems in 170 Patients Followed for a Mean of 17 Months (Adapted from Schwartzman, Reference 15)

Type of Complication	Percentage (%)
Lead dislodgment	4.7
Lead body fracture	3.5
Subcutaneous patch mesh fracture	0.6
Superior vena cava thrombus	1.8
High defibrillation thresholds	5.3
System infection	4.1

Total complication rate = 27/170 (16%), requiring 17/27 (63%) reoperations.

Table 4
Length of Stay in Hospital in Consecutive Patients Having Undergone Three
Different Types of ICD Implant Procedures (Holy Cross Hospital,
Fort Lauderdale, Florida.)

	Thoracotomy	Transvenous with Abdominal Implant	Transvenous with Pectoral Implant
n =	25	25	25
Male/female ratio	22/3	22/3	20/5
Mean age (yrs)	66.1	77.1	68.7
Postoperative stay in hospital (days)	8.3	5.7	3.8
Postoperative stay in intensive care unit (days)	3.2	0.5	0

some type of reoperation. Lead dislodgments and fractures as well as DFTs accounted for a large number of these reinterventions. Fortunately, a lower complication rate is expected in future reports with pectoral implants, since shorter leads, fewer or no lead connectors, and absence of lead tunneling are the hallmarks of these newer implant techniques.

Shorter Hospital Stays with Endocardial Lead Systems

We recently reported our observation of significantly shorter hospital stays in patients with transvenous lead systems when compared to traditional epicardial implants.[16] In our most recent comparison, we have similarly found additional shortening of the hospital stay (from 5.7 days to 3.8 days postoperatively) when the data for pectoral implants was analyzed (Table 4). This is largely attributed to shorter pectoral leads, absence of tunneling, less postoperative pain, and smaller device size.

Conclusion

The automatic ICD has undergone significant changes in its brief reign among treatment options for potentially lethal arrhythmias. The changes are not purely technical or cosmetic, but have provided real solutions to problems occurring with earlier generations of device technology. Reduction in ICD size, widespread availability of pectorally implanted generators, and simplified but effective nonthoracotomy lead systems have all resulted in placing the

ICD on a level par with other modalities of therapy. Ongoing clinical trials which randomize between ICD or drug therapy have been designed in a manner that places the implantable defibrillator as a therapeutic option of first resort. This is in sharp contrast to the first decade of ICD therapy in which this device was frequently and unfairly relegated to therapy of last resort. We all look forward to continuing enhancements in this exciting area of medical therapeutics.

References

1. Mirowski M, Reid PR, Mower MM, et al. Termination of malignant ventricular arrhythmias with an implanted automatic defibrillator in human beings. *N Engl J Med* 1980;303:322–324.
2. Wever EF, Hauer RN, Van Capelle FL, et al. Randomized study of implantable defibrillator as first-choice therapy versus conventional strategy in post infarct sudden death survivors. *Circulation* 1995;91:2195–2203.
3. Greene HL. Antiarrhythmic drugs versus implantable defibrillators: the need for a randomized controlled study. *Am Heart J* 1994;127:1171–1178.
4. Winkle RA, Mead RH, Ruder MA, et al: Long-term outcome with the automatic implantable cardioverter-defibrillator. *J Am Coll Cardiol* 1989;16:1353.
5. Thomas A, Moser SA, Smutka ML, et al. Implantable defibrillation: eight years' clinical experience. *PACE* 1988;11:2053–2058.
6. Moore SL, Maloney JD, Edel TB, et al. Implantable cardioverter defibrillator implanted by non-thoracotomy approach: initial clinical experience with the redesigned transvenous lead system. *PACE* 1991;14:1865.
7. Moser S, Troup P, Saksena S, et al. Non-thoracotomy implantable defibrillator system. *PACE* 1988;11:887.
8. Neuzner J, Pitschner HF, Steinmetz F, et al. 100% successful implantation of non-thoracotomy lead systems with biphasic cardioverter/defibrillator: European multicenter results in 832 patients. *PACE* 1994;17(Pt 11):760 (Abstract).
9. Bardy GH, Dolack GL, Kudenchuk PJ, et al. Prospective randomized comparison in humans of a unipolar defibrillation system with that using an additional superior vena cava electrode. *Circulation* 1994;89:1090–1093.
10. ELA Medical, Montrouge, France. Personal communication.
11. Kall JG, Kopp D, Lonchyna V, et al. Implantation of a subcutaneous lead array in combination with a transvenous defibrillation electrode via a single infraclavicular incision. *PACE* 1995;18:482–485.
12. Luceri RM, Zilo P, and the United States and Canadian Enguard Investigators: Initial clinical experience with a dual lead endocardial defibrillation system with atrial pace/sense capability. *PACE* 1995;18:163–167.
13. Bardy GH, Bradley H, Johnson G, et al. Implantable transvenous cardioverter-defibrillators. *Circulation* 1993;87:1152–1168.
14. Ong JJC, Hsu PC, Lin L, et al. Arrhythmias after cardioverter-defibrillator implantation: comparison of epicardial and transvenous systems. *Am J Cardiol* 1995;75:137–140.
15. Schwartzman D, Nallamothu N, Callans DJ, et al. Postoperative lead-related complications in patients with non-thoracotomy defibrillation lead systems. *J Am Coll Cardiol* 1995;26:776–786.

16. Luceri RM, Zilo P, Habal SM, David IB. Cost and length of hospital stay: comparisons between non-thoracotomy and epicardial techniques in patients receiving implantable cardioverter defibrillators. *PACE* 1995;18:168–171.
17. Bocker D, Block M, Isbruch F, et al. Do patients with an implantable defibrillator live longer? *J Am Coll Cardiol* 1993;21:1638–1644.
18. Hauser RG, Kurschinski DT, McVeigh K, et al. Clinical results with non-thoracotomy ICD systems. *PACE* 1993;16:141–148.
19. Sra JS, Natale A, Axtell K, et al. Experience with two different non-thoracotomy lead systems for implantable defibrillator in 170 patients. *PACE* 1994;17:1741–1750.
20. Raviele A, Gasparini G, et al. Italian multicenter clinical experience with endocardial defibrillation: acute and long-term results in 307 patients. *PACE* 1995;8:599–608.

Chapter 18

Comparison of Burst Pacing, Autodecremental (RAMP) Pacing, and Universal Pacing for Termination of Ventricular Tachycardia

John D. Fisher, MD, Zhi Zhang, MD, Soo G. Kim, MD, Kevin J. Ferrick, MD, James A. Roth, MD, Debra R. Johnston, RN

Introduction

The advent of later generation implantable cardioverter defibrillators (ICDs) has been accompanied by a renewed interest in pacing for termination of ventricular tachycardia (VT). Several ICDs are able to provide a menu of antitachycardia pacing patterns. Although rapid pacing is more effective than one or multiple extrastimuli for terminating VT,[1] it has remained uncertain whether any one of the rapid pacing patterns is superior. The present study discussed in this chapter addresses this issue, by comparing three patterns in a randomized prospective fashion during electrophysiological studies in patients with VT.

Methods

A total of 38 patients participated in this study, in two series; 23 were receiving antiarrhythmic drugs.

First Series (Series 1)

For Series 1 patients, synchronized adaptive burst pacing (SBP), and autodecremental pacing (ADP) (see Figure 1, and below) were compared in

From *Practical Management of Cardiac Arrhythmias* edited by Nabil El-Sherif, and Jean Lekieffre. Futura Publishing Co., Armonk, NY, © 1997.

Antitachycardia Pacing Patterns:
Bursts; Autodecremental (Ramps); and Universal

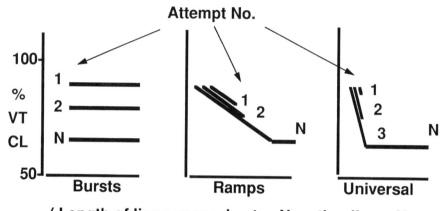

(Length of lines approximates No. stimuli used)

Figure 1. Antitachycardia pacing patterns: bursts; autodecremental (ramps); and universal. The three graphs indicate the essential difference among these three techniques. Bursts are generally delivered with a constant number of stimuli for each successive attempt at termination. With ramps, the number of stimuli is successively increased with each attempt, to a preset upper limit. In addition, the cycle length of each successive stimulus is shorter than its predecessor. The decrement is modest, resulting in a gradual slope as shown in the graft. This slope then plateaus when a minimum predetermined cycle length is reached. Universal pacing is somewhat similar, but the ramp is steeper. Beginning with a single stimulus, successive extrastimuli are added with significantly greater decrements in cycle length for the first three stimuli, after which a plateau is again reached. VT = ventricular tachycardia; CL = cycle length; N = the final attempt.

a randomized sequence. Manual (nonsynchronized) burst pacing was also tested in Series 1 in a nonrandomized fashion: it was used if the randomized methods failed, or in a subsequent induction. These 27 patients in Series 1 consisted of 23 males and 4 females, aged 46 to 78 (mean 64); 22 with coronary disease, 4 cardiomyopathy, and 1 with rheumatic valvular disease. Patients were included in this series if sustained well-tolerated monomorphic VT could be induced. If successfully terminated by pacing, further inductions were immediately performed, with comparison between pacing techniques limited to episodes that were matched in VT morphology and approximate rate.

Second Series (Series 2)

These patients were included only if they had matched episodes of VT induced to allow for comparison of rate adaptive SBP, ADP, and universal pacing, delivered in a randomized sequence. In this series of 11 patients, seven were male. Ages ranged from 45 to 78 (mean 62); eight had coronary disease and three had cardiomyopathy.

For both the first and second series, only one of the test methods was used on any given episode of tachycardia. If VT was not terminated, other techniques including manual burst pacing and cycle length incremental ramp pacing were used.

Manual (Nonsynchronized) Burst Pacing (NBP)[2]

Burst pacing at a constant cycle length was delivered by a Medtronic 5320® (Rochester, MN, USA) external pacemaker, set at 10 to 20 mA, and 2-msec pulse duration. As soon as the rate of the tachycardia was determined, stimulation was begun approximately 25 beats per minute faster, and the operator attempted to achieve seven to ten captures. Subsequent attempts, if needed, were in increments of 25 beats per minute. No specific upper-rate limit was specified, but there was reluctance to exceed 300 beats per minute (200 msec). This represents the simplest type of rapid pacing technique, and can be employed in many clinical settings where more sophisticated equipment is not available.

Rate-Adaptive Synchronized Burst Pacing (SBP)

For Series 1 patients, SBP was delivered using a Savita® Orthorhythmic pacemaker (Paris, France) at 10 MA and 1-ms pulse duration. Initially, five stimuli were delivered at 85% of the VT cycle length CL). All subsequent attempts used 10 stimuli, the sequence being 85%, 80%, 75%, 70%, 67.5%, 65%, and 60%. For Series 2 patients, a Medtronic 1946® (Rochester, MN, USA) Prescription Formulator was used. Stimuli were delivered at 5 Volts and 1.2-msec pulse duration. Ten stimuli were delivered with each termination attempt, the sequence being 88% of the VT cycle length, then 81%, 75%, 69%, 62% and 56%.

Autodecremental Pacing (ADP) or Ramp Pacing[3]

Autodecremental Pacing or Ramp Pacing also known as Cycle Length Decremental Ramp Pacing: (Figure 1). Pacing was delivered using a Medtronic® SP3056, programmed to an output of 10 mA and 1-msec pulse duration for Series 1, and 5 Volts and 1 msec for Series 2. Pacing was initiated with 5 stimuli, the first of these coupled to the last sensed VT beat with a coupling interval of 97% of the VT cycle length, decrementing thereafter by 3% for each of the remaining stimuli. Each successive attempt to terminate the tachycardia involved an increase in the number of stimuli by one. This sequence was repeated to a maximum of ten attempts (14 stimuli). The minimum cycle length was set at 200 msec; if this limit was reached prior to termination of the tachycardia and prior to the delivery of 15 stimuli, the cycle length of the remaining stimuli plateaued at 200 msec.

Universal Pacing (UNI)[4]

Pacing was delivered by a Medtronic SP3056 at an output of 5 Volts and 1.0 msec. (Figure 1). This pattern involves a steep cycle length decremental ramp followed by an early plateau. For the first attempt, a single extrastimulus was delivered at 91% of the VT cycle length. Each successive attempt added an additional extrastimulus, the second at 81%, the third at 75%, and all the remaining at 66% for a maximum of 10 attempts. If tachycardia persisted, the sequence was repeated but with stimuli at 75%, 69%, and then 66% of the VT cycle length, again for up to 10 attempts.

There were two possible end-points to each termination attempt: (1) termination; and (2) ineffective, includes changes in morphology with or without acceleration.

Statistical Analysis

This study involved the matched comparison of similar tachycardias in the same patient on the same day. Because three rather than two comparisons were being made, the repeated measures ANOVA was used initially, rather than paired t-tests which were used only if ANOVA $p = 0.05$ or less. When the paired t-test was used, it was considered significant only at $p = 0.025$ or less, versus $p = 0.05$ or less for other comparisons. Because of the small sample size, the standard error (SE) was used rather than the standard deviation. In Series 2, the number of stimuli used with SBP was constant at 10, and the nonparametric Kruskal-Wallis ANOVA was used for the global test. The Kappa test for concordance was used for determining the comparative efficacy of the pacing modalities for VT termination.

Results

All pacing modalities proved comparable in their ability to terminate VT (Table 1).

Table 1
Termination of Ventricular Tachycardia

	Series 1			Series 2		
	ADP	SBP	OBP	ADP	SBP	UNI
Terminated	23	24	20	10	9	9
Failed	4	3	7	1	2	2
		Kappa = 0.53269			Kappa = 0.76429	
		P = 0.0000008*			P = 0.0000057*	

ADP = Autodecremental Pacing; NBP = Nonsynchronized Manual Burst Pacing; SBP = Synchronized Burst Pacing; UNI = Universal Pacing.
* with the Kappa test, $p < 0.05$ = concordance, or *no* evidence of difference or discordance.

Additional details are provided in Tables 2 and 3, and in Figure 2. These tabulate the relationships among tachycardia cycle length, mean paced cycle length, and the number of stimuli, captures, and attempts needed for each modality to terminate VT. UNI required significantly fewer stimuli to achieve capture than the other methods. Both forms of burst pacing required fewer attempts to achieve termination, although the difference was significant only with respect to ramp pacing. In this study, ADP was therefore the least efficient method, although the ultimate results were comparable. The *mean* pacing cycle length or percentage of the tachycardia cycle length was similar for all modalities. The *shortest* pacing cycle length was found with ramp (ADP) and UNI pacing. As indicated in Table 2, it required an average of seven attempts to termination the arrhythmia using ramp (ADP) pacing; by the 11th stimulus, decrementing in 3% steps from an initial 97%, the final interval was at 67% of the pacing cycle length. With UNI pacing, after four attempts the pacing cycle length was at 66% of the tachycardia cycle length. Both of these are shorter (faster) than for bursts, where the pacing cycle length was constant for each attempt, and averaged 78% to 79% of the tachycardia cycle length at the time of termination.

Discussion

Early reports indicated that extrastimulus[5] and burst pacing[6] could be useful in termination of tachycardia. These findings were later confirmed[2] and expanded, as recently reviewed.[7] Using burst pacing as the gold standard, subsequent papers[8–15] have compared this modality to ADP, or UNI. In most instances, results have been comparable for all these methods, although some studies can be found that show an advantage for each of these methods. In the present study, three major antitachycardia pacing algorithms were compared

Table 2
Details of Tachycardia and Termination

	ADP		SBP		MBP		ANOVA	
Series 1								
	Mean	*SE*	*Mean*	*SE*	*Mean*	*SE*	*Mean*	*SE*
TCL	356.81	15.92	363.52	14.29	332.70	15.41	1.1335	0.3272
PCL	285.74	12.44	285.74	12.80	260.93	10.68	1.4235	0.2471
%	79.22	1.36	79.15	1.88	79.07	2.48	0.0014	0.9986
No. Stimuli	10.81	0.47	9.07	0.38	10.52	0.78	2.6838	0.0746
No. Captures	8.07	0.54	7.56	0.45	6.89	0.76	0.9949	0.3744
No. Attempts	6.93	0.45	2.52	0.31	3.41	0.39	36.0787	<0.000001

	ADP		SBP		MBP		ANOVA	
Series 2								
	Mean	*SE*	*Mean*	*SE*	*Mean*	*SE*	*Mean*	*SE*
TCL	343.36	23.01	345.82	19.38	356.18	23.98	0.0938	0.9107
PCL	247.91	17.59	259.00	21.24	262.64	19.29	0.1841	0.8328
%	78.18	1.35	75.91	3.33	73.91	1.30	0.2148	0.8080
No. Stimuli	11.00	0.54	10.00	0.00	4.09	0.81	$\chi^2 = 20.18$	0.000042
No. Captures	8.73	0.76	8.09	0.69	3.64	0.68	15.1464	0.000028
No. Attempts	7.27	0.45	2.91	0.48	4.09	0.81	14.0076	0.000051

PCL = Pacing Cycle Length in msec; TCL = Tachycardia Cycle Length in msec. Data are given in mean and standard error (SE). Other abbreviations are the same as for Table 1.

Table 3
Intergroup Comparisons

	ADP v SBP		ADP v NBP		SBP v OBP	
Series 1						
	t	*P*	*t*	*P*	*t*	*P*
No. Attempts	8.0827	<0.000001	6.4116	<0.000001	1.6301	0.1071

	ADP v SBP		ADP v UNI		SBP v UNI	
Series 2						
	t	*P*	*t*	*P*	*t*	*P*
No. Stimuli	1.2541	0.2195	8.8080	<0.000001	7.5331	<0.000001
No. Captures	0.6313	0.5326	5.1342	0.000015	4.4929	0.000092
No. Attempts	5.1168	0.0000168	3.7927	0.000648	1.3858	0.1760

Limited intergroup paired t tests were performed after completing the ANOVA. Other abbreviations are the same as for Tables 1 and 2.

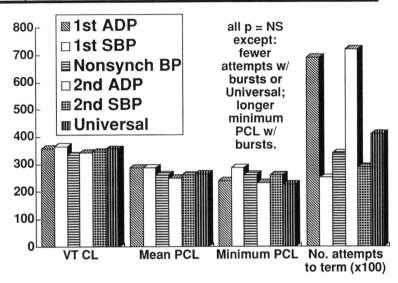

Figure 2. Ventricular tachycardia cycle length, minimum paced cycle length, and number of attempts needed for termination. These grafts illustrate the remarkable comparability of the ventricular tachycardia cycle lengths (VT, CL) and the minimum paced cycle lengths (min PCL) needed for termination. It is also clear from the grafts that more attempts were needed using autodecremental pacing (ADP or ramps). 1st ADP, 2nd ADP, and 2nd SBP refer to the first and second series of patients, as described in the text.

prospectively, in a matched random sequence cross-over study. It should be noted that the specific algorithms or setting used for ramp and UNI were those recommended by the authors who described the techniques.[3,4] All methods proved to be of similar efficacy, although the ramp method was least efficient. The final effective pacing cycle lengths were longest (slowest) with burst pacing. These results may relate to recent studies of the relative refractory period of the tachycardia circuit, and the number and cycle length of stimuli necessary for termination.[16] Of interest, no disadvantage was found for nonsynchronized manual burst pacing.

Conclusion

For a group of patients, burst pacing, ADP, and UNI have similar efficacy. For individual patients, one method may be preferable. The settings for implantable devices should be made on the basis of the clinical response of the individual patient.

Acknowledgment: The authors are grateful to Barouh V. Berkovits, IngEE, for his advice, and for setting up the SP3056 Stimulator for this protocol.

References

1. Fisher JD, Kim SG, Matos JA, Ostrow E. Comparative effectiveness of pacing techniques for termination of well-tolerated sustained ventricular tachycardia. *PACE* 1983;6:915–922.
2. Fisher JD, Mehra R, Furman S. Termination of ventricular tachycardia with bursts of ventricular pacing. *Am J Cardiol* 1978;41:94–104.
3. Charos GS, Haffajee CI, Gold RL, et al. A theoretically and practically more effective method for interruption of ventricular tachycardia: self-adapting autodecremental overdrive pacing. *Circulation* 1986;73:309–315.
4. den Dulk K, Kersschot IE, Brugada P, Wellen HJJ. Is there a universal antitachycardia pacing mode? *Am J Cardiol* 1986;57:950–955.
5. Coumel Ph, Motte G, Gourgon R, Fabiato A, Slama R, Bouvrain Y. Les Tachycardies supre-ventriculaires par rythme reciproque in dehors du syndrome de Wolff-Parkinson-White. *Arch Mal* Coeur 1970;63:35.
6. Fontaine G, Frank R, Beneton H, et al. Interet D'une sonde endocavitaire temporaire pour le diagnostic et l'interruption d, une crise de tachycardie ventriculaire apres infarctus du myocarde. *Ann Cardiol Angeiol* (Paris) 1973;22:321–329.
7. Fisher JD, Kim SG, Ferrick KJ, Roth JA. Antitachycardia pacing for hemodynamic support and arrhythmia termination. In: Josephson ME, Wellens HJJ (eds). *Tachycardias: Mechanisms and Management*. Mount Kisco, New York: Futura Publishing Co., Inc., 1993, pp 421–455.
8. Porterfield JG, Porterfield LM, Bray L. Ninety-six episodes of spontaneous ventricular tachycardia in 1 week: success of ramp pacing by a pacer-cardioverter-defibrillator. *PACE* 1991;14:1440–1442.
9. Cook JR, Kirchhoffer JB, Fitzgerald TF, Lajzer DA. Comparison of decremental and burst overdrive pacing as treatment for ventricular tachycardia associated with coronary artrey disease. *Am J Cardiol* 1992;70:311–315.
10. Kantoch MJ, Green MS, Tang ASL. Randomized cross-over evaluation of two adaptive pacing algorithms for the termination of ventricular tachycardia. *PACE* 1993;16:1664–1672.
11. Newman D, Dorian P, Hardy J. Randomized controlled comparison of antitachycaria pacing algorithms for termination of ventricular tachycardia. *J Am Coll Cardiol* 1993;21:1413–1418.
12. Calkins H, El-Atassi R, Kalbfleisch S, Langberg J, Morady F. Comparison of fixed burst versus decremental burst pacing for termination of ventriuclar tachycardia. *PACE* 1993;16:26–32.
13. Gillis AM, Leitch JW, Sheldon RS, et al. A prospective randomized comparison of autodecremental pacing to burst pacing in device therapy for chronic ventricular tachycardia secondary to coronary artery disease. *Am J Cardiol* 1993;72:1146–1151.
14. Wietholt D, Block M, Isbruch F, et al. Clinical experience with antitachycardia pacing and improved detection algorithms in a new implantable cardioverter-defibrillator.

15. Hammill SC, Packer DL, Stanton MS, Fetter J, and the Multicenter PCD Investigator Group. Termination and acceleration of ventricular tachycardia with auto-decremental pacing, burst pacing, and cardioversion in patients with an implantable cardioverter defibrillator. *PACE* 1995;18:3–10.
16. Callans DJ, Hook BG, Mitra RL, Josephson ME. Characterization of return cycle responses predictive of successful pacing-mediated termination of ventricular tachycardia. *J Am Coll Cardiol* 1995;25:47–53.

Chapter 19

Present and Future Indications for Therapy with Implantable Cardioverter Defibrillators

Michael Block, MD, Dieter Hammel, MD,
Dirk Böcker, MD, Martin Borggrefe, MD,
Günter Breithardt, MD, FESC, FACC

Introduction

When the implantable defibrillator was inaugurated in 1980 by Michel Mirowski, the prevention of sudden cardiac death by defibrillation of hemodynamically, and nontolerated ventricular tachyarrhythmias (VT) was the primary goal of treatment.[1] Within the last 15 years, low energy cardioversion and antitachycardia pacing have extended the treatment to patients with frequent recurrences of hemodynamically tolerated VT. In these patients, improvement of the quality of life has often become another goal of treatment by avoiding hospitalizations and/or side effects of antiarrhythmic drugs.[2] Therapy with the implantable cardioverter defibrillator (ICD) has developed from a last resort therapy to a first-line treatment[3] due to a remarkable evolution of ICD functions[1,4-7] (Table 1) and the surgical approach[1, 8-11] (Table 2). Using a single pectoral skin incision for implantation instead of median thoracotomy and an abdominal device pocket, a significant reduction of the perioperative mortality[12,13] costs less for hospitalization,[14,15] and better cosmetic and functional results have been achieved. Tiered therapy defibrillators can be allowed to tailor the ICD to the arrhythmia characteristics of each patient to achieve prompt termination of VT, avoiding pain due to high energy shocks as often as possible.[6,16]

Current Status of ICD Therapy

Currently, ICDs can be implanted in the pectoral region like pacemakers in combination with one or two endocardial leads in most patients[17,18] (Fig-

From *Practical Management of Cardiac Arrhythmias* edited by Nabil El-Sherif, and Jean Lekieffre. Futura Publishing Co., Armonk, NY, © 1997.

Table 1
Evolution of ICD functions

Year	Programmability	Detection	Therapy
1980[1]	None	PDF	Defibrillation
1982[4]	None	Rate (PDF optional)	+ CV
1988[5]	4 Parameters*	Rate (PDF optional)	+ Low Energy CV
1989[6]	Multiple Zones	Rate, Onset, Stability	+ Pacing (VVI, ATP)
1995[7]	Multiple Zones	+ A-V Relation	+ DDD-Pacing

Abbreviations: ATP = antitachycardia pacing; A-V = atrium-ventricle; CV = cardioversion; DDD = paces and senses in both atrium and ventricle; synchronizes with atrial activity and paces ventricle after a preset interval; PDF = probability density function; VVI = noncompetitive ventricular pacing, inhibition by sensed ventricular signals; * = rate, PDF, detection delay, first shock energy.

ures 1 and 2). The procedure is no longer confined to an operating theater and has also been performed in the catheterization laboratory in local anesthesia.[18,19] It lasts about 1 hour. Usually, the first defibrillation configuration that is tested defibrillates successfully.[17,18] Additional subcutaneous electrodes positioned at the left lateral chest are only needed in a small percentage of patients[10] (Figure 1). The infection rate within the first year had been approximately 2% for the original lead system including a subcutaneous defibrillation patch,[13] but seems to be below 1% for newer lead systems incorporating only transvenous leads.[20] However, rates of reoperations have been as high as 10% after 3 years, mainly due to lead failures.[21] Additionally, high energy shocks cause patient discomfort, even high states of anxiety,[22] and 10% of patients experience syncope within the first year after implantation. Inappropriate ICD therapies, mostly due to atrial fibrillation with a fast ventricular response and sinus node tachycardias, occur in 10% to 20% of patients with tiered therapy ICDs. As a result frequent visits to the outpatient clinic, and even hospitalizations, often cause painful shocks and are potentially proarrhyth-

Table 2
Evolution of Surgical Approach for ICD Implantation

Year	Thoracotomy	Leads	Device
1980[1]	Median sternotomy	Epicardial	Abdominal
1982[8]	Subxiphoidal	Epicardial	Abdominal
1986('89)[9]	No	Transvenous-subcutaneous	Abdominal
1991[10]	No	Transvenous	Abdominal
1993[11]	No	Transvenous	Pectoral

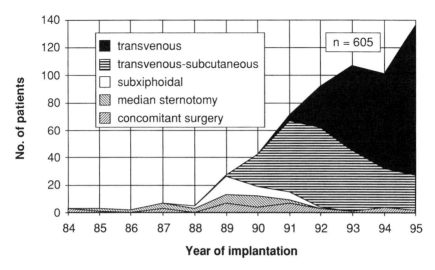

Figure 1. Frequency of ICD lead systems implanted by our group from 1984 to 1995. The surgical approach of choice for implantation of ICD leads has changed over the years.

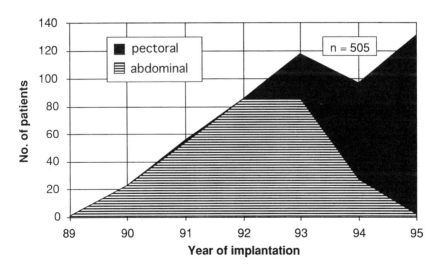

Figure 2. Choice of pocket for ICD devices implanted in combination with transvenous (subcutaneous) lead systems by our group from 1989 to 1995.

mic.[23,24] Battery longevity is approximately 3½ to 5 years,[25] and annual hardware costs of ICD therapy are high.[26]

Present Indications

Guidelines

International and national societies have published guidelines on the indications for ICD implantation,[27-32] analogous to those published for pacemaker implantations. Guidelines for other treatment modalities for VT have been only published for catheter ablation,[33] but not for antiarrhythmic drugs or antitachycardia surgery. However, ICD guidelines are approximately 4- to 5-years old, and do not consider the progress made in ICD technology or recent studies conducted in patients with VT (e.g., the ESVEM study).[34] Revisions of the guidelines are mandatory and only the German Cardiac Society has recently published updated guidelines.[29,35] These guidelines have been issued in the absence of any prophylactic data comparing ICD therapy to placebo or nonantiarrhythmic therapy, or to alternatives such as catheter ablation or antitachycardia surgery. Thus, the guidelines are based on historical controls without antiarrhythmic drug therapy,[36] showing a 47% recurrence of sudden death and cardiac arrests within 2 years, and are also based on results that were published until 1991 on the long-term outcome for patients selected for treatment with ICDs, antiarrhythmic drugs, or antitachycardia surgery. Patients with ICDs have shown a rate of ventricular recurrences in the same order of magnitude as historical controls without treatment, but a low rate of sudden death[12,37,38] (Figure 3). Patients in whom antiarrhythmic drugs reduced the rate of ventricular couplets, nonsustained or sustained VTs during ambulatory and/or exercise,[39-41] or made VTs noninducible during the electrophysiologic study,[42,43] experienced less frequent recurrences of VT, but still showed a substantial rate of sudden death. Patients selected for antitachycardia surgery showed a significantly reduced rate of recurrences of VT and sudden death, but a high perioperative mortality.[44,45]

Guidelines for ICD implantation usually classify the indications in three categories: those on which general agreement exists (indication accepted: Table 3); those frequently used, but where there is no consensus with the respect to the necessity of ICD implantation (possible indications: Table 4); or indication not justified (Table 5). Prophylactic indications are not covered by the current guidelines.

All patients considered for ICD implantation should have experienced at least a single episode of a spontaneous, nonhemodynamically or not well-tolerated VT. In patients with a cardiac arrest without documentation of the rhythm before defibrillation leading to restoration of circulation, a hemody-

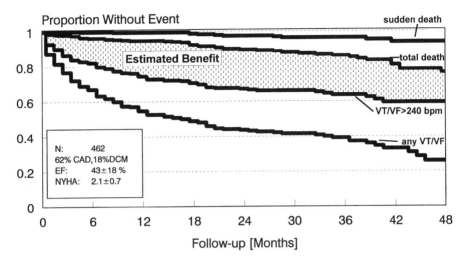

Figure 3. Freedom of sudden death, total death, fast ventricular tachyarrhythmias (> 240 bpm; circles) and any ventricular tachyarrhythmias after implantation of a third generation ICD in combination with transvenous (subcutaneous) defibrillation leads. P value of log rank (Mantel-Cox) test < 0.0001. (Adapted from Böcker et al.[51])

namically nontolerated VT is assumed despite the absence of any documentation. Additionally, an otherwise unexplained syncope in a patient with inducible hemodynamically significant VT is regarded as a possible indication, despite the absence of a documented spontaneous VT. Thus, currently, guidelines recommend that all patients who might receive an ICD should have had at least one episode of a hemodynamically significant VT or an event of circulatory collapse (syncope, cardiac arrest) most probably caused by a VT

Table 3
Accepted Indications for ICD Therapy[35]

• Primary ventricular fibrillation
or
• Ventricular tachycardia that is hemodynamically not tolerable
  and
  • either inducible but not controlled by antiarrhythmic drug therapy
  • or not inducible off-drug and ejection fraction below 40%
  • or VT recurrence during follow-up
    —despite initial suppression of VT by antiarrhythmic drug therapy
    —or non-inducibility in the presence of good left ventricular function

Abbreviations: VT = ventricular tachycardia

Table 4
Possible Indications for ICD Therapy[35]

- VT that is non-inducible off-drug and ejection fraction $\geq$ 40%
- after antitachycardia surgery if VT is still inducible
- not tolerated VT/VF with a potential ischemic cause that cannot be reliably treated
  or
  arrhythmia still inducible after revascularization
- well tolerated VT, reliably terminated by antitachycardia pacing
- syncope with VT/VF as a potential cause
  if monomorphic VT is inducible and ventricular dysfunction present

---

Abbreviations: VF = ventricular fibrillation; VT = ventricular tachycardia.

although not documented. Additionally, recurrent hemodynamically toler-ated VT which can be terminated reliably by antitachycardia pacing, has be-come another possible indication for ICD implantation in the revised version of the guidelines of the German Cardiac Society.

Current guidelines require prerequisites before resuming ICD implanta-tion. The VT should not have occurred during the first 48 hours of an acute myocardial infarction and has no remediable cause of the VT. However, fu-ture prevention of VT should be safe (e.g., quinidine caused torsades de pointes tachycardia),[46] and not rely on causes which most likely have only functioned as a trigger mechanism in the presence of an arrhythmic substrate (e.g., hypokalemia or exacerbation of heart failure in the presence of a severely depressed myocardial function).[47] If the coronary angiogram shows a high grade lesion supplying noninfarcted myocardium, ischemia has to be consid-

Table 5
No Indications for ICD Therapy[35]

- VT/VF during the first 48 hours of acute myocardial infarction
- VT/VF with a remediable cause
  (e.g. drug-induced VT/VF
  or VF in presence of a main stem stenosis and good ventricular function)
- VT which can be cured by map-guided surgery with low risk
  (e.g. monomorphic VT and large anterior wall aneurysm)
- incessant or very frequent VT
- sustained VT without major symptoms that can be controlled by antiarrhythmic drugs
- non-sustained VT
- accelerated idioventricular rhythm
- in the presence of severe concomitant disorders

Abbreviations: VF = ventricular fibrillation; VT = ventricular tachycardia.

ered as a cause of VT. Currently, no study in postinfarct patients showed that revascularization alone could prevent sudden death in comparison to the ICD. However, the rate of VT recurrences has been reduced in patients who have been revascularized.[48,49] An ischemic cause of VT and thus a prevention of VT by revascularization should be assumed if the left ventricular function is normal or near normal, VT is not reproducibly inducible, but polymorphic, and VT is triggered by exercise. However, assuming an ischemic cause of VT in postinfarct patients is due only to the presence of high grade coronary lesions, is unsafe.[50]

A further prerequisite before resuming ICD implantation, is that any other treatment modality suppressing or curing the VT should not be applicable. Current policy of most guidelines is to require that the VT is refractory to drugs, with the only exception being the patient in whom VT is noninducible, and in whom no serial electrophysiological drug testing can be performed. This also applies if there is only a low frequency of nonsustained VTs during monitoring which cannot be used to predict drug responses. Drug refractoriness is defined as a spontaneous recurrence of the VT, persistent inducibility during electrophysiological studies, or nontolerated side effects on oral antiarrhythmic drug therapy with the appropriate dosage. The revised version of the guidelines of the German Cardiac Society requires the test of class III antiarrhythmic drugs before drug refractoriness can be declared. However, patients with a low left ventricular ejection fraction ($\leq 40\%$) might receive an ICD without drug refractoriness.[35]

Recent Results of ICD Treatment

The information on the rate and type of tachycardia causing ICD shocks as stored in present generation devices can be used to assess the frequency of otherwise life-threatening arrhythmic events. Böcker et al used this information of 462 patients (62% with coronary artery disease) to calculate the projected survival by assuming that every VT with a rate > 240 beats per minute would cause sudden cardiac death, if not terminated by the device[51] (Figure 3). Due to the occurrence of fast VT, the projected survival after 4 years was 58%, significantly lower than the actual mortality of 76%. The sudden death rate at 1 year was 6%. This suggests that the ICD is life-saving in patients with accepted or possible indications for ICD implantation. Most of the patients received no antiarrhythmic drugs. Subsequently, a subgroup of 50 patients with coronary artery disease who received an ICD capable of antitachycardia pacing because of hemodynamically tolerated VT, was analyzed in the same way.[52] None of the patients had a history of syncope, cardiac arrest, or nonsustained VT. Nevertheless, one-fifth of all patients experienced a fast VT (> 240 bpm) during a follow-up of an average of 17 months; and at 1 year the difference between projected and total mortality was 12%. This suggests that even patients presenting with hemodynamically tolerated VT may not only benefit from antitachycardia pacing, but they may also need cardioversion defibrillation, because despite a history of hitherto stable VT, fast, and thus, life-threatening VT may occur during longer follow-up.

The influence of the ICD on the long-term prognosis of survivors of out-of-hospital cardiac arrest has been retrospectively analyzed by Powell et al.[53] The majority (72%) of these patients had coronary artery disease. An ICD was implanted if serial drug testing based on electrophysiological studies could not suppress, slow down, or render the arrhythmia to be more difficult to induce. The cardiac mortality rate in patients with an ICD was lower than in patients without an ICD: by 2% at 1 year; 8% at 5 years, for patients with preserved left ventricular function (ejection fraction $\geq$ 40%); 12% at 1 year; and 24% at 5 years, in patients with reduced left ventricular function (ejection fraction < 40%). This reduced cardiac mortality rate in patients with an ICD was observed despite the fact that the clinical characteristics showed that patients receiving an ICD were "more ill" (lower left ventricular ejection fraction, higher pulmonary capillary wedge pressure), and would thus have been expected to have a higher cardiac mortality rate than the remaining patients. Interpretation of these data should be done with caution, because the patients were not randomized, and were retrieved from two institutions, of whom one was only contributing ICD recipients. This study supports the "possible" indication of the revised guidelines for ICD implantations of the German Cardiac Society, allowing ICD implantations without drug refractoriness in patients with a reduced left ventricular ejection fraction. Another similar retrospective analysis of 282 patients with coronary artery disease found a nonsignificant 8% improved survival with the ICD at 1 year, and 6% at 3 years.[54] This study did not analyze the influence of left ventricular ejection fraction on improvement in survival by the ICD. The only randomized study comparing ICD therapy to other treatment modalities presently available is the Cardiac Arrest Study Hamburg (CASH). The treatment arm of propafenone was terminated prematurely due to higher mortalities in comparison to ICDs, empiric amiodarone, or empiric beta-blocker therapy.[55] In addition, a randomized comparison of empiric amiodarone to therapy with class I drugs, guided by Holter monitoring, or electrophysiological studies, had shown that amiodarone is superior to class I antiarrhythmic drugs.[56] Another retrospective study used a case-control design and compared ICD recipients with those treated with amiodarone.[57] Seventy-eight percent of the patients had coronary artery disease, and 12% had dilated cardiomyopathy. Survival in ICD recipients was better by 17% after 1 year, and 16% after 3 years. Retrospectively, the ESVEM study has suggested that sotalol might be superior to class I antiarrhythmic drugs in patients who had both inducible VT and frequent ventricular arrhythmias.[58] Another retrospectively matched case-control study has compared ICD recipients and patients treated with sotalol who showed a complete suppression of VTs on sotalol during electrophysiological testing.[59] Survival in ICD recipients was higher than for patients treated with sotalol; 25% higher at 1 year and 15% at 3 years.

Thus, these studies suggest that ICD therapy may be superior to treatment with class I and III antiarrhythmic drugs, and may question whether drug refractoriness should be considered as a prerequisite before ICD implantation. A prospective randomized study in postinfarct sudden cardiac death survivors, compared the ICD as first-choice therapy with a conventional strategy that included serial drug testing, catheter ablation, or map-guided surgery.[3] The authors concluded that ICD implantation should be used as first choice as conventionally treated patients are likely to end up with an ICD or have a high risk of death, regardless of efficacy assessment, including electrophysiological studies.

As the vast majority of malignant VTs occur in patients with a low ejection fraction, owing to coronary artery disease, the studies on ICDs quoted above are reflecting this special disease state.[51,53,55-57] Some of the studies have even been restricted to patients with coronary artery disease.[3,52,54,59] Information on clinical results of ICD patients with dilated cardiomyopathy, the second largest group of patients presenting with malignant VT, is limited. Grimm and Marchlinski analyzed the shock occurrence and survival in 49 patients with dilated cardiomyopathy.[60] Total mortality was 14%, 39%, and 49% during 1, 3 and 5 years of follow-up, respectively, while the incidence of appropriate shocks was 16%, 49%, and 72% at 1, 3 and 5 years respectively, suggesting a survival benefit by the ICD. Chen et al retrospectively compared 70 patients with dilated cardiomyopathy treated without an ICD with 32 patients who received an ICD.[61] At 1 year, patients without an ICD showed a 9% higher sudden death rate than patients with an ICD. Thus, benefit of ICD therapy seems to also exist in patients with dilated cardiomyopathy.

For other types of heart disease (arrhythmogenic right ventricular cardiomyopathy, hypertrophic cardiomyopathy, postoperative congenital heart disease, acquired valve disease, and primary electrical disease) that also cause VT, only preliminary data with a small number of implantations are available. Due to their preserved left ventricular function, the medium-term mortality of these patients is overwhelmingly caused by sudden death.[32] Multicenter data collection and longer follow-up has to be awaited to define the role of ICD in these rare indications of ICD implantation.

As an alternative to ICDs, catheter ablation can be used in selected patients. Preliminary results indicate that for certain VTs and underlying cardiac disorders, VT recurrences are rare after catheter ablation.[62,63] However, studies proving prevention of sudden deaths during long-term follow-up have not been published yet. Current guidelines consider catheter ablation for treatment of hemodynamically tolerated VT which can be localized by mapping.[33] As a treatment of first choice, catheter ablation should be used in patients with incessant VT, bundle branch reentry VT, or idiopathic VT.

Future Indications

Ongoing Studies Comparing ICD Therapy and Other Antiarrhythmic Therapies

Many reports have questioned the benefit from ICDs in comparison to other antiarrhythmic treatment modalities, and requested the randomization of the best medical management against the ICD.[64–67] Three large trials are in progress: (1) the CASH[55], comparing ICD therapy to empiric therapy with beta-blocking agents; empiric therapy with propafenone; and empiric therapy with amiodarone; (2) the Canadian Implantable Defibrillator Study (CIDS[68]), comparing ICD therapy to empiric amiodarone; and (3) the Antiarrhythmic Versus Implantable Defibrillators (AVID[69]) study, comparing ICD therapy to empiric amiodarone or guided sotalol. These studies might restrict the ICD to patients who are not suppressed on sotalol (AVID) or have recurrences on class III antiarrhythmic drugs (CASH, CIDS, AVID), or metoprolol (CASH), or might establish the ICD as the first choice therapy for cardiac arrest survivors. Prospective studies comparing ICD therapy to catheter ablation or map-guided antitachycardia surgery in candidates for these alternative interventional antiarrhythmic therapies have not been initiated.

Ongoing Studies on Prophylactic ICD Indications

Several prospective randomized studies have been started to evaluate the role of ICDs in patients who have not experienced a sustained VT, such as syncope or cardiac arrest, but are considered to be at a high risk for a cardiac arrest. These studies differ with respect to the underlying cardiac disease and the risk predictors for sudden death. The CABG Patch study compares ICD therapy to nonantiarrhythmic therapy in patients in whom coronary artery bypass surgery is performed, and who have a low ejection fraction ($\leq 35\%$) and positive late potentials.[70] The enrollment of 900 patients was finished in January 1996. The Cardiomyopathy Trial (CAT) originally termed the German Dilated Cardiomyopathy Study compares ICD therapy to nonantiarrhythmic therapy in patients with a recent onset of dilated cardiomyopathy who have an ejection fraction below 30%.[71] The enrollment of 100 patients in the pilot study was finished in 1995. The Multicenter Automatic Defibrillator

Implantation Trial (MADIT) compares ICD therapy to nonantiarrhythmic treatment in patients with coronary artery disease, low ejection fraction ($\leq$ 35%), spontaneous nonsustained VTs, and inducible-nonsuppressible VTs.[72] Enrollment has not been finished in 1995. Further studies evaluating the role of prophylactic ICDs in high-risk patients awaiting heart transplantation, and after an acute infarction will be initiated based on pilot studies.

References

1. Mirowski M, Reid PR, Mower MM, et al. Termination of malignant ventricular arrhythmias with an implanted automatic defibrillator in human beings. *N Engl J Med* 1980;303:322–324.
2. Schöhl W, Trappe H, Lichtlen P. Acceptance and quality of life after implantation of the automatic cardioverter defibrillator. *Z Kardiol* 1994;83:927–932.
3. Wever EFD, Hauer RNW, van Capelle FJL, et al. Randomized study of implantable defibrillator as first-choice therapy versus conventional strategy in postinfarct sudden death survivors. *Circulation* 1995;91:2195–2203.
4. Reid PR, Mirowski M, Mower MM, et al. Clinical evaluation of the internal automatic cardioverter-defibrillator in survivors of sudden cardiac death. *Am J Cardiol* 1983;51:1608–1613.
5. McVeigh K, Mower MM, Nisam S, Voshage L. Clinical efficacy of low energy cardioversion in automatic implantable cardioverter/defibrillator patients. *PACE* 1991;14:1846–1849.
6. Fromer M, Brachmann J, Block M, et al. Efficacy of automatic multimodal device therapy for ventricular tachyarrhythmias as delivered by a new implantable pacing cardioverter-defibrillator. *Circulation* 1992;86:363–374.
7. Saoudi N, Henry C, Nitzsche R, et al. Accuracy of rapid automatic arrhythmias identification using atrioventricular interval analysis during induced tachycardias. *PACE* 1995;18(Pt II):901 (Abstract).
8. Watkins L, Mirowski M, Mower MM, et al. Implantation of the automatic defibrillator: the subxiphoid approach. *Ann Thorac Surg* 1982;34:515–520.
9. Saksena S, Parsonnet V. Implantation of a cardioverter/defibrillator without thoracotomy using a triple electrode system. JAMA 1988;259:69–72.
10. Neuzner J, for the European Ventak P2 Investigator Group. Clinical experience with a new cardioverter/defibrillator capable of biphasic waveform pulse and enhanced data storage: results of a prospective multicenter study. *PACE* 1994;17: 1243–1255.
11. Hammel D, Block M, Geiger A, et al. Single-incision implantation of cardioverter-defibrillators using nonthoracotomy lead systems. *Ann Thorac Surg* 1994;58: 1614–1616.
12. Block M, Breithardt G. Long-term follow-up and clinical results of implantable cardioverter-defibrillators. In: Zipes DP, Jalife J (eds): *Cardiac Electrophysiology: From Cell to Bedside.* Philadelphia: WB Saunders Company, 1995, pp 1412–1425.
13. Zipes DP, Roberts D, for the Pacemaker-Cardioverter-Defibrillator Investigators. Results of the international study of the implantable pacemaker cardioverter-defibrillator. *Circulation* 1995;92:59–65.
14. Kleman JM, Castle LW, Kidwell GA, et al. Nonthoracotomy-versus thoracotomy-implantable defibrillators: Intention-to-treat comparison of clinical outcomes. *Circulation* 1994;90:2833–2842.

15. Luceri RM, Zilo P, Habal SM, David IB. Cost and length of stay: comparisons between nonthoracotomy and epicardial techniques in patients receiving implantable cardioverter/defibrillators. *PACE* 1995;18:168–171.

16. Wietholt D, Block M, Isbruch F, et al. Clinical experience with antitachycardia pacing and improved detection algorithms in a new implantable cardioverter/defibrillator. *J Am Coll Cardiol* 1993;21:885–894.

17. Bardy GH, Dolack GL, Kudenchuk PJ, et al. Prospective comparison in humans of a unipolar defibrillation system with that using an additional superior vena cava electrode. *Circulation* 1994;89:1090–1093.

18. Strickberger SA, Hummel JD, Daoud E, et al. Implantation by electrophysiologists of 100 consecutive cardioverter/defibrillators with nonthoracotomy lead systems. *Circulation* 1994;90:868–872.

19. Tung RT, Bajaj AK. Safety of implantation of a cardioverter-defibrillator without general anesthesia in an electrophysiology laboratory. *Am J Cardiol* 1995;75: 908–912.

20. Block M, Hammel D, Bänsch D, et al. Prevention of ICD complications. In: Allessie M, Fromer M (eds). *Atrial and Ventricular Fibrillation—Mechanisms and Device Therapy.* Armonk, New York: Futura Publishing Company, 1995.

21. Böcker D, Block M, Hammel D, et al. Re-operations after implantation of automatic defibrillators with endocardial leads: long-term results in 348 patients. *Eur Heart J* 1995;16(Suppl):262 (Abstract).

22. Morris PL, Badger J, Chmielewski C, et al. Psychiatric morbidity following implantation of the automatic implantable cardioverter/defibrillator. *Psychosomatics* 1991;31:58–64.

23. Pinski SL, Fahy GJ. The proarrhythmic potential of implantable cardioverter-defibrillators. *Circulation* 1995;92:1651–1664.

24. Weber M, Block M, Brunn J, et al. Proarrhythmic effects of inappropriate implantable cardioverter/defibrillator therapies: incidence, causes and prevention . *Eur Heart J* 1995;16(Suppl):221 (Abstract).

25. Block M, Breithardt G. Implantable cardioverter defibrillator technology in the next ten years: what can be expected? In: Raviele A (ed). *Cardiac Arrhythmias 1995.* Milano: Springer, 1995, pp 91–95.

26. Kupperman M, Luce BR, McGovern B, et al. An analysis of the cost-effectiveness of the implantable defibrillator. *Circulation* 1990;81:91–100.

27. Dreifus LS, Gillette PC, Fisch C, et al. Guidelines for implantation of cardiac pacemakers and antiarrhythmic devices. A report of the American College of Cardiology /American Heart Association Task Force on assessment of diagnostic and therapeutic cardiovascular procedures (Committee on Pacemaker Implantation). *J Am Coll Cardiol* 1991;18:1–13.

28. Lehman MH, Saksena S. Implantable cardioverter/defibrillators on cardiovascular practice: report of the policy conference of the North American Society of Pacing and Electrophysiology. *PACE* 1991;14:969–979.

29. Steinbeck G, Meinertz T, Andresen D, et al. Empfehlungen zur Implantation von Defibrillatoren der Kommission für Klinische Kardiologie unter Mitwirkung der Arbeitsgruppe "Interventionelle Elektrophysiologie" der Deutschen Gesellschaft für Herz- und Kreislaufforschung. *Z Kardiol* 1991;80:475–478.

30. Crijns HJ, Hauer RNW, Kingma JH, Smeets JL. Cardiological guidelines. Cardioverter/defibrillator implantation. *Neth J Cardiol* 1991;4:234–235.

31. Raviele A, Bellocci F, Capucci A, et al. Guidelines for the use of implantable

defibrillators. Italian Group of Arrhythmology. Italian Association of Cardiac Pacing Task Force. *New Trends Arrhythm* 1992;8:555–567.

32. Breithardt G, Camm AJ, Campbell RWF, et al. Guidelines for the use of implantable cardioverter/defibrillators. *Eur Heart J* 1992;13:1304–1310.

33. American College of Cardiology/American Heart Association Task Force on Practice Guidelines (Committee on Clinical Intracardiac Electrophysiologic and Catheter Ablation Procedures) in collaboration with the North American Society of Pacing and Electrophysiolgy. Guidelines for clinical intracardiac electrophysiological and catheter ablation procedures. *J Am Coll Cardiol* 1995;26:555–573.

34. Mason JW, for the ESVEM Investigators. A comparison of electrophysiologic testing with Holter monitoring to predict antiarrhythmic-drug efficacy. N Engl Med 1993;329:445–451.

35. Andresen D, Block M, Borggrefe M, et al. Empfehlungen zur Implantation von Defibrillatoren der Kommission für Klinische Kardiologie unter Mitwirkung der Arbeitsgruppe "Interventionelle Elektrophysiologie" der Deutschen Gesellschaft für Herz- und Kreislaufforschung. *Z Kardiol* 1993;82:242–246.

36. Cobb LA, Baum RS, Alvarez H III, et al. Resuscitation from out-of-hospital ventricular fibrillation: 4 years follow-up. *Circulation* 1975;52(Suppl III):223–229.

37. Mirowski M, Reid PE, Winkle RA, et al. Mortality in patients with implanted automatic defibrillators. *Ann Intern Med* 1983;98:585–588.

38. Winkle RA, Mead RH, Ruder MA, et al. Long-term outcome with the automatic implantable cardioverter-defibrillator. *J Am Coll Cardiol* 1989;13:1353–1361.

39. Lown B, Graboys TB. Management of patients with malignant ventricular arrhythmias. *Am J Cardiol* 1977;39:910–918.

40. Graboys TB, Lown B, Podrid J, et al. Long-term survival of patients with malignant ventricular arrhythmia treated with antiarrhythmic drugs. *Am J Cardiol* 1982; 50:437–443.

41. Hohnloser SH, Raeder EA, Podrid PJ, et al. Predictors of antiarrhythmic drug efficacy in patients with malignant ventricular tachyarrhythmias. *Am Heart J* 1987; 114:1–7.

42. Mitchell LB, Duff HJ, Manyari DE, et al. A randomized clinical trial of the noninvasive and invasive approaches to drug therapy of ventricular tachycardias. *N Engl J Med* 1987;317:1681–1687.

43. Wilber DJ, Garan H, Finkelstein D, et al. Use of electrophysiologic testing in the prediction of long-term outcome. *N Engl J Med* 1988;318:19–24.

44. Borggrefe M, Podczeck A, Ostermeyer J, Breithardt G, and the Surgical Ablation Registry. Long-term results of electrophysiologically guided antitachycardia surgery in ventricular tachyarrhythmias: a collaborative report on 665 patients. In: Breithardt G, Borggrefe M, Zipes DP (eds). *Nonpharmacological Therapy of Tachyarrhythmias*. Mount Kisco: Futura Publishing Company, 1987, pp 109–132.

45. Ostermeyer J, Borggrefe M, Breithardt G, et al. Direct operations for the management of life threatening ischemic ventricular tachycardia. *J Thorac Cardiovasc Surg* 1987;6:848–865.

46. Haverkamp W, Shenasa M, Borggrefe M, Breithardt G. Torsades de Pointes. In: Zipes DP, Jalife J (eds). *Cardiac Electrophysiology: From Cell to Bedside*. Philadelphia: WB Saunders Company, pp 885–899.

47. Stevenson WG, Middlekauf HR, Stevenson LW, et al. Significance of aborted cardiac arrest and sustained ventricular tachycardia in patients referred for treatment therapy of advanced heart failure. *Am Heart J* 1992;124:123–130.

48. Autschbach R, Falk V, Gonska BD, Dalichau H. The effect of coronary bypass

graft surgery for the prevention of sudden cardiac death: recurrent episodes after ICD implantation and review of literature. *PACE* 1994;17:552–558.

49. Wiesfeld ACP, Crijns HJGM, Hillege HL, et al. The clinical significance of coronary anatomy in post-infarct patients with late sustained ventricular tachycardia or ventricular fibrillation. *Eur Heart J* 1995;16:818–824.

50. Natale A, Sra J, Axtell K, et al. Ventricular fibrillation and polymorphic tachycardia with critical coronary artery stenosis: does bypass surgery suffice? *J Cardiovasc Electrophysiol* 1994;12:988–998.

51. Böcker D, Block M, Isbruch F, et al. Do patients with an implantable defibrillator live longer? *J Am Coll Cardiol* 1993;21:1638–1648.

52. Böcker D, Block M, Isbruch F, et al. Benefits of treatment with implantable cardioverter-defibrillators in patients with stable ventricular tachycardia without cardiac arrest. *Br Heart J* 1995;73:158–163.

53. Powell AC, Fuchs T, Finkelstein DM, et al. Influence of implantable cardioverter-defibrillators on the long-term prognosis of survivors of out-of-hospital cardiac arrest. *Circulation* 1993;88:1083–1092.

54. Choue CW, Kim SG, Fisher JD, et al. Comparison of defibrillator therapy and other therapeutic modalities for sustained ventricular tachycardia or fibrillation associated with coronary artery disease. *Am J Cardiol* 1994;73:1075–1079.

55. Siebels J, Kuck KH. Implantable cardioverter/defibrillator compared with antiarrhythmic drug treatment in cardiac arrest survivors (the Cardiac Arrest Study Hamburg). Am Heart J 1994;127:1139–1144.

56. The CASCADE Investigators. Randomized antiarrhythmic drug therapy in survivors of cardiac arrest (the CASCADE Study). *Am J Cardiol* 1993;72:280–287.

57. Newman D, Sauve MJ, Herre J, et al. Survival after implantation of the cardioverter defibrillator. *Am J Cardiol* 1992;69:899–903.

58. Mason JW, for the ESVEM Investigators. A comparison of seven antiarrhythmic drugs in patients with ventricular tachyarrhythmias. *N Engl Med* 1993;329:452–458.

59. Böcker D, Haverkamp W, Block M, et al. Comparison of d,l-sotalol and implantable defibrillators for treatment of sustained ventricular tachycardia or fibrillation in patients with coronary artery disease. *Circulation* 1996 (In press).

60. Grimm W, Marchlinksi FE. Shock occurrence and survival in 49 patients with idiopathic dilated cardiomyopathy and an implantable cardioverter-defibrillator. *Eur Heart J* 1995;16:218–222.

61. Chen X, Shenasa M, Borggrefe M, et al. Role of programmed ventricular stimulation in patients with idiopathic dilated cardiomyopathy and documented sustained ventricular tachyarrhythmias: inducibility and prognostic value in 102 patients. *Eur Heart J* 1994;15:76–82.

62. Haverkamp W, Chen X, Kottkamp H, et al. Radiofrequency-current catheter ablation of ventricular tachycardia. *Z Kardiol* 1995;84(Suppl 2):83–102.

63. Gonska BD, Cao K, Schaumann A, et al. Catheter ablation of ventricular tachycardia in 136 patients with coronary artery disease: results and long-term follow-up. *J Am Coll Cardiol* 1994;24:1506–1514.

64. Connolly SJ, Yusuf S. Evaluation of the implantable cardioverter/defibrillator in survivors of cardiac arrest: the need for randomized trials. *Am J Cardiol* 1992;69:959–962.

65. Epstein AE. AVID necessity. *PACE* 1993;16:1773–1775.

66. Green HL. Antiarrhythmic drugs versus implantable defibrillators: the need for a randomized controlled study. *Am Heart J* 1994;127:1171–1178.

67. Zipes DP. Implantable cardioverter-defibrillator: lifesaver or a device looking for a disease? *Circulation* 1994;89:2934–2936.
68. Conolly SJ, Jent M, Roberts RS, et al. Canadian Implantable Defibrillator Study (CIDS): study design and organization. *Am J Cardiol* 1993;72:103F-108F.
69. Hallstrom AP, Greene HL, Wyse DG, et al. Antiarrhythmics versus implantable defibrillators (AVID)—rationale, design, and methods. *Am J Cardiol* 1995;75: 470–475.
70. The CABG Patch Trial Investigators and Coordinators. The coronary artery bypass graft (CABG) patch trial. *Progr Cardiovascular Dis* 1993,36:97–114.
71. The German Dilated Cardiomyopathy Study Investigators. Prospective studies assessing prophylactic therapy in high risk patients: The German Dilated Cardio-Myopathy Study (GDCMS)-study design. *PACE* 1992;15:697–700.
72. MADIT Executive Committee. Multicenter automatic defibrillator implantation trial (MADIT): design and clinical proposal. *PACE* 1991;14:920–927.

Chapter 20

New Generations of Implantable Pacemaker Defibrillators for Ventricular and Atrial Tachyarrhythmias

Sanjeev Saksena, MD, FACC,
Atul Prakash, MD, MRCP,
Nandini Madan, MBBS, MD,
Irakli Giorgberidze, MD, Anand N. Munsif, MD,
Philip Mathew, MS, Ryszard B. Krol, MD

Introduction

Implantable defibrillation devices have now been extensively applied to patients requiring cardioversion and defibrillation of sustained ventricular arrhythmias. Technology for these devices is in its fourth generation of development.[1] The current device is a hybrid pacemaker defibrillator capable of bradycardia and antitachycardia pacing, low and high energy cardioversion, and defibrillation, all of which are performed in the ventricle. Future development of this device is focused along the lines of increasing technological versatility, improving physiological performance, and finding new patient populations that may benefit from its application.

New Technology

The focus of new developments in technology has been on improving lead systems and their performance, reducing defibrillator generator size and output, and achieving physiological operation in both the atrium and ventricle. Lead-related complications constitute the major morbidity after implantable cardioverter defibrillator (ICD) insertion.[2] In a recent multicenter study,

From *Practical Management of Cardiac Arrhythmias* edited by Nabil El-Sherif, and Jean Lekieffre. Futura Publishing Co., Armonk, NY, © 1997.

Fourth Generation ICD System

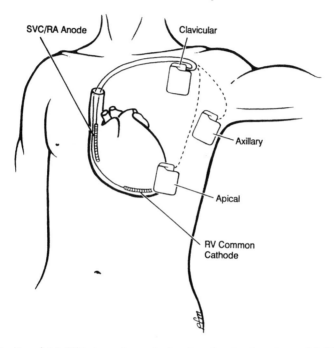

Figure 1. Panel 1A. This is a schematic drawing showing locations of defibrillation electrodes, with a fourth generation implantable cardioverter defibrillator system. Electrodes are located at the right ventricular apex, superior vena cava /right atrium, and axilla. The generator can also be used as an electrode in the locations as shown with the left pectoral site being preferred.

these occurred in 10.9% of patients and lead dislodgment was by far the most common complication. In an effort to address this and simplify the insertion procedure, a single lead system with an active can electrode has been developed by several manufacturers. Figure 1A is a schematic of such a system in situ. Insertion of the single lead with a cephalic vein access and proper attention to suturing and active fixation have been emphasized to minimize the problems with lead function. With an active can system, the left pectoral location has been preferred. A recent study from our center confirmed the efficacy of several left thoracic electrode locations in defibrillation.[3] Thus, an axillary or apical location as well as pectoral sites can be considered. Retro-mammary implants or submammary locations for an active can system are thus feasible. In patients with left-sided access or pectoral site difficulties, right pectoral locations can be employed. Figure 1B shows mean defibrillation

JOULES

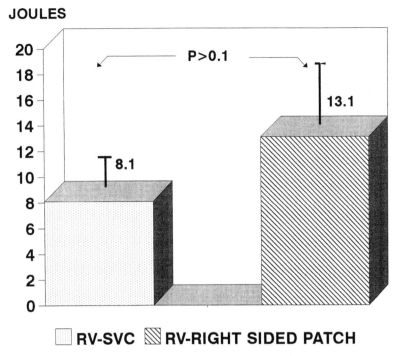

☐ **RV-SVC** ☒ **RV-RIGHT SIDED PATCH**

Figure 1. *(continued)* **Panel 1B.** Comparison of the mean defibrillation thresholds using the RV cathode to SVC anode and the RV cathode to a right-sided patch (simulating active can). Note that the difference was not statistically significant. ICD = implantable cardioverter defibrillator; RA = right atrium; RV = right ventricle; SCV = superior vena cava.

thresholds (DFTs) with a right ventricular (RV) cathode and a right-sided pectoral patch (to simulate an active can) compared to the standard alternative, the RV to superior vena cava (SVC) dual-electrode configuration. These thresholds are well within the capability of a 25 to 35-Joule ICD generator in the vast majority of patients.

However, active can unipolar systems are not invariably effective in achieving transvenous implants. DFTs with the RV to can configurations do not permit transvenous implants in 5% to 10% of patients receiving Medtronic® 7219C devices (Rochester, MN, USA). Other lead configurations may be employed in newer more flexible models such as the Medtronic® 7219SP18, the Angeion Sentinel 2000 or the CPI Mini. These devices permit use of both transvenous leads, active can electrode, and left thoracic electrodes (either an array or a patch lead). This flexibility results in multiple lead configuration

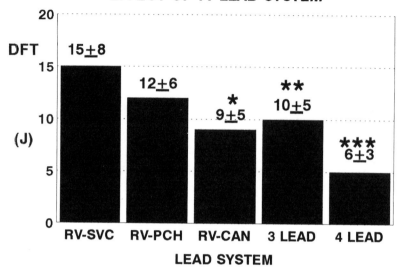

Figure 2. Defibrillation thresholds with a variety of lead systems are depicted. Note that the lowest defibrillation threshold was seen for the quadruple electrode array using the Right ventricle-superior vena cava + patch + can. PC = patch; RA = right atrium; RV = right ventricle; SVC = superior vena cava.

options. In an effort to clarify the relative benefits of each option, we recently studied biphasic shock DFTs with five different lead configurations.[4] In this study, we evaluated three dual-electrode configurations (RV-can, RV-axillary patch, and RV-SVC), one triple lead system (RV-SVC + patch), and one quadruple lead array (RV-SVC + patch + can). In all these systems, the RV electrode was a cathode and asymmetric biphasic shocks were used with a 65% tilt, 120 microfarad capacitors, with the trailing edge voltage of the first phase equaling the leading edge voltage of the second phase. Mean defibrillation energy was lowest for the quadruple electrode array at 5.7 Joules, with the RV-can system coming in next at 9.2 Joules (Figure 2). The triple lead system was comparable to the RV-can system with the highest DFTs being seen with the RV-SVC configuration. In contrast, current thresholds were lowest for the RV-can configuration suggesting greatest efficiency for this approach. This finding was explainable based on a 50% difference in impedance between the two most efficient configurations. The mean impedance in the unipolar system was 68 ohms, while it was 41 ohms for the array. These findings result in a family of defibrillation efficacy curves. As can be seen in the figure, 50% and 80% of the population are defibrillated at varying energies, depending on the lead system. The implications of these findings bear on lowering the maximum output of ICD generators. Lower output devices can decrease size. However, to preserve a sufficient safety margin, for example 10 Joules , maximum outputs of 25 to 30 Joules will be needed for unipolar systems, while 20 Joules would suffice for quadruple lead arrays in > 90% of patients. Thus, in clinical practice lower output ICDs such as the Sentinel would utilize the option of adding leads to a dual-electrode system in selected patients to avoid thoracotomy or to increase defibrillation safety margins.

While lower output ICDs are being evaluated to reduce generator size, other approaches such as new capacitor technologies or a smaller capacitance have been pursued. The former is still to be clinically applied. The latter has been and shows potential for some modest decreases in defibrillation energy.[5] Examination of the effect of generator volume on DFT shows only a modest effect. In fact, reduction in can size to as little as 15 cc may be tolerable for defibrillation in animals.[6]

Physiological Performance

The newest generation of ICD technology under investigation (the fifth generation) also includes the capability of dual-chamber sensing and pacing. The benefits of dual-chamber ICD systems are outlined in Table 1. In view of the well-known coexistence of moderate and severe left ventricular dysfunction in ICD patients, the availability of atrial pacing could benefit hemodynamics and survival.[7] Benefits of programming different atrioventricular delays could thus be studied. Recent studies on the sensing capabilities of such

Table 1
Benefits of Dual-Chamber ICD Systems

1. Electrical
   —Permits atrial or atrioventricular pacing without the need for another pulse generator or other leads
   —Can improve discrimination between supraventricular and ventricular tachyarrhythmias
   —Reduces pacemaker-ICD interactions that could have potential for proarrhythmic effects
   —Could prevent atrial fibrillation by atrial pacing
   —Atrial or dual-chamber defibrillation may be considered in the future
2. Hemodynamic
   —Atrioventricular pacing may improve hemodynamics in patients with compromised left ventricular function

systems have measured the sensitivity and specificity of ventricular tachycardia (VT) ventricular fibrillation detection algorithms in such systems. DiCarlo et al examined a contextual analysis of atrial and ventricular electrograms.[8] Timing intervals of two successive cycles were identified and classified. In a second analysis, this was compared to six preceding cycles. The accuracy of this method was 99.2% for supraventricular and ventricular arrhythmia diagnosis. A simpler analysis that used only rate and timing of atrial and ventricular electrograms was also highly successful. However, atrial rate, behavior at arrhythmia onset, and loss of atrioventricular activation snapshots alone are inadequate and result in periodic misdiagnosis of these arrhythmias. Sensing atrial electrograms consistently present challenges. In single wavefront reentrant arrhythmias such as junctional tachycardias or type 1 atrial flutter, the atrial electrogram may have an equivalent or somewhat lower amplitude than sinus rhythm, but it generally exceeds 0.5 mV. However, in atrial fibrillation, electrograms with amplitudes < 1 mV are common. Sensing thresholds in automatic gain control devices may vary between 0.15 to 0.2mV and these would in general be adequate for amplitude detection. However, slew rates may also decrease greatly and further impede detection. Nevertheless, dual-chamber sensing and pacing is an inevitable development and may, in fact, soon become the standard device.

New Patient Populations

Ongoing clinical trials and feasibility studies are enrolling new patient populations for ICD therapy. Two major groups are high-risk patients for sudden cardiac death with structural heart disease, and patients with refractory atrial fibrillation. In the MADIT (Multicenter Automatic Defibrillator Implantation Trial) study, coronary heart disease patients with nonsustained VT are randomized to drug or ICD therapy.[9] We have been risk stratifying patients with nonsustained VT at our center using noninvasive and invasive methods including electrophysiological testing for over 5 years. In our experience, with 72 patients with nonsustained VT and coronary disease, 25 patients (35%) had inducible sustained VT. These patients were then treated with drugs (types 1, 2 or 3) or implantable defibrillators. Their long-term outcome shows 20% mortality at 2 years. Another patient population under study includes high-risk individuals with dilated cardiomyopathy. Two trials in progress or in development examine the role of these devices in the prevention of sudden death and the improvement on the survival of these patients. In the German dilated cardiomyopathy trial and the SCD-HeFT trial, a randomized comparison of device and drug therapy is planned.[10] End-points in these trials are total mortality.

Atrial fibrillation constitutes the largest new population segment under study. The feasibility of atrial defibrillation has long been demonstrated but

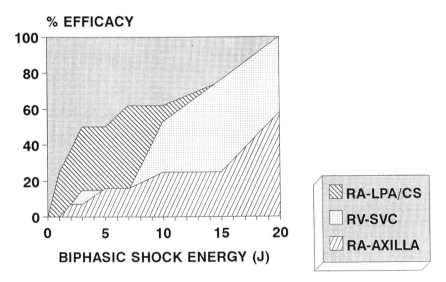

Figure 3. This shows a percent efficacy curve for each lead configuration used for internal atrial defibrillation. At 5 Joules, the right atrium to coronary sinus (CS)/left pulmonary artery (LPA) had higher efficacy whereas at energies > 10 Joules there was no significant difference. CS = coronary sinus; LPA = left pulmonary artery; RA = right atrium; RV = right ventricle; SVC = superior vena cava.

systematic studies of optimal methods are lacking. In one uncontrolled series, a right atrial to coronary sinus (CS) electrode configuration achieved biphasic DFTs of 6.7 Joules for induced atrial fibrillation.[11] We recently completed a prospective randomized comparison of atrial DFTs with several different lead systems.[12] Figure 3 shows a percent efficacy curve for three of the four preferred systems. In two of these configurations (right atrium [RA]-coronary sinus [CS]/left pulmonary artery or RV-SVC), all patients could be defibrillated at 20 Joules but mean DFTs varied from 8 to11Joules. While there was no significant difference at > 10 Joules, the RA-CS/left pulmonary artery leads had higher efficacy at 5 Joules.[12] However, both systems are well above pain thresholds for endocardial shocks. Thus, at the present time, atrial defibrillation shocks, regardless of lead configuration, are suitable for infrequent application as backup therapy for atrial fibrillation recurrences. Prevention of atrial fibrillation assumes larger proportions as the mainstay of treatment in this condition. Prevention may be achieved by the treatment of the primary heart disorder if present, antiarrhythmic drug therapy, or pacing devices. Lone atrial fibrillation occurs in 10% to 15% of most representative reports. Thus, the large proportion of atrial fibrillation patients do have a primary disorder requiring therapy. Hypertension, primary myocardial disease, coronary disease, and valvular heart disease usually account for the bulk of these patients. Of these diseases, only hypertension is generally treatable early enough for an attempt to delay the onset of atrial fibrillation. The time course of ischemic or hemodynamic complications of coronary or valvular disease, warranting intervention, frequently permits the substrate for recurrent or chronic atrial fibrillation to develop independently. Thus, treatment as currently undertaken for these complications (revascularization or valvular surgery) frequently fails to prevent atrial fibrillation recurrences.

More recent efforts have focused on pacemaker therapy. Initially performed for primarily bradycardia-dependent atrial fibrillation with good results, more recent data shows positive results in the absence of a primary bradyarrhythmic disorder. In early studies, Attuel et al demonstrated excellent results with the suppression of recurrent atrial fibrillation in vagally mediated arrhythmias.[13] The concept of preexcitation of critical elements of a reentrant circuit to prevent arrhythmia induction or recurrence by simultaneous pacing of two sites was first applied to supraventricular tachycardias, due to atrioventricular nodal and atrioventricular reentry.[14] Subsequently, it was investigated without extensive clinical application in VTs.[15] It has recently been applied to patients with atrial fibrillation.[16,17] Daubert and colleagues[16] have performed biatrial pacing using a high right atrial electrode and a distal or mid-CS electrode in the triggered mode, in patients with advanced intra-atrial conduction defects, often in the setting of hypertrophic cardiomyopathy. In their report, recurrent atrial fibrillation was observed in 8 of 19 patients (42%) at a follow-up period of 21 months. Lead dislodgment with pacing failure was observed with the CS or another lead in six patients. This was often the cause of atrial fibrillation recurrence, and the replacement of the lead was associated with reestablishment of atrial fibrillation suppression. They considered benefits of this pacing modality to be due to reduction in P wave duration and simultaneous activation of both atria, improving atrial hemodynamic performance.

We have developed a novel method of dual-site right atrial pacing using high right atrial and CS ostial electrodes. A wide atrial bipole constituted by the distal high right atrial and coronary ostial electrodes is used with a ventricular lead in the DDDR pacing mode (Figure 4). In this system, continuous atrial pacing is established with a lower rate of 80 to 90 beats per minute, and a rapid rate response with a upper rate as high as 140 or 150 beats per minute. Concomitant antiarrhythmic drug therapy with a previously ineffec-

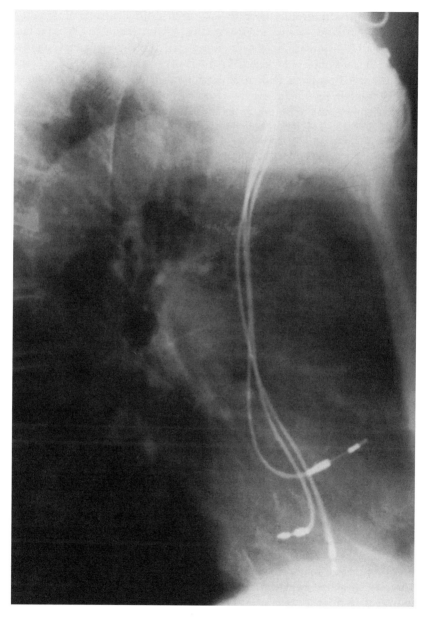

Figure 4. A lateral radiograph of a dual-site pacing system with two atrial leads in situ. The lead in the right atrial appendage is seen pointing superiorly, while a second atrial lead positioned at the coronary sinus ostium is directed posteriorly. The third lead is at the right ventricular apex.

tive agent was continued. In the initial 17 patients with drug refractory paroxysmal atrial fibrillation receiving this pacing system, during the 3-month period prior to the system implant, the mean arrhythmia-free interval on drug therapy alone was 14 + 14 days. The interval from the last atrial fibrillation recurrence to the system implant averaged 5.2 days. In the first 6 months, the arrhythmia-free interval increased to a mean of 89.9 days in the dual-site right atrial mode, and to 71 days in high right atrial pacing alone (p < 0.02). At 1 year, > 80% of all patients are in atrial paced rhythm. Transient recurrences occurred in the dual-site mode when drug therapy was discontinued or reduced but were usually brief, spontaneously terminating, and usually resolved after drug resumption. Only one patient required cardioversion for such a recurrence. Atrial fibrillation recurrences due to drug-related difficulties were most often seen with disopyramide.

Our recent studies have been devoted to elucidating the electrophysiological effects of each atrial pacing mode, as well as relative benefit of dual-site right atrial pacing. We have examined atrial activation using regional atrial mapping at cardiac surgery or catheter endocardial mapping procedures.[18] We examined atrial activation times in four different pacing modes. High right atrial pacing results in relatively late activation (> 130 msec) in the CS, particularly at the distal left atrium. In contrast, coronary ostial pacing activates the left atrium along the sinus within 40 msec, but is markedly delayed in lateral RA or left atrial appendage activation. However, dual-site right atrial pacing activates RA and left atrium excluding the left atrial appendage within 60 to 80 msec. Left atrial appendage activation in this mode may take up to 100 msec. In contrast, biatrial pacing will activate the left atrium and appendage relatively quickly but is delayed in the inferior and lateral RA. Critical to understanding antiarrhythmic effect is the behavior of extrastimuli in these pacing modes. During acute electrophysiological studies, there was no significant difference in effective refractory period of high RA or CS.[19] However, a dual-site drive train suppressed 56% of reproducibly inducible atrial fibrillation elicited using a single site drive. Patients demonstrating atrial fibrillation suppression had a higher dispersion in atrial effective refractory period between the two atrial sites as compared to those who failed to suppress. This may imply that the former group had conditions for reentrant rhythms in proximity to the pacing electrodes or may simply reflect a more generalized dispersion in refractory periods. It raises important questions as to site of arrhythmia initiation (RA or left atrium) versus maintenance. During regional atrial mapping, P wave duration is noted to be abbreviated with both biatrial and dual-site right atrial modes. Finally, initiation of atrial fibrillation is being examined. In some instances, the earliest site of reentrant excitation is located in the CS ostial region with inferior to superior activation of the high right atrium and probable bystander activation of the left atrium.

Conclusions

Progress in ICD technology will further simplify implementation of this therapy. Devices for ventricular application will be increasingly user-friendly, cosmetically desirable, and address quality of life issues for patients. Dual-chamber pacing, sensing, and defibrillation capabilities can be anticipated. Newer patient populations will include selected high-risk patients. Atrial application will be feasible in a patient group with paroxysmal atrial fibrillation when atrial pacing is combined with a higher energy defibrillation unit, capable of both atrial and ventricular defibrillation.

References

1. Saksena S, Krol RB, Kaushik RR. Innovations in pulse generator and lead systems: balancing complexity with clinical benefit and long-term results. *Am Heart J* 1994; 127(Suppl):1010–1021.
2. Saksena S and the PCD Investigator Group: Clinical outcome of patients with malignant ventricular tachyarrhythmias and a multiprogrammable cardioverter-defibrillator implanted with or without thoracotomy: an international multicenter study. *J Am Coll Cardiol* 1994;23:1521–1530.
3. Saksena S, DeGroot P, Krol RB, Raju R, Mathew P, Mehra R. Low-energy endocardial defibrillation using an axillary or a pectoral thoracic electrode location. *Circulation* 1993;88:2655–2660.
4. Saksena S, Krol R, Kaushik R, et al. Endocardial defibrillation with dual, triple and quadruple nonthoracotomy electrode systems using biphasic shocks. *PACE* 1994;17(II):743 (Abstract).
5. Swerdlow CD, Kass RM, Chen PS, Hwang C, Raissi S. Effect of capacitor size and pathway resistance in defibrillation threshold for implantable defibrillators. *Circulation* 1994;90:1840–1846.
6. Heil JE, Liu Y, Dreifus DL, Lang DJ. Future ICD size reductions may not impact defibrillation efficacy of transvenous lead plus can electrode systems. *PACE* 1995; 18:807 (Abstract).
7. Rosenqvist M, Brandt J, Shuller H. Long-term pacing in sinus node disease: effects of stimulation mode on cardiovascular morbidity and mortality. *Am Heart J* 1988;116:16–22.
8. DiCarlo L, Jenkins JM, Caswell S, Morris M, Pariseau B. Tachycardia detection by antitachycardia devices: present limitations and future strategies. *J Interven Cardiol* 1994;7:459–472.
9. Kolettis TM, Saksena S. Prophylactic implantable cardioverter defibrillator therapy in high-risk patients with coronary artery disease. *Am Heart J* 1994; 127(Suppl):1164–1170.
10. Borggrefe M, Chen X, Martinez-Rubio A, et al. The role of implantable cardioverter defibrillators in dilated cardiomyopathy. *Am Heart J* 1994;127(Suppl): 1145–1150.
11. Murgatroyd FD, Slade AKB, Sopher M, Rowland E, Ward DE, Camm AJ. Efficacy and tolerability of transvenous low energy cardioversion of paroxysmal atrial fibrillation in humans. *J Am Coll Cardiol* 1995;25:1347–1353.
12. Saksena S, Prakash A, Mangeon L, et al. Clinical efficacy and safety of atrial

defibrillation using biphasic shocks and current nonthoracotomy endocardial lead configurations. *Am J Cardiol* 1995;76:913–921.

13. Attuel P, Pellerin D, Mugica J, Coumel P. DDD pacing: an effective treatment modality for recurrent atrial arrhythmias. *PACE* 1988;11:1647–1654.
14. Akhtar M, Gilbert CJ, Al-Nouri M, Schmidt DH. Electrophysiologic mechanisms for modification and abolition of atrioventricular junction tachycardia with simultaneous and sequential atrial and ventricular pacing. *Circulation* 1979;60: 1443–1449.
15. Mehra R, Gough WB, Zeiler R, El-Sherif N. Dual ventricular stimulation for prevention of reentrant ventricular tachyarrhythmias. *J Am Coll Cardiol* 1984;3: 472 (Abstract).
16. Daubert C, Mabo P, Berder V. Permanent dual atrium pacing in major interatrial conduction blocks: a four years experience. *PACE* 1993;16(II):885 (Abstract).
17. Prakash A, Saksena S, Hill M. Dual site atrial pacing for the acute and chronic prevention of atrial fibrillation: a prospective study. *J Am Coll Cardiol* 1995;25: 230A (Abstract).
18. Prakash A, Saksena S, Kaushik R, Krol RB, Munsif AN. Regional atrial activation during single and multisite atrial pacing. *J Am Coll Cardiol* 1995.
19. Prakash A, Saksena S, Krol RB, et al. Electrophysiology of acute prevention of atrial fibrillation and flutter with dual site right atrial pacing. *PACE* 1995;18(II): 803 (Abstract).

Index

333